AF245556

THE NEUROMUSCULAR JUNCTION

edited
by

Roger A. Brumback, M.D.
Division of Neuropathology
Department of Pathology
University of Rochester Medical Center
Rochester, New York

and

Jeffery W. Gerst, Ph.D.
Department of Zoology
North Dakota State University
Fargo, North Dakota

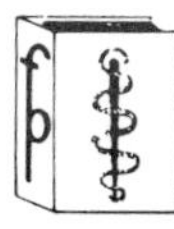

FUTURA PUBLISHING COMPANY
Mount Kisco, New York
1984

Copyright © 1984
Futura Publishing Company, Inc.

Published by
Futura Publishing Company, Inc.
295 Main Street
Mount Kisco, New York 10549

LCCN: 83-082876
ISBN: 0-87993-210-4

All rights reserved.
No part of this book may be translated or produced in
any form without written permission of the publisher.

To

Mary
   Diane
      Darryl
         Audrey
            Owen
               Christopher
                  Kathryne

for
understanding
and
support

Contributors

Roger A. Brumback, M.D.
Division of Neuropathology
Department of Pathology
University of Rochester
 Medical Center
Rochester, New York

Michael R. Carry, Ph.D.
Departments of Neurology
 and Anatomy
University of Colorado School
 of Medicine
Denver, Colorado

Jeffery W. Gerst, Ph.D.
Department of Zoology
North Dakota State University
Fargo, North Dakota

Michael K. Greenberg, M.D.
Wilford Hall Medical Center
Lackland Air Force Base, Texas

Joseph J. McArdle, Ph.D.
Department of Pharmacology
University of Medicine &
 Dentistry of New Jersey
Newark, New Jersey

Robert G. Miller, M.D.
Clinical Service of Neurology
Children's Hospital of San
 Francisco
San Francisco, California

Michio Morita, Ph.D.
Department of Physiology
 and Biophysics
Colorado State University
Colorado Springs, Colorado

Donald B. Saunders, M.D.
Division of Neurology
Duke University Medical
 Center
Durham, North Carolina

Frank G. Standaert, M.D.
Department of Pharmacology
Georgetown University School
 of Medicine
Washington, D.C.

Thomas R. Swift, M.D.
Department of Neurology
Medical College of Georgia
Augusta, Georgia

Preface

Knowledge of the basic mechanisms of neuromuscular transmission is critical to physicians dealing with neuromuscular disorders. In order to diagnose and develop effective therapy, we have assumed responsibility for understanding pathogenesis, including major and recent advances in ultrastructure, physiology, pharmacology, biochemistry, and immunology.

In 1934, at a meeting of the Physiological Society in England, Dale and Feldberg presented experimental evidence that acetylcholine (ACh) was responsible for the transmission of nerve impulses in voluntary muscle. On the same day, Mary Walker submitted evidence to the editors of *Lancet* that intramuscularly administered physostigmine, a cholinesterase inhibitor, was temporarily effective in treating myasthenia gravis (MG). Dale, Feldberg, and Vogt attributed the effectiveness of physostigmine to its inhibition of acetylcholinesterase, the enzyme that hydrolyzes ACh. Dale was awarded the Nobel Prize for Medicine and Physiology in 1936.

The true neurophysiologic significance, however, was not determined until 1948, when Eccles' work was reported by Kuffler. Eccles won the Nobel Prize for Medicine and Physiology in 1963. Katz, at the University College, London, contributed the concept of quantal release of ACh from motor nerve endings; for his investigations, he was awarded the Nobel Prize in 1970. The physiologic disorder of MG in humans was demonstrated by Harvey and Masland in Baltimore, using the "macro" technique of electromyography. On motor nerve stimulation the muscle fiber action potential amplitude decreased rapidly in MG—a reaction similar to that produced in normal persons by curare, and reversed by neostigmine.

In the early 1960s, Elmqvist, Johns and Thesleff, and their associates in Sweden used micro techniques to demonstrate the normal physiology of neuromuscular transmission in humans, then demonstrated that the amplitude of miniature endplate potentials in patients with MG was greatly reduced. Their studies favored the concept that there were subnormal amounts of ACh in each quantum released. That could be explained either by defective binding of ACh in each vesicle, or by the presence of some false transmitter in the vesicles. Depolarization of the post-junctional membrane by ACh agonists, carbacol or decamethonium, appeared normal, but the investigators emphasized that their study of the post-junctional membrane lacked precision.

In 1939, Blalock in Baltimore empirically demonstrated improvement of MG following thymectomy. That therapy became popular, yet the immunologic significance of the thymus was not established until 1960. Also at that time, Simpson in Scotland suggested that MG might occur on an immune basis, partly because of its association with other autoimmune diseases such as rheumatoid arthritis. Strauss and Nastuk demonstrated antibodies to muscle striations in the serum of 30% of patients with MG, and in almost all patients with MG and thymoma. It became apparent that those antibodies, however, were not the immediate cause of MG.

In the late 1960s Chang and Lee in Taiwan isolated α-bungarotoxin from a cobra, and found it to interact irreversibly with the motor endplate, causing paralysis. In the early 1970s, Miledi and Potter, in England, and Changeux and Lee, in France, used the toxin to isolate and purify ACh receptors from the electric organ of electric eels or rays. Then Fambrough and Drachman used labelled α-bungarotoxin in an autoradiographic study of human endplates, demonstrating that, in MG, the number of reacting sites was decreased. Then, in 1973 and 1975, Lindstrom and Patrick in La Jolla, Lambert and associates in Rochester, Minnesota, and Sanders, Eldefrawi, Johns and associates at Virginia produced an experimental model of myasthenia gravis, with all the physiologic, pharmacologic, and anatomic characteristics of the human disease. Experimental autoimmune myasthenia gravis (EAMG) was produced by injecting acetylcholine receptors (AChR) from eel or ray electroplax into rabbits or rats. EAMG was responsive to thymectomy and treatment with corticosteroids.

In 1976, Albuquerque and his associates in Baltimore demonstrated electrophysiologically that there was decreased post-junctional receptor responsiveness in human myasthenic intercostal muscle.

Many questions remain: What causes the production of antibodies to AChR? How do the antibodies cause the muscle weakness? Why are antibodies not demonstrated in all patients, and why is the titer not always related to the severity of weakness? What is the role of the thymus in MG? Why are some muscles involved, others not, and why are there remissions and exacerbations?

It is obvious that some of our discoveries have been empiric, or serendipitous, yet we are achieving ultimate understanding of neuromuscular disorders because of scientists' and physician scientists' thorough knowledge of the basic principles so well set forth in this volume on *The Neuromuscular Junction*.

T. R. Johns, II, M.D.
Alumni Professor and Chairman,
Department of Neurology,
University of Virginia School of Medicine

Foreword

The important interrelationships of basic medical science and clinical patient care are never more apparent than in studies of the neuromuscular junction. This book is an attempt to review the basic anatomy, physiology, and pharmacology of the neuromuscular junction and relate these to the pathological processes affecting this structure. Even though the peripheral motor nerves (and the skeletal muscle fibers they innervate) are among the most readily accesssible structures of the nervous system, it was not until almost forty years ago that the chemical basis of neuromuscular transmission was clarified. The studies that in a century propelled our understanding from hardly more than Galen's "animal spirits" to the quantal release of acetylcholine are outlined by Drs. Gerst and Brumback in Chapter 1. The discovery of the nature of synaptic transmission at the neuromuscular junction initiated an intense investigative effort aimed at fully understanding this structure.

In Chapter 2, Drs. Carry and Morita depict the structural relationships at the neuromuscular junction. The elegant light and electron microscopic studies reviewed by these authors have permitted us to visualize the morphological correlates of the chemical transmission process. Anatomic studies have also demonstrated that, even though chemically similar, there are many variations in neuromuscular junction morphology, not only among different animal species, but also among different muscles in the same animal.

The physiological changes that underlie neuromuscular transmission are thoroughly reviewed by Dr. McArdle in Chapter 3. In a clear and understandable step-wise fashion, Dr. McArdle derives the equations that have allowed physiologists to discover and quantitate such neuromuscular junction parameters as endplate potentials, miniature endplate potentials, quantal acetylcholine content, and the sodium, potassium, and calcium ion currents in membrane channels. In the following chapter, Chapter 4, Dr. Standaert defines the effects of pharmacologic agents on the membrane ion channels and other parts of the neuromuscular junction. The muscle relaxants used in surgical anesthesia, the cholinesterase inhibitors used in treating myasthenia gravis, and the cholinesterase inhibitors used as insecticides and as wartime "nerve gases" are all carefully described. In addition, Dr. Standaert provides cautions about the "incidental" effects on the function of the neuromuscular junction of a number of other commonly prescribed drugs—effects that under certain circumstances can be detrimental to the patient.

Both structural and functional changes occur in the neuromuscular junction whenever the ability of the nerve to supply its presumed trophic influence on the muscle is compromised. In Chapter 5, Dr. Miller elucidates the disturbances in the muscle membrane, synapse, and nerve terminal that become apparent after structural damage or toxic-metabolic injury to the motor nerve.

The most important clinical disease of the neuromuscular junction is myasthenia gravis. During the past twenty years, there have been remarkable advances in the understanding of the changes in the neuromuscular junction in this disorder, but the immunopathologic disturbances, including the thymic abnormalities, have not yet been clarified. In his review of myastenia gravis in Chapter 6, Dr. Sanders points out the varying clinical symptoms of this disorder and the difficulties in diagnosis despite electromyography, edrophonium (Tensilon) tests, oculography, tonometry, and stapedial reflex fatigue tests. Based upon his extensive clinical experience, Dr. Sanders provides us with a workable approach to the evaluation and treatment of patients afflicted with myasthenia gravis. In Chapter 7, Drs. Swift and Greenberg provide a comprehensive summary of the other major disorders that affect the neuromuscular junction, including the myasthenic (Lambert-Eaton) syndrome, congenital myasthenia, botulism, tetanus, and snake and arthropod envenomation.

Acknowledgments

In recent years there has been a profusion of clinical and research interest in the neuromuscular junction, sparked in part by a desire to understand the basic pathophysiology of the disabling disease, myasthenia gravis. While a clinical associate under Dr. W. King Engel at the National Institutes of Health, one of us (RAB) had the opportunity to participate in studies of neuromuscular junction physiology and in the evelution of new treatment regimens for myasthenia gravis. Subsequently, thanks to the efforts of Dr. William Olson, formerly Chairman of Neurology, University of North Dakota School of Medicine, the two editors of this text at the University of North Dakota and the North Dakota State University began collaborative studies of the neuromuscular junction. In addition to our research efforts, we prepared various teaching materials for our medical students and graduate assistants. It quickly became apparent to us that no single textbook adequately reviewed neuromuscular junction structure, function, pharmacology, and disease states. Therefore, when Mr. Steven E. Korn, Chairman of the Board of Futura Publishing Company, approached us with the idea of producing such a volume, we immediately agreed to the project. We were fortunate to obtain the assistance of experts in the fields of neuromuscular junction anatomy, physiology, pharmacology and pathology who promptly prepared chapters for inclusion in the text. Throughout this project we have been aided by the valuable support of the Department of Neuroscience, University of North Dakota School of Medicine, the Department of Zoology, North Dakota State University, and the Department of Pathology, University of Rochester Medical Center. We hope this book will serve as a source for both the clinician dealing with disorders affecting the neuromuscular junction and the investigator pursuing studies of neuromuscular function.

Roger A. Brumback, M.D.
Jeffery W. Gerst, Ph.D.

xi

Contents

Chapter 1

Neuromuscular Transmission: Early Historical Development of the Concept

Jeffery W. Gerst, Ph.D. and
Roger A. Brumback, M.D.

According to these results of morphological research, it appears that contact of the muscle substance with the non-medullated nerve suffices to allow the transfer of the excitation from the latter to the former. The only strange thing is that in the reverse order excitation of the muscle never extends to its own nerve.

—W. Kuhne, 1888

The ability of today's scientists to estimate single ion channel conductances,[72] and to clone acetylcholine receptor protein subunits,[73] obscures the fact that our basic understanding of neuromuscular transmission has only really been clear since 1948. For nearly 1500 years, Galen's gaseous "animal spirits," thought to be produced in the base of the brain and carried throughout the body through hollow nerves, were believed to cause muscle contraction.[4] In the late 1600's, Giovanni Borelli slit the muscle of an animal that was submerged in water. He observed no release of bubbles from the contracting muscle and suggested that the animal spirits were liquid, not gaseous, humors that caused contraction of muscle by inducing an explosive fermentation. William Croone, a founding member of the Royal Society of London, believed that the "spiritous liquid" of the nerve mixed with the "nourishing juice of the muscle," causing the muscle to swell like an inflating balloon. The works of John [Jan] Swammerdam, translated into English in 1738, almost 70 years after his death, demonstrated that muscle contraction was accompanied only by a change in muscle shape, and not by an increase in muscle volume. He noted the importance of understanding the functional anatomic relationship of the nerve to the muscle and ". . . what that very subtle matter properly is which is undoubtedly conveyed to the muscle through the nerve."[5] Albrecht von Heller, in the mid 1700's, considered and then rejected the idea that the nerve's influence on muscle was electrical since he felt nerves lacked sufficient insulation for nerve conduction, which was thought to occur in the same manner as electric conduction down a wire. However, the works of Luigi Galvani, in the late 1700's, and of Carlo Matteucci, in the mid 1800's, laid the foundation for an electrical basis of nerve and muscle physiology.

The mechanism underlying "the transfer of the excitation" from motoneuron to skeletal muscle fiber required more than half a century (from the late 1800's to the mid 1900's) to be fully elucidated. Throughout much of this period, two strongly competing ideas helped sharpen the focus and force the accumulation of more detailed evidence. In the end, each idea found justification. This chapter will provide a brief historical review of the early years of the quest for the mechanism of neuromuscular transmission.

The necessity of an intimate anatomic association between the nerve and the muscle was readily accepted by nearly all investigators. Kuhne,[53] using gold chloride staining techniques, describes the motor nerves as terminating beneath the sarcolemma, and ". . . clothed with nothing else than the axolemma." (Fig. 1.1) In skeletal muscle, the nerve ending contacts an "unstriped," highly nucleated area of protoplasm, the motor endplate. These nuclei were believed to have been derived from muscle fiber nuclei,[44] a proposition supported subsequently by embryological studies.[78] Tello[78] pointed out that in embryonic and neonatal material, single motor endplates were formed by the termination of a number of nerve fibers.[43,12]

Pelouze and Bernard[74] demonstrated that the arrow poison, curare, used by certain South American Indian tribes, abolished the effect of nervous stimulation on muscle. This toxin blocked neuromuscular transmission, but did not affect the excitability of either the nerve or the muscle, suggesting to Bernard that the toxin worked on some intermediate structure or process.[3] Du Bois-Reymond[22] speculated that the nature of the transmission process might be either electrical or chemical, and referring to the possibility of chemical transmission, he suggested that substances capable of exciting the muscle, such as ammonia or lactic acid, might be liberated by the motor nerve.

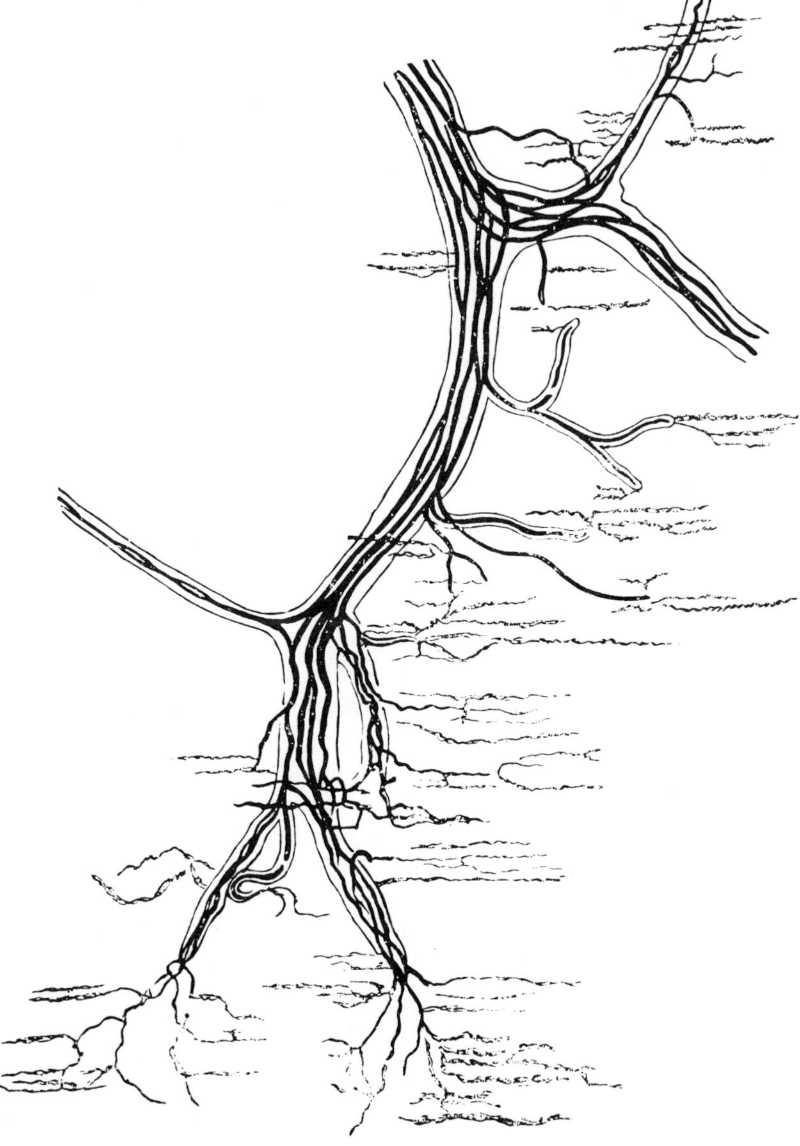

Figure 1.1. Motor nerve endings in a frog pectoral muscle prepared by the gold chloride staining technique. The restriction of nerve endings to discrete "fields of innervation" suggested to Kuhne that muscle fibers must share with nerves the ability to propagate their own excitation. (From Kuhne, 1888,[53] by permission of the Royal Society of London.)

Pollitzer,[75] using an array of platinum-stimulating electrodes spaced at 2 mm intervals along the frog sartorius muscle from the knee end to the hip end, associated the differences in irritability of muscle segments with the distribution of the motor nerve. Since curarization failed to alter this association, Pollitzer, entering the "region of pure speculation . . . ," suggested that curare acted on the cement substance of the last node of Ranvier, modifying it "in such a way that the nervous impulse can no longer pass through." Langley[54] addressed the question of site of action of nicotine and curare (Fig. 1.2). Both compounds blocked neuromuscular transmission in the gastrocnemius of the chicken without affecting the contractile response of the muscle to direct stimulation. Intrajugular injection of nicotine elicited slow contractions of long duration. Curare, injected during the rise in muscle tension of a nicotine-induced contraction, caused a fall in muscle tension, and nicotine injected after curare elicited only "a trace of contraction." This apparent mutual antagonism of the two drugs suggested to Langley that they worked on the same "protoplasmic substance or substances." The mutual antagonism persisted following denervation of the gastrocnemius, although the denervated muscle appeared to be more sensitive to nicotine and less sensitive to curare. Langley concluded that "nicotine and curare do not act on the axon endings but on the muscle itself." He concluded further that the drugs "do not act directly on the contractile substance, but on other substances in the muscle which may be called receptive substances." The receptive substance was believed "to receive the nervous stimulus and, by transmitting it, cause contraction."[55] Langley[55] pointed out that such an hypothesis demanded that the nervous impulse not directly affect the contractile substance of the muscle, recalling du Bois-Reymond's earlier speculation. Elliot[35] had, two years before, proposed the existence of an intermediary in the transmission of nervous stimuli to smooth muscle. He suggested that in order for adrenalin to evoke a response in smooth muscle, the muscle must have been innervated by the sympathetic nervous system. He postulated that "perhaps a mechanism developed out of the muscle cell in response to its union with the synapsing sympathetic fiber, the function of which is to receive and transform the nervous impulse. Adrenalin might then be the chemical stimulant liberated on each occasion when the impulse arrives at the periphery."[35] The myoneural junction was the site of the proposed mechanism, and the site of action of adrenalin.[36]

Attempts to establish the physico-chemical nature of isolated nerve and isolated muscle excitability occupied most of the attention of scientists in the early 1900's,[69] although some observations pertinent to understanding the nature of their functional interconnection (neu-

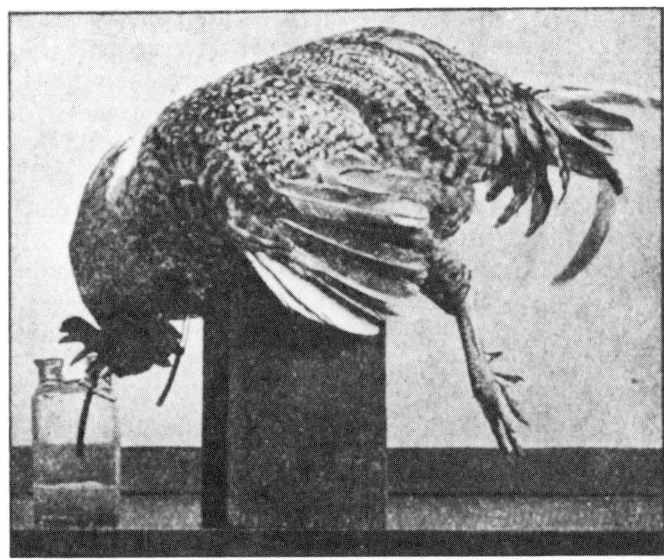

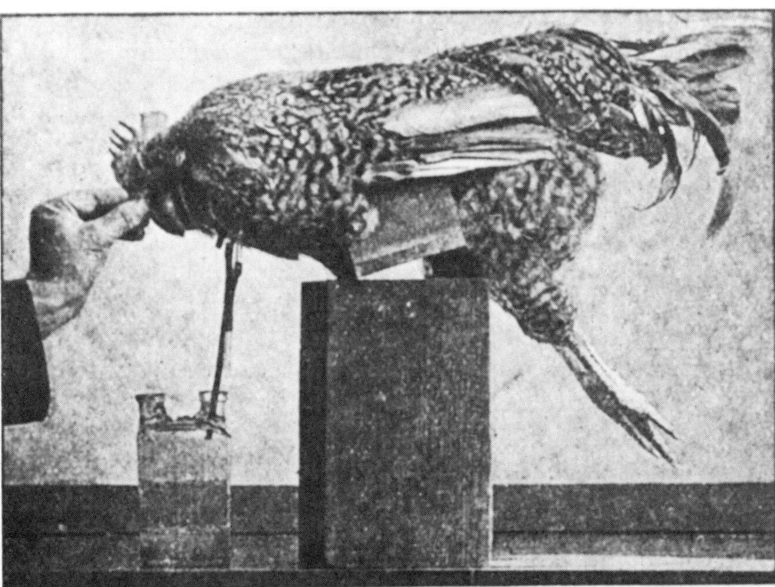

Figure 1.2. An anesthetized chicken supported on a wooden, V-shaped form (upper panel). The neck and legs hang flaccidly, and the eyelids are closed. Two minutes after tran intrajugular injection of 5 mg nicotine, the neck is retracted and twisted, the legs are extended and eyelids are open (lower panel). These tonic contractions were maintained for 15 minutes or longer, and could be induced in chickens whose motor nerves were severed. (From Langley, 1906,[55] by permission of the Royal Society of London.)

romuscular transmission) continued to be published. Using condensor discharges of variable duration, Lucas[66] observed that the optimal electrical stimulus for contraction of the sartorius muscle of the frog and the toad varied with the local placement of the stimulating electrode. Three "excitable substances" were recognized by Lucas—the alpha substance in nerve-free regions of the muscle fibers, the beta substance in regions of the muscle fibers containing nerve endings, and the gamma substance found in the sciatic nerve trunk. The beta substance exhibited the greatest excitability. Using direct current stimulation, Lucas demonstrated all three substances in single experiments.[67,68] Estimating the "liminal" stimulus current strength at various stimulus durations, he found that doses of curare capable of blocking the excitation of muscle by its motor nerve left the beta substance "still excitable and in functional connection with the muscle." Slightly higher levels of curare abolished beta excitability. Lucas speculated that the beta substance might serve as "an intermediate in the conduction of excitation from nerve to muscle."[68] Of the early experiments, those of Langley and Lucas, while supporting the existence within the muscle of an intermediate link in the process of neuromuscular transmission, did not argue for or against either the electrical or chemical nature of the link. Elliot[35] alone spoke of a "chemical excitant."

The process of conduction, ". . . the excitation of one region of a continuous element by some process occurring in the adjacent active region. . . ," was addressed by Lillie in a series of papers.[59,60,61] The positive correlation between the rate of change in electrical variation in an excitable tissue and the velocity of propagation of excitation in that tissue was presented[59] as evidence supporting the hypothesis that the electrical variation, the "action current," is the "essential change on which the conduction depends." Commenting on the ability of electrical variation in one excitable tissue acting as the stimulus for another irritable tissue, Lillie indicated that the temporal variation in the action current in the stimulating tissue must correspond with the temporal change of electrical excitation in the responding tissue. The absence of such temporal correspondence suggested to Lillie "a possible basis for the irreciprocality of conduction between motor and sensory nerve-cells in the reflex arc." On the basis of his hypothesis, Lillie believed that muscle cells were electrically stimulated by the action current of the motor nerve that branched over the muscle at the motor endplate.

The chronaxie, the stimulus duration necessary to obtain a threshold response when the stimulus intensity was twice the liminal strength (rheobase intensity), was a unit of time used by the Lapicques in explaining the action of curare.[57,58] The Lapicques' law of isochronism held that the chronaxie of a motor nerve and the muscle that it innervated must be closely similar. Curare, they believed, lowered the chronaxie of the muscle so as to result in a heterochronic relationship; that is, the ratio of chronaxie of the nerve and muscle approached 1:2. Such heterochronism was believed to be the cause of the block in neuromuscular transmission. While the observations of Lucas[66,67,68] failed to support the Lapicques' idea of isochronism, the latter hypothesis received much support and was variously formulated mathematically.[40] Major criticisms of the hypothesis were presented, particularly by Grundfest[42] and Rushton[76] (see reviews[77,56,21]). Grundfest,[42] making use of the widely separated muscle fibers in the retrolingual membrane of the frog's tongue, demonstrated that the chronaxie of the nerve fiber was always smaller than that of the muscle fiber. Furthermore, the chronaxie of the muscle fiber could be increased by increasing the size of the stimulating electrode. Not only did heterochronism appear to be the usual case, but curarization failed to affect the chronaxie of the muscle fiber. Rushton[76] confirmed the observations of Grundfest and questioned whether strichnine could restore the excitability of a veratrine (cevadine) blocked myoneural junction. The Lapicques had observed that strichnine blocked neuromuscular transmission by shortening the chronaxie of the motor nerve while not affecting the chronaxie of the muscle. Veratrine, on the other hand, shortened the chronaxie of the muscle, but not that of the nerve. Rushton applied both drugs in the ratio of concentrations recommended by the Lapicques, and in ratios up to nine times higher than recommended. He found that ". . . there is never restoration of conduction, no matter which drug is applied first. . . ." While extant, the Lapicques' law of isochronism favored the electrical nature of the neuromuscular transmission process. Even with its eventual loss of support, electrophysiologists retained a kinship with the idea.

In 1913, Henry Dale, later Sir Henry Dale, a research scientist in the Wellcome Physiological Laboratories, received "an ordinary liquid extract of ergot" in order to perform a routine determination of its activity.[16] The intravenous injection of a conventional dose into an anesthetized cat caused "a profound inhibition of the heart-beat; I suspected, indeed, a fatal accident of injection, till recovery set in, and successive repetitions of the injection then caused the same sequence at every trial." A full account of the activities of this extract appeared the following year.[14] Comparison of the activity of the ergot extract was made with a variety of choline esters, including "acetyl-choline." Prominent in his results is the description of a dual action of the choline esters on the heart and circulation: ". . . the depressor, car-dioinhibitor 'muscarine' type of action, unaltered by nicotine, but abolished by atropine, and a pressor action of the nicotine type, unaffected by atropine, but abolished by large doses of nicotine." The latter action could be observed only after the abolition of the former action with atropine. Feldberg in his "reminiscences of an eye wit-ness,"[37] points to this article by Dale as the starting point for the history of the role of acetylcholine in neuromuscular transmission.

Otto Loewi, in 1921, published the results of the first of a series of experiments that were both straightforward in design and far-reaching in consequence. Loewi[62] stimulated the vagus nerve of a frog heart containing a small volume of Ringer solution in the ventricles. He observed the expected decrease in heart activity, and then trans-ferred fluid from the stimulated heart into a second test heart that lacked vagal innervation. This second test heart also exhibited a decrease in activity. The transferred fluid contained a vagus sub-stance, "Vagusstoff," that transmitted the effect of vagal stimulation to the test heart. The vagus substance had biochemical characteris-tics of an unstable choline ester, and was thought possibly to be acetylcholine. The effect of the vagus substance was blocked in previ-ously atropinized test hearts, and it was quickly shown that atropine acted by preventing the effect of the vagus substance directly on the heart, and not by interferring with release of vagus substance.[63] Eserine prolonged the inhibitory effects of vagal stimulation, of vagus substance, and of acetylcholine on the frog heart.[64,65] The experiments of Loewi and his co-workers had demonstrated unam-biguously that nervous system activity could be transmitted to its effector indirectly, through the release of a chemical mediator. Ace-tylcholine, the presumed mediator of vagal activity, was not known to occur naturally in animal tissue until Dale and Dudley in 1929,[17] while looking for the presence of a vasodilating substance, isolated it from horse spleen. The following year, the destruction of acetylcho-line by blood was shown to be due to a hydrolytic enzyme whose activity was inhibited by eserine.[37,71] Chang and Gaddum[11] extended the list of tissues containing acetylcholine, and proposed a series of pharmacological criteria for the differentiation of acetylcholine from other physiologically active substances. Evidences, although subject to interpretation, quickly accumulated relating the release of acetyl-choline to stimulation of preganglionic autonomic, and postgangli-onic parasympathetic nerves.[1,23]

The enigmatic "pseudomotor" response of the denervated tongue to parasympathetic stimulation[17] was investigated by Dale and Gaddum[20] after the initial isolation and identification of acetylcholine as a natural animal product. The hypoglossal nerve, the normal motor innervation of the dog tongue, was sectioned on one side and allowed to degenerate for 10 to 24 days. Stimulation of the chorda-lingual nerve, a known parasympathetic vasodilator, resulted in contracture of the denervated half of the tongue, causing "the whole tongue to rise from the roof of the mouth. . . ." At a fixed stimulus strength, varying the frequency of chorda-lingual stimulation from 4 to 20 Hz resulted in marked decreases in the latency and increases in the strength of the contracture. At stimulus rates of 20 Hz or more, relaxation commenced prior to the cessation of stimulation, and continued monotonically after stimulation was withdrawn. The authors pointed out that such results can not easily be explained by the direct transmission of the nerve impulse to the muscle. "On the other hand, they, together with all the observations made on these phenomena by earlier workers, become easy to interpret, if we suppose the direct effect of the nerve impulses to be the liberation, at their peripheral endings in relation to the blood vessels, of a labile, diffusible substance, which stimulates contracture in the sensitized muscle."[20] Eserine potentiated the effects of either chorda-lingual stimulation or arterial injection of acetylcholine, but not the arterial injection of the non-esteric tetramethylammonium iodide. Antagonism by atropine of the parasympathetic nervous system effects—and its "less potent" antagonistic effects in denervated mammalian skeletal muscle—were discussed by the authors, who cautioned those who "accept the evidence of the atropine action as deciding the nature of the transmitter" since the mechanism of its antagonism was not known.

On May 12, 1934, two important events occurred: Mary Walker, a resident physician, submitted a letter to the editors of *The Lancet*, and on the same day, Dale and Feldberg made a presentation to the Physiological Society. Walker's letter,[79] published in June 1934, reported "striking though temporary" relief of fatigability in a myasthenia gravis patient given hypodermic injections of eserine (Fig. 1.3). The clinical improvement, she stated, ". . . supports the opinion that the fatigability is due to a poisoning of the motor end-organs, or 'myoneural junctions,' rather than to an affection of the muscle itself. It may be significant that physostigmine [eserine] inhibits the action of the esterase which destroys acetylcholine." The presentation by Dale and Feldberg[18] provided the first experimental evidence of a role of acetylcholine at the myoneural junction of voluntary muscle when they reported, "We have perfused the tongue of the cat with warm,

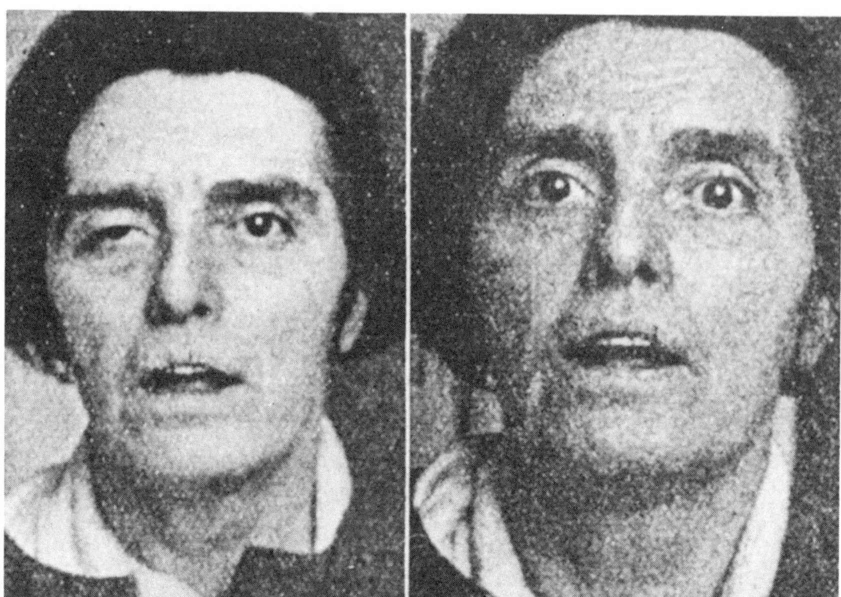

Figure 1.3. Dr. Mary Walker's myasthenia gravis patient before (left panel) and 30 minutes after (right panel) hypodermic injection of physostigmine salicylate. Prior to treatment, the patient was unable to raise her left eyelid. (From Walker, 1934,[79] by permission of the *The Lancet*.)

oxygenated Locke's solution containing a little eserine. On rhythmically stimulating the (motor) hypoglossal nerve, we have regularly observed the appearance in the venous fluid, inactive in the resting interval, of a substance having the usual properties by which we now recognize acetylcholine."

The initial evidence for the role of acetylcholine in neuromuscular transmission was quickly reaffirmed and extended.[19] Stable in acid, labile in dilute alkali, protected from destruction in blood by eserine, and equipotent with pure acetylcholine when assayed on eserinized leech muscle and on the cat's blood pressure, the latter potency being annulled by atropine, the substance collected in the eserine–containing perfusion solution was identified as acetylcholine. Stimulation of the hypoglossal nerve, after separation from sympathetic fibers and degeneration of the parasympathetic chorda-lingual nerve, regularly resulted in the appearance of acetylcholine. Curare, added to the perfusion fluid, blocked the response of the tongue to hypoglossal stimulation. However, as assayed on the cat's blood pressure, curare failed to affect the release of acetylcholine.

While these pharmacological evidences for the role of acetylcholine in neuromuscular transmission appeared compelling, Dale[15] pointed to "a gap in the chain of evidence, owing to the apparent lack of response of the normally innervated mammalian muscle to acetylcholine, when injected or otherwise applied artificially." That "gap" was soon filled by the introduction of a "close-range" injection technique.[9] When acetylcholine was injected into the tibial artery of the cat gastrocnemius, at close range, while temporarily halting normal circulation, 2.5 micrograms of acetylcholine, in 0.5 ml of saline, produced a contraction slightly higher in tension than that elicited by supramaximal nerve stimulation[10] (Fig. 1.4). The amount of muscle tension developed in response to acetylcholine injection was positively correlated with the speed of injection. The effects of close-range acetylcholine injection were diminished by curare, and potentiated by eserine. The quick, twitch-like contractions were shown to be accompanied by "an irregular outburst of [muscle spike] activity shortly preceding and during the mechanical response. . . ."[6] Brown[6]

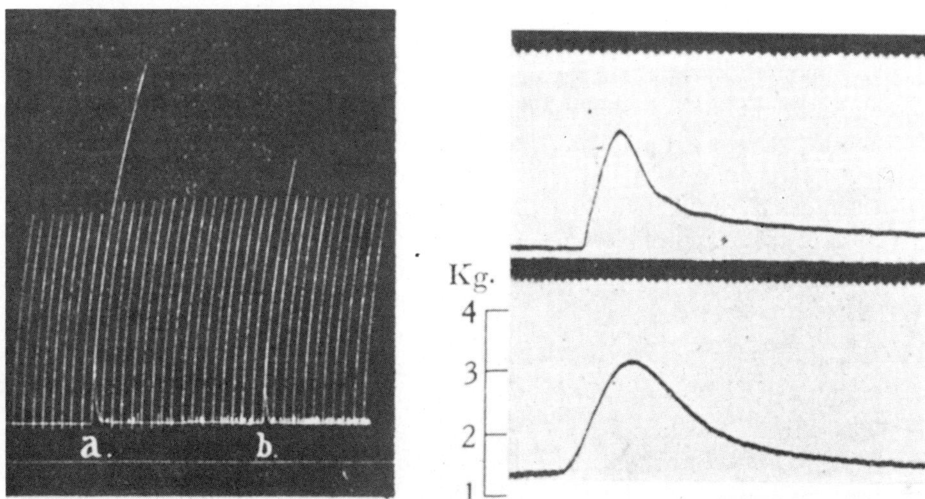

Figure 1.4. Isometric records from naturally perfused gastrocnemius of a spinal cat. Indirectly stimulated, maximal muscle twitches were elicited at 10-second intervals (left panel). Close arterial injection of acetylcholine (5 micrograms at point a, 2.5 micrograms at point b) replaced nerve stimulation at points a and b. Optical myograms (right panel) display response to indirectly stimulated twitch, upper frame, and to close arterial injection of 2.5 micrograms of acetylcholine, lower frame. Time marks calibrated at 10 milliseconds. (From Brown, Dale and Feldberg, 1936,[10] by permission of the *Journal of Physiology*).

also noted that in heavily eserinized preparations, close-range injection of acetylcholine caused a depression in muscle response to indirect stimulation. Similar observations were made on denervated mammalian and frog muscle, and on normally innervated frog muscle.[7] Cowan[13] reported that application of acetylcholine to isolated, prostigmin-treated frog sartorius muscle caused a temporary decrease in a burn-induced injury potential. Curare, while without effect on the injury potential, decreased the sensitivity of the muscle to acetylcholine.[13] Referring to the lack of information concerning the minimal change in local potential necessary to elicit a propagated response in a muscle, Cowan[13] stated, "If it is justifiable to extend this inference to muscle, then it appears that the amount of ACh. used by Brown *et al.* in their 'short range' arterial injection experiments would be sufficient to give the required depolarization."

The pharmacological evidence for acetylcholine's role as transmitter at skeletal muscle neuromuscular junctions was compelling.[8] However, many electrophysiologists remained skeptical, and pointed out apparent weaknesses in the hypothesis of chemical mediation. A major objection concerned the action of eserine. The potentiating action of eserine on acetylcholine-induced or nerve volley-induced muscle contraction was associated with repetitive discharge of muscle spike potentials. Since eserine inhibited the hydrolysis of acetylcholine, it was argued that the repetitive discharge was caused by a persistence of acetylcholine.[10,6] This explanation was supported by Bacq and Brown,[2] who used a series of choline esterase inhibitors having graded potencies. Yet, use of the anti-esterases resulted in the appearance of "small irregular [mechanical] twitchings" of the muscle fibers.[2] Eccles[23] suggested that the anti-esterase–induced twitching originated in the region of the motor endplate, and represented an increase in sensitivity of the endplate. Furthermore, the long duration of repetitive spike discharge in eserinized muscle suggested the existence within the endplate of "some self-re-exciting mechanism. . . ."[29] Thus, eserine or other anti-esterases might potentiate neuromuscular transmission by prolonging the action of acetylcholine on the motor endplate, or by increasing the sensitivity of the motor endplate to whatever the neurotransmitter might be, either acetylcholine liberated by the motor nerve or action currents produced by the motor nerve. A second criticism concerned the rate of hydrolysis of acetylcholine at neuromuscular junctions, estimated by Marnay and Nachmansohn[70] in intact and finely cut muscle. The rate was considered to be too slow to account for destruction of the supposed transmitter within the refractory period of the muscle. Brown and co-workers[9] had realized this difficulty and had suggested the presence of "a local concentration at the nerve ending, on surfaces in relation to which acetylcholine is liberated by nerve impulse" could account for the necessarily rapid rate of hydrolysis. Eccles[24] would later point out that the estimated quantity of acetylcholine liberated by a single nerve volley, stated by Brown, Dale and Feldberg[10] to be 0.02 micrograms, was in error and should have been reported as 0.02 nanograms. Marnay and Nachmansohn[70] had used the erroneous value in drawing their conclusion. While some electrophysiologists remained unconvinced of the chemical–mediation hypothesis, the electrical-mediation hypothesis remained, in Eccles'[24] words, "largely untested."

Focal localization of extracellular recording electrodes at the motor endplates permitted Eccles and O'Connor[27,28] to record "two kinds of action potentials" in curare-blocked soleus muscles of the cat. While both potential changes were localized to the region of the motor endplate, they could be differentiated by varying the level of curarization. Indirect stimulation of deeply curarized muscle resulted in slow negative potentials, less than 10% of the normal muscle spike, whose amplitude grew in response to a second nerve volley. Indirect stimulation of less deeply curarized muscle resulted in "a brief sharp spike" superimposed on the early phase of the slow potential. The sharp spike propagated less than 5 mm from the endplate was referred to as an "abortive impulse," and resulted in no detectable muscle contraction. A nerve volley, 0.8–2.0 ms after an initial volley, failed to elicit a muscle action potential in normal soleus muscle. However, the second volley did result in a negative potential change whose shape, although twice as large, was identical to the slow potentials recorded from deeply curarized soleus muscle.[29] Eccles and O'Connor[29] referred to this negative potential change as the "endplate potential," and indicated that if the stimulus interval was increased from 1.5 to 2.0 ms, the size of the endplate potential (epp) was increased as abortive impulses are produced. "The second nerve volley is setting up 'new-born' muscle impulses so early in the muscle's refractory period that they quickly die out."[29] A fuller description of these nerve-evoked skeletal muscle responses focused, in part, on the elaboration of the new-born impulses.[31] While the new-born impulses and epps were consistently observed together, the former were not considered to be a consequence of the latter. The new-born impulse potential was estimated to begin "slightly earlier than the endplate potential."[31] Thus the new-born impulse and the epp were believed to represent independent responses to the nerve impulse, the excitatory action of the motor nerve capable of producing the former lasting for less than 1 ms. Feng,[39] referring to the changes in responsiveness of the endplate and adjacent regions of the muscle during the refractory period, indicated that "it need not cause surprise if the 'new-born impulse' obtained later in the refractory period should appear to begin slightly sooner than the endplate potential obtained earlier in the refractory phase." He was, however, ". . . inclined to agree with Eccles and O'Connor in thinking that it would not generally be correct to regard the 'new-born impulse' as set up by the endplate potential. . . ."

The nature of the epp in curarized frog sartorius and cat soleus muscle was described by Eccles, Katz and Kuffler.[32] The local nature of the epp was confirmed, and its decremental spread was likened to "the spread of electric charge along a leaky capacitive cable."[32] The latency of the epp (the delay between the arrival of the nerve stimulus and the start of the epp) was insensitive to curarization, although increasing levels of curarization greatly diminished the epp amplitude. The decay of the epp was exponential, and was believed to represent the passive decay of a membrane potential similar to those observable in nerve or muscle at the end of a subthreshold, depolarizing current pulse. Endplate potentials, set up simultaneously with, or a few milliseconds prior to the arrival of an antidromic muscle spike, summed with the initial foot of the muscle spike, and then apparently disappeared ". . . since neither the summit nor the descending phase of the action potential shows any addition or any alteration apart from a slight speeding."[32] Whatever had been the cause of the epp must have been removed prior to the epp's collapse or decay. No mention of new-born impulses was made by Eccles and co-workers;[32] in fact, the authors state that "when above a certain critical level, an e.p.p. gives rise to a propagated action potential. . . ." The nature of the transmitter giving rise to the epp was not addressed. However, the ability of curare to reduce the sensitivity of the endplate to acetylcholine, and to reduce the amplitude of the epp, favored the acetylcholine-mediated theory of neuromuscular transmission. This theory was further strengthened when it was shown that eserine lengthened the local, negative potential changes recorded at motor endplates in response to nerve stimulation.[33] Eserinized frog sartorius and cat soleus muscle appeared to exhibit two imperfectly separated waves of local, endplate negativity: (1) a lengthened epp, and (2) a slow wave exhibiting a slow rise and a much slower decay. The slow wave was most easily observed in frog muscle and was accentuated by higher doses of eserine. Curare antagonized the effects of eserine, with subparalytic doses shortening the period of endplate negativity, and with higher doses completely eliminating the slow wave component. Eserine, 10 micromolar, increased the size and the duration of the rising phase of the epp in previously curarized frog muscle. However, the rate of the voltage change during the rising phase was unchanged when compared to controls, and suggested that the increase in epp amplitude was associated with an increase in the duration of transmitter action. Eserine levels above 10 micromolar resulted in a reduction in epp amplitude, while only slightly decreasing the rate of voltage rise. Discussing their results, the authors stated, "If there is any special process at the junctional region, it would concern the setting up of the catelectrotonus by the transmitting agent, and it is this process which is lengthened by eserine, and diminished and shortened by curare."[33] The mechanism by which curare shortened the epp and obliterated the slow-wave component of the eserine-lengthened endplate negativity was still unknown. The authors concluded that "by making plausible assumptions, the observed curarine and eserine actions may readily be reconciled with the hypothesis that ACh, liberated by nerve impulse, is responsible for all the local potential changes at the neuromuscular junctions."[33] The use of an isolated, single nerve-muscle fiber preparation would provide a clearer picture of the neuromuscular transmission process.

The first attempts at isolating a single nerve and muscle fiber from a frog were described by Kato[45] in his book, *The Microphysiology of Nerve.* He stated: "After severe patience and trials the triumph was crowned to T. Kamaya toward the end of December, 1929, and in May the next year, T. Shimizu succeeded in the isolation of a single nerve fibre from a sciatic nerve which required by far the finer technique than the isolation of a single muscle fibre." Stephen Kuffler, without reference to Kato's work, succeeded in isolating single muscle fibers, along with their motor nerve, from the adductor longus muscle of a frog.[47] Recording from the fiber after lifting it into paraffin or at the saline-paraffin interface, he was able to record epp's whose amplitudes were "so large that no spike could be detected rising above it." Confirming previous observations, Kuffler[47] demonstrated curare's ability to diminish the rate of rise and the amplitude of the epp, to lengthen the muscle spike latency, and to finally leave only a diminished, pure epp (Fig. 1.5). The voltage threshold for muscle spike initiation did not appreciably change during the progress of curarization. He suggested that muscle spike propagation began in a region of the muscle adjacent to the endplate whenever the

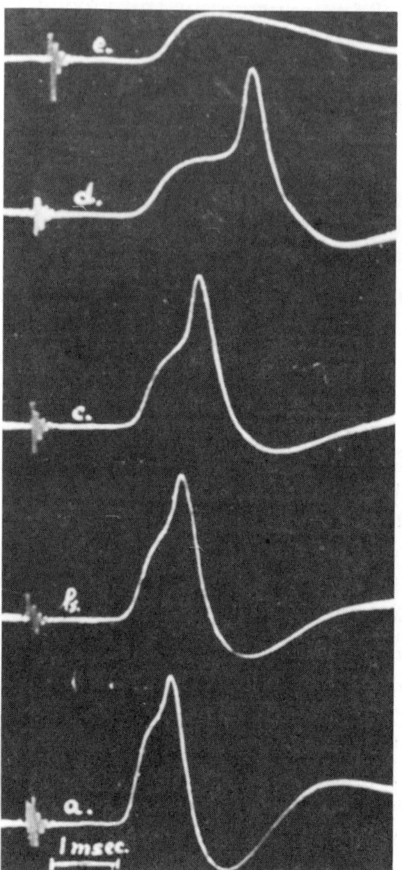

Figure 1.5. Extracellular recordings from the endplate region of a single nerve-muscle fiber preparation from the *adductor longus* muscle of the frog (*Hyla aurea*). Records taken prior to (record a) and following the addition of curare to the saline bath. Records b thru e display the effect of progressive curarization over a 20–30 minute period. Depression of endplate potential amplitude and increase in muscle spike latency are clearly visible. Neuromuscular blockade is demonstrated in record e where only a diminished endplate potential is recorded. (From Kuffler, 1942,[47] by permission of the *Journal of Neurophysiology*).

endplate became depolarized to approximately 30% of the spike amplitude. Referring to "abortive impulses," Kuffler[48] demonstrated that the refractory period of the motor endplate is lengthened by a nerve-stimulated muscle spike, when compared with an antidromic muscle spike (Fig. 1.6). Thus, abortive impulses set up following a conditioning nerve impulse are passively conducted away from the endplate only about half the distance of those set up following an antidromic conditioning spike. The single nerve-muscle fiber preparation also permitted the accurate estimation of the duration and the intensity of transmitter action. The peak of a nerve-induced muscle spike was followed by a rise in the electronegativity of the endplate, reaching an amplitude of about 55% of the spike amplitude. The amplitude of this late potential decreased as the recording electrode was moved away from the endplate. Comparing the potentials of nerve-stimulated muscle spikes recorded at the endplate with those recorded a few millimeters away, and comparing the potentials of nerve-stimulated and antidromically stimulated muscle spikes recorded at the endplate permitted Kuffler[49] to derive accurate estimates of the epp's time course. The transmitter action was found to last at least 2 ms at 28°C, and Kuffler inferred that the transmitting agent produced by the nerve "outlasts the spike and builds up a potential in the refractory muscle." Furthermore, the action of the transmitting agent persisted for up to 4 ms in muscle fibers treated with a just-paralytic dose of curare.[49] Finally, Kuffler[49] was able to mimic all of the actions of the transmitting agent by means of constant current, catelectrotonic pulses.

Measuring the transverse impedance changes in fully curarized frog sartorius muscle, Katz[46] showed that the epp is accompanied by small, localized permeability changes in the endplate region. The time courses of the two events were "very consistent . . . ," and both were lengthened by eserine. There was "no evidence for a rapid component of impedance loss concurrent with the period of extrinsic [motor nerve] current flow. . . ."[46] Meanwhile, Kuffler continued to exploit the opportunities afforded by his single nerve-muscle fiber technique.

The endplate region of normal frog muscle fibers exhibited special sensitivity to the application of acetylcholine, nicotine and caffeine. Application of 10 micromolar acetylcholine to the endplate resulted in the production of muscle spikes, while application of 10 millimolar acetylcholine "failed to produce more than a small local contracture at an endplate free region."[50] Nicotine and caffeine exhibited similar regional differences in activity. Chronically denervated muscle fibers, lacking observable motor endplates, exhibited marked increases in the sensitivity to drug application, while retaining the regional differences in activity exhibited by normal muscle fibers. Paralytic levels of curare decreased the sensitivity of the fibers to drug application. The reduction of the calcium concentration in Ringer solution to one-third the normal concentration resulted in the production of a neuromuscular block and the recording of pure epps.[51] Twin nerve stimuli, spaced 2–5 ms apart, resulted in summation of the epps and the production of muscle spikes. Further depletion of the calcium concentration resulted in the ultimate disappearance of epps, although directly elicited muscle spike potentials remained unaltered in low calcium Ringer solution. Excess calcium also resulted in neuromuscular blockade. However, this effect appeared to be mediated by a lowering of the excitability of the muscle fiber.[51]

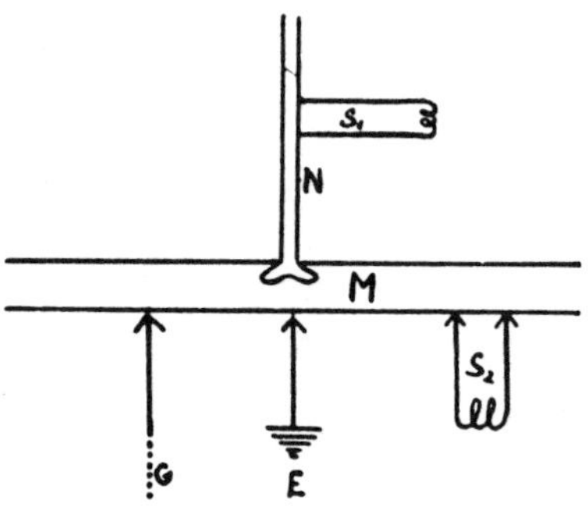
S₁
N
M
S₂
G
E

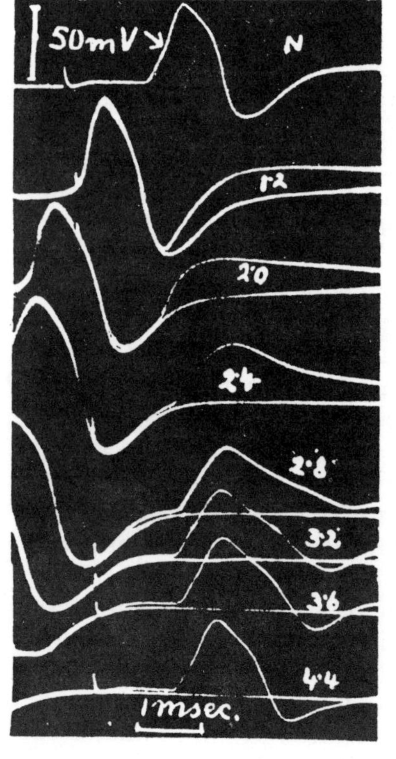
50mV
N
1·2
2·0
2·4
2·8
3·2
3·6
4·4
1 msec.

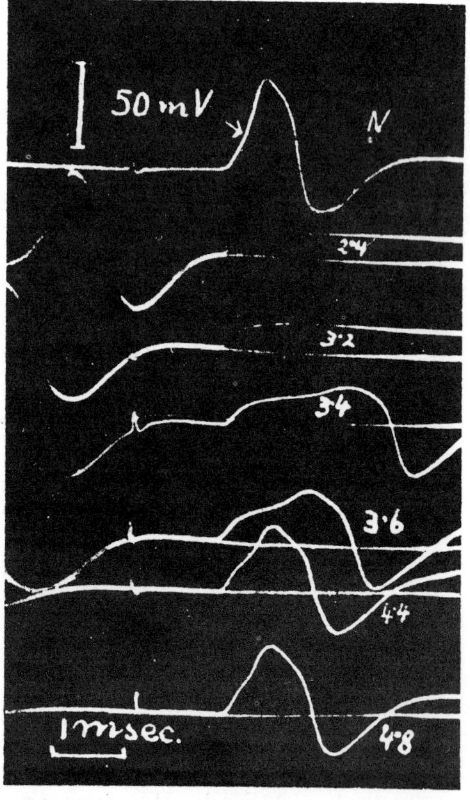
50 mV
N
2·4
3·2
3·4
3·6
4·4
4·8
1 msec.

In 1948, Kuffler[52] discussed "the 'transmitter' problem," presenting the contemporary ideas concerning the chemically mediated and the electrically mediated theories of neuromuscular transmission. An addendum to the article announced that, "Since this symposium was held a communication from Dr. Eccles has been received, stating that the electrical hypothesis cannot be reconciled with more recent experimental results on neuromuscular transmission. Eccles and his co-workers now believe that their evidence favors acetylcholine as the sole mechanism (*Ann. Rev. Physiol.*, 1948)."[25] Eccles and MacFarlane (1949)[34] presented the evidence in a study concerning the effects of varied anticholinesterases on the epps of fully curarized frog sartorius muscle. Dose-response relationships were derived by means of graphical analysis and provided measures of activity independent of the absolute magnitudes of the epps. Summarizing their finding, the authors state: "The ACh hypothesis of neuromuscular transmission is fully in accord with all observations, which themselves throw light on the detailed mechanisms involved in the transmission. . . ."[34]

The reconciliation of pharmacological and electrophysiological evidences brought to a close a remarkable epoch in biological investigation. Personal recollections by Dale,[16] Feldberg[38] and Eccles[26] provide readers with an opportunity to vicariously share in the excitement of

---

Figure 1.6. Extracellular recordings from the endplate region of a single nerve-muscle fiber preparation from the *adductor longus* muscle of the frog (*Hyla aurea*). The recording method (upper panel) permitted indirect stimulation (S_1) through the motor nerve (N) and direct, antidromic stimulation (S_2) of the muscle fiber (M). The bottom left panel displays records of action potentials recorded at the neuromuscular junction at the indicated millisecond interval following an antidromic muscle action potential. The top record of the panel records the response to a single nerve stimulus, and the arrow indicates the contribution of the endplate potential to action potential. The nerve stimulus in each record was delivered at a fixed interval following the start of the oscilloscope sweep, and is indicated by the stimulus artifact in the records. The bottom right panel displays action potential recorded at the neuromuscular junction in response to stimulus N_2 at the indicated millisecond interval following a conditioning stimulus (N_1). The nerve stimulus N_2 in each record was delivered at a fixed interval following the start of the oscilloscope sweep, and is indicated by the stimulus artifact in the records. A comparison of the records in the bottom panels at comparable delay intervals reveals that the refractory period at the endplate region following a conditioning nerve stimulus (N_1) is longer than the refractory period recorded following an antidromic muscle spike. (From Kuffler, 1942,[48] by permission of the *Journal of Neurophysiology*).

the 1930's and 1940's. The Nobel Prize in Physiology and Medicine was awarded to Sir Henry H. Dale and Otto Loewi in 1936 for their contributions to the understanding of the chemical transmission of the nerve impulse. Sir John C. Eccles, in 1963, and Bernard Katz, in 1971, were also honored as Nobel Prize Laureates in Physiology and Medicine for their contributions to the understanding of nerve cell function, and the chemistry of nerve impulse transmission. As for the electrical-mediation theory of neuromuscular transmission, Furshpan and Potter[41] were the first to demonstrate the existence of an electrically mediated synapse. The synapse, found in a crayfish, coupled a lateral giant axon with a large motor neuron.

References

1. Bacq ZM: La transmission chimique des influx dans le système nerveux autonome. *Ergebn Physiol* 37:82–185, 1935.
2. Bacq ZM, Brown GL: Pharmacological experiments on mammalian voluntary muscle, in relation to the theory of chemical transmission. *J Physiol* 89:45–60, 1937.
3. Bernard C: *Leçons sur les effets des substances toxiques et medicamenteuses*. Paris, J-B Bailliere et fils, 1857.
4. Brazier MAB: The historical development of neurophysiology. In Feild J (Editor-in-Chief): *Handbook of Physiology*, Vol. I. Washington, American Physiological Society, 1959, pp 1–58.
5. Brazier MAB: The problem of neuromuscular action: Two 17th century Dutchmen. In Rose CF, Bynum WF (eds): *Historical Aspects of the Neurosciences*. New York, Raven Press, 1982, pp 13–22.
6. Brown GL: Action potential of normal mammalian muscle. Effects of acetylcholine and eserine. *J Physiol* 89:220–237, 1937.
7. Brown GL: The actions of acetylcholine on denervated mammalian and frog's muscle. *J Physiol* 89:438–461, 1937.
8. Brown GL: Transmission at nerve endings by acetylcholine. *Physiol Rev* 17:485–513, 1937.
9. Brown GL, Dale HH, Feldberg W: Chemical transmission of excitation from motor nerve to voluntary muscle. *J Physiol* 87:42P–43P, 1936.
10. Brown GL, Dale HH, Feldberg W: Reactions of the normal mammalian muscle to acetylcholine and to eserine. *J Physiol* 87:394–424, 1936.
11. Chang HC, Gaddum JH: Choline esters in tissue extracts. *J Physiol* 79:255–285, 1933.
12. Couteaux R: Contribution a l'etude de la synapse myoneurale. *Rev Canadienne Biol* 6:563–711, 1947.
13. Cowan SL: The initiation of all-or-none responses in muscle by acetylcholine. *J Physiol* 88:3P–5P, 1936.
14. Dale HH: The action of certain esters and ethers of choline, and their relation to muscarine. *J Pharmac Exp Ther* 6:147–190, 1914.
15. Dale HH: Some recent extensions of chemical transmission. *Cold Spring Harbor Symp Quant Biol* 4:143–149, 1936.

16. Dale HH: *Adventures in Physiology With Excursions into Autopharma-cology.* London, Pergamon Press, 1953.
17. Dale HH, Dudley HW: The presence of histamine and acetylcholine in the spleen of the ox and the horse. *J Physiol* 68:97–123, 1929.
18. Dale HH, Feldberg W: Chemical transmission at motor nerve endings in voluntary muscle? *J Physiol* 81:39P–40P, 1934.
19. Dale HH, Feldberg W, Vogt M: Release of acetylcholine at voluntary motor nerve endings. *J Physiol* 86:353–380, 1936.
20. Dale HH, Gaddum JD: Reactions of denervated voluntary muscle, and their bearing on the mode of action of parasympathetic and related nerves. *J Physiol* 70:109–144, 1930.
21. Davis H, Forbes A: Chronaxie. *Physiol Rev* 16:407–441, 1936.
22. Du Bois-Reymond EH: *Gesammelte Abhandlungen zur allgemeinen Muskel- und Nervenphysik*, vol 2. Leipzig, Veit, 1877.
23. Eccles JC: Synaptic and neuro-muscular transmission. *Ergebn Physiol* 38:339–444, 1936.
24. Eccles JC: Synaptic and neuro-muscular transmission. *Physiol Rev* 17: 538–555, 1937.
25. Eccles JC: Conduction and synaptic transmission in the nervous system. *Ann Rev Physiol* 10:93–116, 1948.
26. Eccles JC: The synapse: From electrical to chemical transmission. *Ann Rev Neurosci* 5:325–339, 1982.
27. Eccles JC, O'Connor WJ: Responses evoked by a nerve volley in mammalian striated muscle. *J Physiol* 94:7P–9P, 1938.
28. Eccles JC, O'Connor WJ: Action potentials evoked by indirect stimulation of curarized muscle. *J Physiol* 94:9P–11P, 1938.
29. Eccles JC, O'Connor WJ: Excitatory actions at the neuro-muscular junction. *J Physiol* 95:32P–33P, 1939.
30. Eccles JC, O'Connor WJ: The action of eserine on striated muscle. *J Physiol* 95:36P–38P, 1939.
31. Eccles JC, O'Connor WJ: Responses which nerve impulses evoke in mammalian striated muscles. *J Physiol* 97:44–102, 1939.
32. Eccles JC, Katz B, Kuffler SW: Nature of the "endplate potential" in curarized muscle. *J Neurophysiol* 4:362–387, 1941.
33. Eccles JC, Katz K, Kuffler SW: Effect of eserine on neuromuscular transmission. *J Neurophysiol* 5:211–230, 1942.
34. Eccles JC, MacFarlane WV: Actions of anticholinesterases on endplate potential of frog muscle. *J Neurophysiol* 12:59–80, 1949.
35. Elliot TR: On the action of adrenalin. *J Physiol* 31:xx-xxi, 1904.
36. Elliot TR: The action of adrenalin. *J Physiol* 32:401–467, 1905.
37. Engelhart E, Loewi O: Fermentative Azetylcholinspaltung im Blut und ihre Hemmung durch Physostigmin. *Arch Exp Path Pharmakol* 150:1–13, 1930.
38. Feldberg W: The early history of synaptic and neuromuscular transmission by acetylcholine: Reminiscences of an eye witness. In *The Pursuit of Nature. Informal Essays on the History of Physiology.* Cambridge, Cambridge Univ Press, 1977, pp 65–83.
39. Feng TP: Studies on the neuromuscular junction. XVIII. The local potentials around N-M junctions induced by single and multiple volleys. *Chinese J Physiol* 15:367–404, 1940.
40. Fredericq H: Chronaxie: Testing excitability by means of a time factor. *Physiol Rev* 8:501–544, 1928.

41. Furshpan EJ, Potter DD: Transmission at the giant motor synapse of the crayfish. *J Physiol* 145:289–325, 1959.

42. Grundfest H: Excitability of the single fiber nerve-muscle complex. *J Physiol* 76:95–115, 1932.

43. Hinsey JC: The innervation of skeletal muscle. *Physiol Rev* 14:514–584, 1934.

44. Huber GC, DeWitt LMA: A contribution on the motor nerve-endings and on the nerve-endings in the muscle spindles. *J Comp Neurol* 7:169–230, 1897.

45. Kato G: *The Microphysiology of Nerve.* Tokyo, Maruzen Co., 1934, p 139.

46. Katz B: Impedance changes in frog's muscle associated with electrotonic and "endplate" potentials. *J Neurophysiol* 5:164–184, 1942.

47. Kuffler SW: Electric potential changes at an isolated nerve-muscle junction. *J Neurophysiol* 5:18–26, 1942.

48. Kuffler SW: Responses during refractory period at myoneural junction in isolated nerve-muscle fiber preparation. *J Neurophysiol* 5:199–209, 1942.

49. Kuffler SW: Further study on transmission in an isolated nerve-muscle fiber preparation. *J Neurophysiol* 5:309–322, 1942.

50. Kuffler SW: Specific excitability of the endplate region in normal and denervated muscle. *J Neurophysiol* 6:99–110, 1943.

51. Kuffler SW: The effect of calcium on the neuro-muscular junction. *J Neurophysiol* 7:17–26, 1944.

52. Kuffler SW: Physiology of neuro-muscular junctions: Electrical aspects. *Fed Proc* 7:437–446, 1948.

53. Kuhne W: On the origin and the causation of vital movement (Croonian Lecture). *Proc R Soc* 44:427–448, 1888.

54. Langley JN: On the reaction of cells and of nerve-endings to certain poisons, chiefly as regards the reaction of striated muscle to nicotine and to curare. *J Physiol* 33:376–413, 1905.

55. Langley JN: On nerve endings and on special excitable substances in cells (Croonian Lecture). *Proc R Soc Lond Ser B* 78:170–194, 1906.

56. Lapicque L: La chronaxie en biologie générale. *Biol Rev* 10:483–514, 1935.

57. Lapicque L, Lapicque M: Variations de l'excitabilité du muscle dans la curarisation. *C R Soc Biol* 58:991–993, 1906.

58. Lapicque L, Lapicque M: Action du curare sur les muscles d'animaux divers. *C R Soc Biol* 68:1007–1010, 1910.

59. Lillie RS: The conditions determining the rate of conduction in irritable tissues and especially in nerve. *Am J Physiol* 34:414–445, 1914.

60. Lillie RS: The conditions of conduction of excitation in irritable cells and tissues and especially in nerve. II. *Am J Physiol* 37:348–370, 1915.

61. Lillie RS: The conditions of physiological conduction in irritable tissues. III. Electrolytic local action as the basis of propagation of the excitation-wave. *Am J Physiol* 41:126–136, 1916.

62. Loewi O: Ueber humorale Uebertragbarkeit der Herznervenwirkung. *Pfluegers Arch* 189:239–242, 1921.

63. Loewi O, Navratil E: Ueber humorale Uebertragbarkeit der Herznervenwirkung. VI. Der Angriffspunkt des Atropins. *Pfluegers Arch* 206:123–134, 1924.

64. Loewi O, Navratil E: Ueber humorale Uebertragbarkeit der Herznervenwirkung. X. Ueber das Schicksal des Vagusstoffs. *Pfluegers Arch* 214:678–688, 1926.
65. Loewi O, Navratil E: Ueber humorale Uebertragbarkeit der Herznervenwirkung. XI. Ueber den Mechanismus der Vaguswirkung von Physostigmin and Ergotamin. *Pfluegers Arch* 214:689–697, 1926.
66. Lucas K: On the optimal electric stimuli of muscle and nerve. *J Physiol* 35:103–114, 1907.
67. Lucas K: The analysis of complex excitable tissues by their response to electric currents of short duration. *J Physiol* 35:310–331, 1907.
68. Lucas K: The excitable substances of amphibian muscle. *J Physiol* 36: 113–135, 1907.
69. Lucas K: The process of excitation in nerve and muscle (Croonian Lecture). *Proc R Soc London Ser B* 85:495–524, 1912.
70. Marnay A, Nachmansohn D: Cholinesterase in voluntary frog's muscle. *J Physiol* 89:359–367, 1937.
71. Matthes K: Action of blood on acetylcholine. *J Physiol* 70:338–348, 1930.
72. Neher E, Sakmann B, Steinbach JH: The extracellular patch clamp: A method for resolving currents through individual open channels in biological membranes. *Pfluegers Arch* 375:219–228, 1978.
73. Noda M, Takahashi H, Tanabe T, Toyosato M, Furutani Y, Hirose T, Asai M, Inayama S, Miyata T, Numa S: Primary structure of α-subunit precursor of *Torpedo californica* acetylcholine receptor deduced from cDNA sequence. *Nature* 299:793–797, 1982.
74. Pelouze M, Bernard C: Recherches sur le curare. *C R Acad Sci* 1850: 533–537, 1850.
75. Pollitzer S: On curare. *J Physiol* 7:274–288, 1886.
76. Rushton WAH: Lapicque's theory of curarization. *J Physiol* 77: 337–364, 1933.
77. Rushton WAH: The time factor in electrical excitation. *Biol Rev* 10: 1–17, 1935.
78. Tello JF: Genesis de las terminaciones nerviosas motrices y sensitivas. I. En el sistema locomotor de los vertebrados superiores. *Madrid Univ Lab Invest Biol Trabajos* 15:101–199, 1917.
79. Walker MB: Treatment of myasthenia gravis with physostigmine. *Lancet* 1:1200–1201, 1934.

Chapter 2

Structure and Morphogenesis of the Neuromuscular Junction

Michael R. Carry, Ph.D. and
Michio Morita, Ph.D.

The neuromuscular junction, or motor endplate, is the site of communication between nerve and muscle. Although the motor endplate displays a wide range of structural diversity in different types of vertebrate myofibers, it has features common to all synapses. As with other chemical synapses, the neuromuscular junction has a presynaptic axon terminal with synaptic vesicles containing a neurotransmitter, in this case, acetylcholine. The presynaptic axolemma has specialized sites where the vesicles fuse in response to membrane depolarization, releasing the neurotransmitter into the synaptic cleft or gap which separates the axon terminal and myofiber. The postsynaptic sarcolemma has specialized regions with receptors where the released acetylcholine binds and allows a postsynaptic depolarization which leads to a contraction of the myofiber. Associated with the neuromuscular junction is an extracellular enzyme, acetylcholinesterase, which hydrolyzes the neurotransmitter, causing its deactivation. All neuromuscular junctions have the above components which are necessary for neurotransmission, but there is a wide variation in the gross structure of motor endplates in addition to less obvious differences in the fine structure. The purpose of this chapter is to discuss the structural diversity, and morphogenesis of vertebrate neuromuscular junctions.

Structure of the Neuromuscular Junction

Light Microscopy

The structure of the motor endplate (neuromuscular junction) has been studied in a variety of vertebrate muscles (Table 2.1). Early studies of endplate morphology were limited to the light microscope using reduced silver, gold chloride and methylene blue techniques and these observations have been extensively reviewed elsewhere.[3,29,33,65,121,128] The neuromuscular junction is a cholinergic synapse [34] and more recently, histochemical techniques which localize cholinesterase activity [32,73] have been used for studying the morphology of motor endplates. The motor endplate of most mammalian striated muscle fibers has a typical appearance when stained for either nonspecific cholinesterase or acetylcholinesterase when the appropriate substrates and inhibitors have been utilized.[108] The endplate has an oval shape with the long axis usually parallel to the muscle fiber (Fig. 2.1A). This is the focal type of innervation, the endplate, or "terminaison en plaque" of the classical literature.[65,121] If the muscle is stained for a short enough period of time, numerous internal branches or ramifications are visible within the limits of the endplate. With extended staining periods the reaction product tends to diffuse and fill in the endplate, obscuring the ramifications. When a cholinesterase stain is combined with a stain for axons, it is obvious that the cholinesterase activity follows the same pattern as the terminal branches innervating the muscle fiber.[84]

Most muscle fibers have but a single site of innervation and in teased fiber preparations display only a single cholinesterase positive endplate. Exceptions to this rule are fibers which have multiple sites of contact, classically referred to as "terminaisons en grappe," along the length of the fiber;[65,121] among the examples are myofibers of the chicken anterior latissimus dorsi (ALD) and biventercervicis,[57,113] frog extensor digitorum longus (EDL) and iliofibularis,[30,53,56] and at least one fiber type of all extraocular muscles (EOM) that have been examined.[2,25,58,62,93,96,104,119,131] In the mouse recti muscles (EOM), the small diameter fine fibers have a multi-terminal innervation. Teased fibers display multiple cholinesterase positive sites (Fig. 2.1B) with a mean distance of 73 microns between adjacent sites of innervation.[25] It is unclear whether the multiple sites of innervation are derived from the same axon.[62] There are reports of polyneuronal innervation in adult cat,[103] amphibian,[77] and avian[50] myofibers with multi-terminal innervation. The multi-terminal innervation of the

Table 2.1
Studies of Neuromuscular Junction Morphology

Author(s)	Muscle	Technique(s)
	Amphibian—'T'	
Birks, et al. (14)	Sartorius	EM
Cole (30)	Iliotibialis	LM (gold chloride)
Desaki & Uchara (37)	Sartorius	EM (scanning)
Gray (53)	EDL	LM (methylene blue)
Hess (56)	Sartorius, Iliofibularis	LM (ChE), EM
Heuser & Reese (63)	Sartorius	EM
Kuffler & Yoshikami (78)	Cutaneous pectoris	LM (ZnI-OsO$_4$)
Letinsky & Morrison-Graham (84)	Cutaneous pectoris	LM (ChE, NBT)
Peper, et al. (101)	Cutaneous pectoris	EM (freeze fracture)
	Amphibian—Multi-terminal	
Cole (30)	Iliotibialis	LM (gold chloride)
Gray (53)	EDL	LM (methylene blue)
Hess (56)	Iliofibularis	LM (ChE), EM
Page (98)	EDL, Rectus abdominus	EM
	Avian—Focal	
Cole (30)	Iliotibialis	LM (gold chloride)
Hess (57)	PLD	LM (ChE), EM
Silver (113)	PLD, EOM	LM (ChE)
	Avian—Multi-terminal	
Bennett & Pettigrew (10)	ALD	LM (silver, ChE), electrophysiology
Hess (30)	ALD, Biventercervicis	LM (ChE), EM
Silver (113)	ALD, EOM	LM (ChE)

(Continued)

Table 2.1 *(Continued)*

Author(s)	Muscle	Technique(s)
	Fish—Focal	
Cole (30)	Paravertebral	LM (gold chloride)
	Mammalian—Focal	
Andersson-Cedergren (3)	Intercostal	EM
Cole (30)	Iliotibialis	LM (gold chloride)
Desaki & Uchara (37)	Sternothyroid	EM (scanning)
Ellisman, et al. (40)	EDL, Soleus	EM (freeze-fracture)
Fernard & Hess (44)	Tensor tympani, Stapedius	LM (ChE), EM
Hess (58)	EOM	LM (ChE), EM
Hess & Pilar (62)	EOM	LM (ChE), EM
Manolov (87)	Soleus, Gastrocnemius	LM (ChE)
Namba, et al. (93)	EOM	LM (ChE), EM
Padykula & Gauthier (97)	Diaphragm	EM
Pilar & Hess (104)	EOM	EM
Reger (107)	Intercostal	EM
Rossi & Cortesina (110)	Vocalis	LM (ChE)
Salpeter, et al. (112)	EOM	LM (ChE), EM
Silver (113)	Soleus, Gastrocnemius	LM (ChE)
Teravainen (119)	EOM	LM (ChE), EM
Zacks & Blumberg (129)	Intercostal	EM
Zenker & Anzenbacher (131)	EOM	LM (ChE)

Mammalian—Multi-terminal

Fernard & Hess (44)	Tensor tympani	LM (ChE), EM
Hess (58)	EOM	LM (ChE), EM
Hess & Pilar (62)	EOM	LM (ChE), EM
Namba, et al. (93)	EOM	LM (ChE), EM
Pilar & Hess (104)	EOM	EM
Rossi & Cortesina (110)	Vocalis	LM (ChE)
Salpeter, et al. (112)	EOM	LM (ChE), EM
Silver (113)	EOM	LM (ChE)
Teravainen (119)	EOM	LM (ChE), EM
Teravainen (120)	EOM	EM
Zenker & Anzenbacher (131)	EOM	LM (ChE)

Reptile—Focal

Cole (30)	Iliotibialis	LM (gold chloride)
Hess (59)	Dorsal longitudinal	LM (ChE)
Hess (60)	Segmental	EM
Kuffler & Yoshikami (78)	External oblique	LM (ZnI-OsO$_4$)
Kulchitsky (79)	Segmental	LM (gold chloride)

Reptile—"T"

Cole (30)	Iliotibialis	LM (gold chloride)

Reptile—Multi-terminal

Cole (30)	Iliotibialis	LM (gold chloride)
Hess (59)	Dorsal longitudinal	LM (ChE), EM
Hess (60)	Segmental	EM
Kulchitsky (79)	Segmental	LM (gold chloride)

Abbreviations: ALD = anterior latissimus dorsi; ChE = cholinesterase; EDL = extensor digitorum longus; EM = electron microscopy; EOM = extraocular muscle; LM = light microscopy; PLD = posterior latissimus dorsi.

fine or "Felderstruker" fibers of EOM is commonly referred to as "en grappe." This may not be accurate terminology since the multi-terminal innervation of EOM fibers is not identical to the true "en grappe" sites of innervation described for the slow (Felderstruker) fibers of the tonus bundles of the frog iliofibularis muscle.[119] Rather, the multiple innervation sites of EOM fibers have the appearance of miniature focal endplates.

A third type of innervation occurs on the myofibers of amphibians and some reptiles (Table 2.1). In cholinesterase-stained muscle, this type of innervation appears to be a series of branches from a single axon which run parallel to the long axis of the fiber (rather than forming the oval endplate common to mammalian striated muscle).[84] This type of innervation is referred to as a T-termination or "End-buschel."[121]

When a muscle is sectioned and stained, or stained as a whole mount for cholinesterase activity, it is possible to localize the position of endplates relative to the whole muscle. Most muscles have but a single band of endplates (Fig. 2.1C) extending across the approximate mid-point of the myofibers. The pattern varies, depending upon the arrangement of the fibers (fusiform or pennate) in the muscle. In muscles where the fibers do not extend from tendon to tendon (i.e., sartorius or gracilis), but overlap, multiple bands of endplates occur within the single muscle (Fig. 2.1D).[29,89,122] The multiple bands of endplates in a composite muscle may be confused with myotendonous or myomyous junctions, since all three types of junctions stain positive for cholinesterase activity.[89] In larval *Xenopus laevis*, the developing myofibers of the tail are not innervated at the mid-point, but rather are innervated at both ends. Similarly, the myofibers of the muscular sheets of the thoracic and abdominal cavities are initially innervated at their ends, but the sites of innervation subsequently shift to the mid-point of the fiber.[85]

Electron Microscopy

The fine structure of the neuromuscular junction has been described for different fiber types in various vertebrate muscles (Table 2.1), and excellent reviews have been written.[64,102,105,128] The structural diversity of endplates found in vertebrate striated muscle is summarized in Table 2.1. The basic structure of the neuromuscular junction described below is that of a focally innervated mammalian striated myofiber. Typically, a myelinated axon branch from an intramuscular nerve approaches the myofiber. The axon's myelin sheath ends in

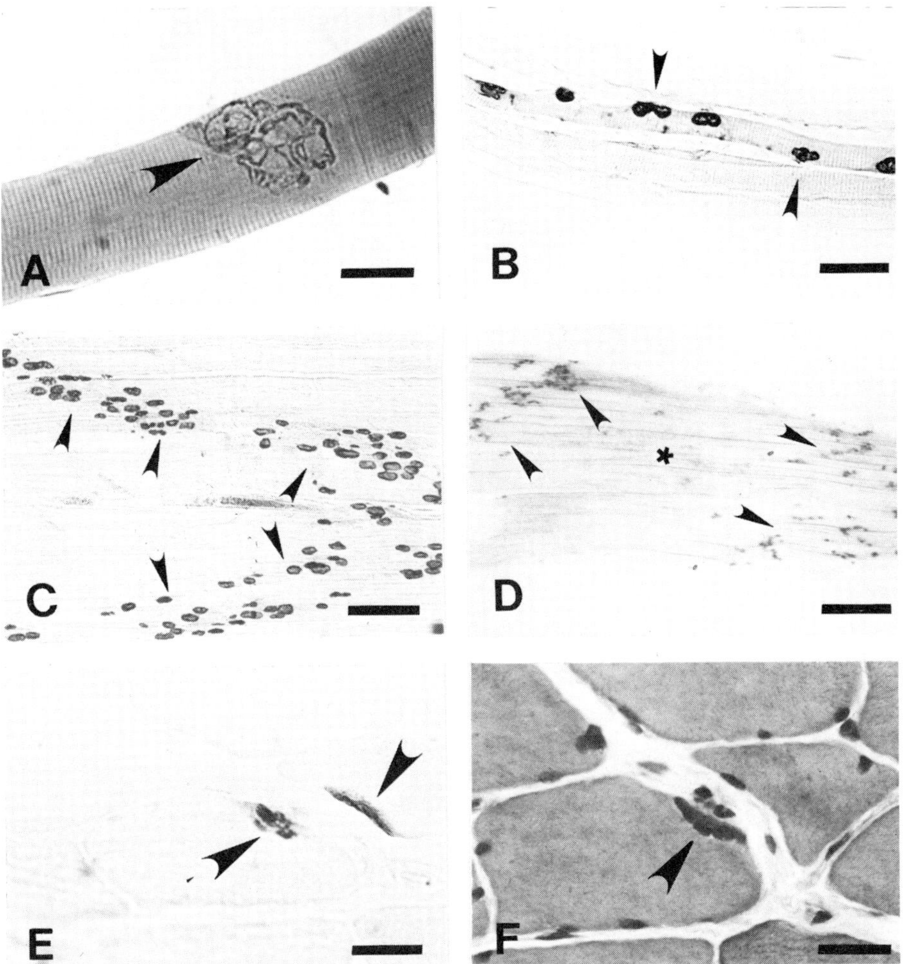

Figure 2.1. A. A myofiber of the mouse lateral rectus muscle with focal innervation. The single motor endplate is stained for cholinesterase activity (arrow). (Bar = 28 microns). **B.** A myofiber of the mouse lateral rectus muscle with multi-terminal innervation. The multiple sites of axonal contact (arrowheads) stain for cholinesterase activity. (Bar = 45 microns). **C.** A cryostat section of the mouse extensor digitorum longus muscle stained for cholinesterase activity. The endplates (arrowheads) are localized to a V-shaped band running across the muscle. (Bar = 150 microns). **D.** A cryostat section of the mouse (14 days postnatal) biceps femoris muscle stained for cholinesterase activity. This muscle displays two bands of endplates (arrowheads) and diffuse staining (*) in the region of overlap between fibers. (Bar = 420 microns). **E.** A cryostat section of the human quadriceps femoris muscle reacted with alpha-bungarotoxin conjugated to horseradish peroxidase. The labelled α-BuTx binds to acetylcholine receptors localized to the motor endplate. (Bar = 25 microns). **F.** A serial cryostat section adjacent to that of Fig. 2.1E stained with the modified trichrome technique. The motor endplate displays numerous myofiber nuclei (arrowhead). (Bar = 25 microns).

Table 2.2
Studies of Neuromuscular Junction Morphogenesis

Author(s)	Muscle	Technique(s)
	Amphibian	
Bennett & Pettigrew (11)	Iliofibularis, Sartorius	LM (silver, ChE), EM, Electrophysiology
Kullberg, et al. (80)	Myotome	EM, Electrophysiology
Lentz (82)	Regenerating limb	LM (ChE), EM
Letinsky & Morrison-Graham (84)	Cutaneous pectoris	LM (ChE, NBT)
Peng, et al. (100)	Myotome	Tissue culture, EM (freeze-fracture)
	Avian	
Atsumi (4)	Intercostal	LM (silver, ChE)
Atsumi (5)	ALD, PLD	LM (silver, ChE), EM
Bennett & Pettigrew (10)	ALD	LM (silver, ChE), EM, Electrophysiology
Burrage & Lentz (20)	ALD, PLD	Tissue culture, EM (AChR)
Burden (21)	PLD	LM (AChR)
Frank & Fischbach (48)	Pectoral	Tissue culture, LM (ChE, AChR), EM, Electrophysiology
Gorden, et al. (51)	ALD, PLD	Curare, LM (ChE)
Hirano (66)	Proximal hindlimb	EM
Ishikawa & Shimada (68)	PLD	LM (ChE, AChR)
Jacob & Lentz (69)	ALD, PLD	EM (AChR)
Sisto-Daneo & Filogamo (114)	EOM	EM
Sisto-Daneo & Filogamo (115)	ALD, PLD, EOM	EM

	Rabbit	
Bennett, et al. (9)	Diaphragm	LM (silver, ChE), EM, Electrophysiology
Bixby (15)	Diaphragm	EM
	Rat	
Bennett & Pettigrew (10)	Diaphragm	LM (silver, ChE), EM, Electrophysiology
Bevan & Steinbach (12)	Diaphragm, Sternomastoid	LM (ChE, AChR)
Bird (13)	Somite	Tissue culture, EM
Brown, et al. (17)	Soleus, Diaphragm	LM (ChE), Electrophysiology
Brzin, et al. (18)	Diaphragm	EM (AChE, BuChE)
Cardasis & Padykula (23)	Soleus	EM
Dennis, et al. (36)	Intercostal	LM (silver, dye injection), Electrophysiology
Duxon (39)	Soleus	LM (AChR), EM
Fagg, et al. (41)	Soleus	LM (ZnI-OsO$_4$)
Gozenback & Wasser (52)	Diaphragm	Regeneration, EM
Juntunen (71)	Anterior tibialis	LM (ChE)
Kelly & Zacks (74)	Intercostal	EM
Korneliussen & Jansen (75)	Soleus	EM
Nakajima, et al. (92)	Forelimb, Hindlimb	Tissue culture, EM, Electrophysiology
Teravainen (117)	Tibialis anterior	LM (ChE)
Teravainen (118)	Intercostal	EM
Tweedle & Stephens (124)	Soleus	LM (silver, ChE)
Weinberg, et al. (126)	Soleus	LM (ChE, AChR, BL-antigens)
Ziskind-Conhaim & Dennis (132)	Thoracic wall	Organ culture, LM (silver, ChE, AChR), Electrophysiology

(Continued)

Table 2.2 *(Continued)*

Author(s)	Muscle	Technique(s)
	Mouse	
Bird (13)	Hindlimb	Tissue culture, EM
Carry (24)	RF, EDL, FHB	LM (ChE, AChR), EM
Carry, et al. (26)	RF, FHB	LM (ChE), EM
Jirmanova (70)	Lumbricals	Regeneration, EM
Slater (116)	Soleus, EDL	LM (ChE, AChR, ZnI-OsO$_4$)
	Human	
Blechschmidt & Daikoku (16)	Tongue	EM
Caujunco (27)	Biceps brachi	LM (silver)
Fidzianska (46)	RF	EM
Fidzianska (47)	RF	EM
Juntunen & Teravainen (72)	Intercostal, Anterior tibialis	LM (ChE)

Abbreviations: AChE = acetylcholinesterase; AChR = acetylcholine receptor; ALD = anterior latissimus dorsi; BL = basal lamina; BuChE = butyrylcholinesterase; ChE = cholinesterase; EDL = extensor digitorum longus; EM = electron microscopy; FHB = flexor hallucis brevis; LM = light microscopy; PLD = posterior latissimus dorsi; RF = rectus femoris.

immediate proximity to the myofiber (Fig. 2.2), and the axon expands into numerous terminal branches. The terminal branches all lie within grooves or primary synaptic gutters on the surface of the myofiber. In the region of the synapse there is a large area of sarcoplasm which is devoid of myofibrils. This area, often referred to as the "sole plate,"[29,33] protrudes above the contour of the remainder of the myofiber and is rich in mitochondria and nuclei. At the neuromuscular junction, both the external myelin sheath and the internal microtubules end as the axon expands into its terminal branches (Fig. 2.3). The axon terminals lie in close apposition to the sarcolemma without any intervening cellular element. The outer surface of the axon terminals is covered by expansions of the Schwann cells associated with the axon. The extensions of the Schwann cells expand to meet the myofiber and the elements of the endomysium, thus surrounding the axon terminal on all surfaces except that adjacent to the sarcolemma. The Schwann cell and endplate are in turn surrounded by a bell-shaped covering of perineural cells which extends toward, but does not quite reach, the myofiber basal lamina.[111]

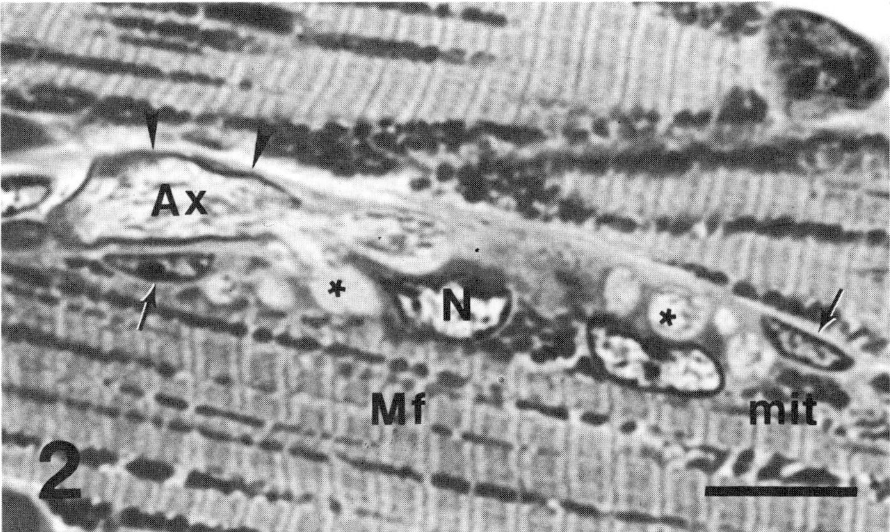

Figure 2.2. A semithin plastic section of the adult mouse inferior rectus muscle. The axon (Ax) loses its myelin sheath (arrowheads) as it splits into numerous terminal branches (*) characteristic of the neuromuscular junction. The axon terminals lie in deep primary synaptic gutters on the surface of the myofiber (Mf). The endplate region of the myofiber has accumulations of mitochondria (mit) and nuclei (N). Schwann cells (arrow) cover the axon terminals. (Bar = 10 microns).

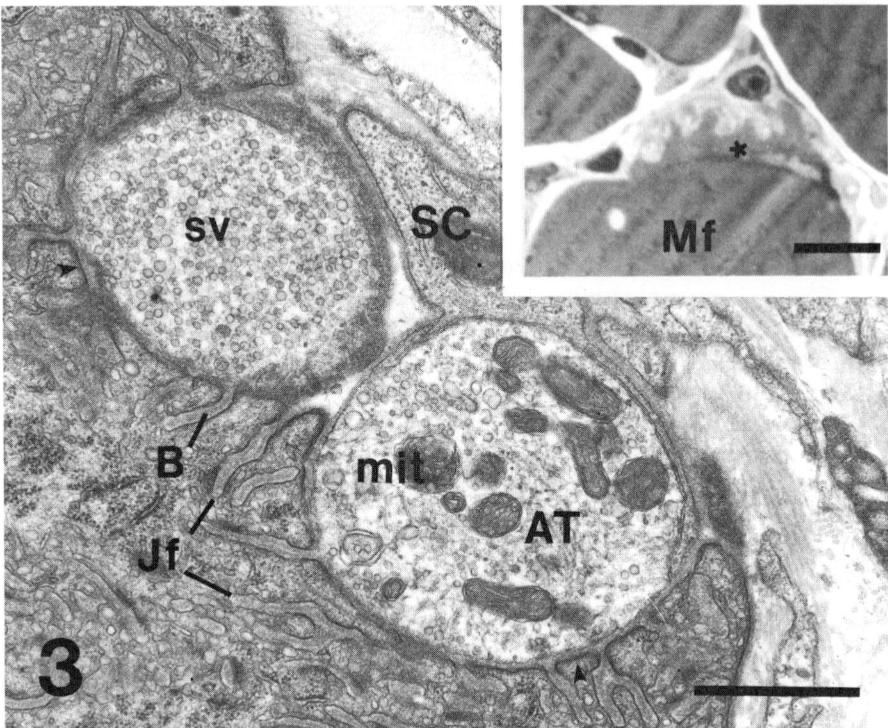

Figure 2.3. An electron micrograph of a neuromuscular junction (insert is a light micrograph of the same fiber) of a myofiber (Mf) of the adult mouse flexor hallucis brevis muscle. Axon terminals (AT), rich in mitochondria (mit) and synaptic vesicles (sv), lie in deep primary gutters in the sarcoplasm of the endplate (*). The external surface of the terminals is capped by a Schwann cell (SC) process. The sarcolemma forms numerous deep secondary postjunctional folds (Jf) with prominent densities (arrowheads) at their crests. Within the synaptic cleft is a distinct basal lamina (B). (Insert bar = 10 microns, bar = 1 micron).

The axon terminals are distinguishable by the absence of microtubules and the presence of numerous acetylcholine-containing 40–50 nm synaptic vesicles.[64] Additional organelles found in axon terminals are mitochondria, neurofilaments, coated vesicles, and cisternae of smooth endoplasmic reticulum. The coated vesicles and smooth endoplasmic reticulum may function in the retrieval of axonal membrane and the replenishment of synaptic vesicles.[38,63,99]

The presynaptic axolemma displays small patches of increased axoplasmic density. These regions are associated with aggregates of synaptic vesicles and are the sites of transmitter release, the active zones.[101] Freeze-fracture and etching techniques have allowed for the study of the internal structure of membranes. Using these techniques, rows of 10 nm intramembranous particles have been observed adjacent to the patches of increased presynaptic membrane density.[40,101] In frog myofibers the patches of increased membrane density and associated intramembranous particles are bar-shaped and parallel to each other, but perpendicular to the long axis of the axon terminal (T-terminal).[101] The rows of particles are localized over the openings to the secondary postjunctional folds (see below). In mammalian twitch fibers the synaptic vesicles are also aggregated over the openings of the secondary postjunctional folds, but the double rows of intramembranous particles which form the active zones are oriented perpendicular to the orientation of the secondary folds.[40]

The pre- and postsynaptic membranes are separated by a 60 nm gap.[102] The postsynaptic (myofiber) membrane is thrown into a series of processes and folds. These secondary postjunctional folds either extend to the myofibrils or into the "sole plate" sarcoplasm if it is present (see below). At the crests of the postjunctional folds are patches of increased sarcolemmal density. As with the presynaptic membrane, the postsynaptic membrane densities are the sites of membrane specialization functioning in neurotransmission. Freeze-fracture microscopy has demonstrated rows of 10 nm intramembranous particles extending perpendicular to the axis of the junctional fold.[40,105] Immediately beneath the membrane densities are located a branching, ladder-like filamentous network associated with the intramembranous particles.[40] More recently, the use of saponin treatment to remove all soluble cytoplasmic proteins has allowed for the resolution of a submembranous meshwork located immediately beneath the postsynaptic membrane which connects the membrane to bundles of intermediate filaments that course through the postsynaptic processes.[67] The filamentous network most likely functions to maintain the intramembranous particles at the crests of the secondary postjunctional folds.

The 10 nm intramembranous particles are believed to be acetylcholine receptors or proteins associated with receptor complexes.[40,67,105] Acetylcholine receptors have been localized with the aid of alpha-bungarotoxin (α-BuTx), a neurotoxin isolated from the Formosan banded krait, a species of snake belonging to the extremely venemous genus *Bungarus*.[28] This neurotoxin is believed to bind irreversibly to acetylcholine receptors since it blocks the action of acetylcholine and is itself competitively inhibited by curare.[90] The α-BuTx is typically labelled with horseradish peroxidase, a fluorescent label or ^{125}I to allow for the visualization of the binding sites. At the light microscopic level (Fig. 2.1E) the area binding the labelled α-BuTx approximates the same area as that which stains for cholinesterase activity.[126] Electron microscopic studies demonstrate that the α-BuTx binding sites are localized at the crests of the postjunctional folds, but do not extend into the depths of the secondary folds.[35,45] The area of α-BuTx binding overlaps that of the 10 nm intramembranous particles, and the evidence linking the two has been extensively reviewed by Rash and his co-workers.[105]

Myofibers and non-migrating Schwann cells,[19] but not axons, are surrounded by a single basal lamina. The basal lamina extends into the synaptic cleft of the neuromuscular junction, including the depths of the secondary postjunctional folds. The basal lamina material appears as a fuzzy-coat between the opposing membranes. Fine wisps extend from the basal lamina to the regions of increased membrane density,[67] and may serve to anchor the pre- and postsynaptic membranes, since synapses in general display a high degree of membrane adhesion.[64] The enzyme acetylcholinesterase is localized to the basal lamina at the neuromuscular junction.[86] The basal lamina may also play an important role in the recognition process between axon and myofiber during the formation of the neuromuscular junction (see chapter 5). The basal lamina of the junctional region has specific antigenic characteristics[126] and in frog muscle serves as a recognition site for regenerating axons[88] and the localization of new acetylcholine receptors in regenerating myofibers.[22]

Variation in Structure

The basic arrangement of axon and myofiber at the neuromuscular junction displays a wide variation depending upon the vertebrate class and fiber type (Figs. 2.3, 2.4, 2.5). In the rat diaphragm, a total of three fiber types are found: red (slow twitch, type I); white (fast twitch, type IIb); and intermediate (fast twitch, type IIa). The neuromuscular junctions of the red fibers have small axonal profiles lying in a moderately deep primary synaptic gutter. The secondary postjunctional folds are sparse, shallow, irregular in distribution, and branched at their depths.[97] The white fibers have longer, flatter axon terminals in deep primary synaptic gutters. The secondary postjunctional folds are regularly arranged and deeper than those of the red fibers. The bottom of the folds are closer to the myofibrils than in the red fibers, because the white fibers have less accumulation of subsynaptic mitochondria and nuclei. The intermediate fibers have neuromuscular junctions with the deepest postjunctional folds of the

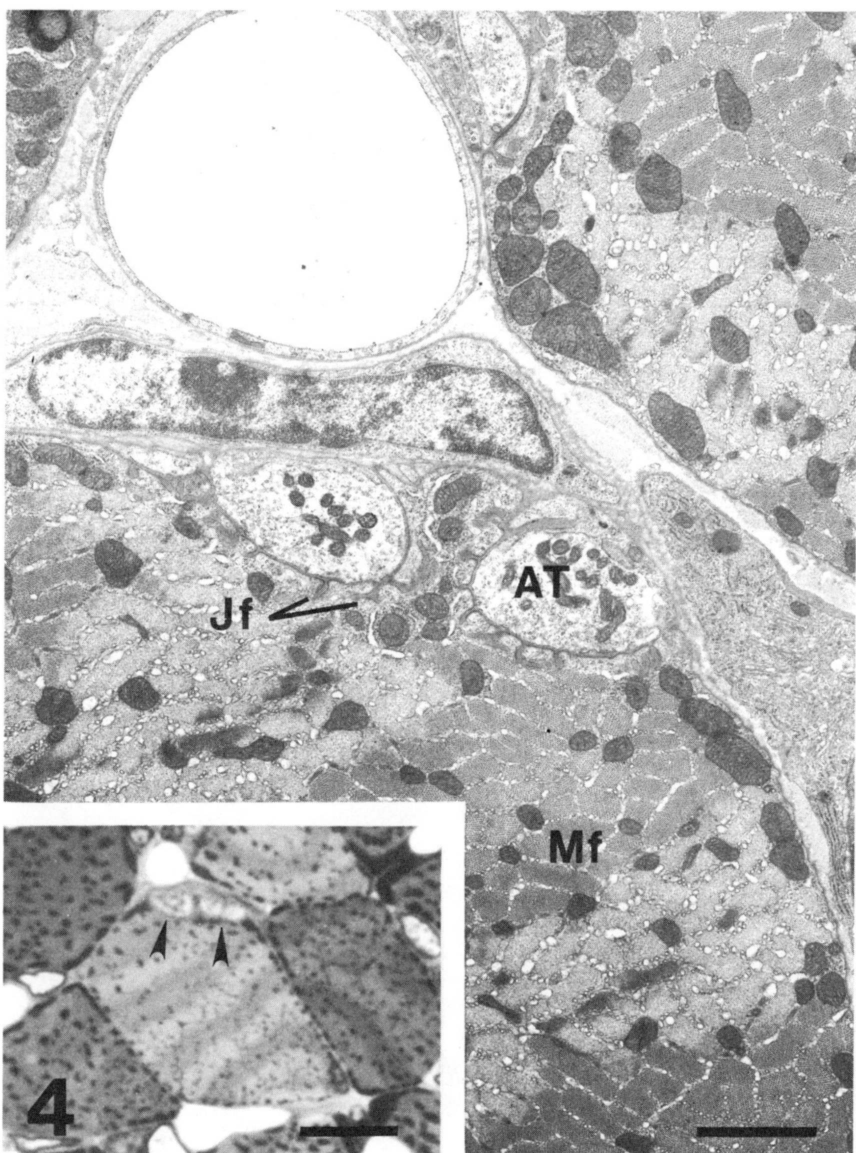

Figure 2.4. An electron micrograph of a granular fiber (Mf) from the adult mouse lateral rectus muscle. The axon terminals (AT) of the neuromuscular junction lie in a deep primary synaptic gutter, but the secondary postjunctional folds (Jf) are less frequent and shallow when compared with those of limb twitch fibers (Fig. 2.3). The lack of 'sole plate' (arrowhead) sarcoplasm (mitochondria and nuclei) is evident in the light micrograph of an adjacent section (insert, compare with Fig. 2.3). (Insert bar = 10 microns, bar = 2 microns).

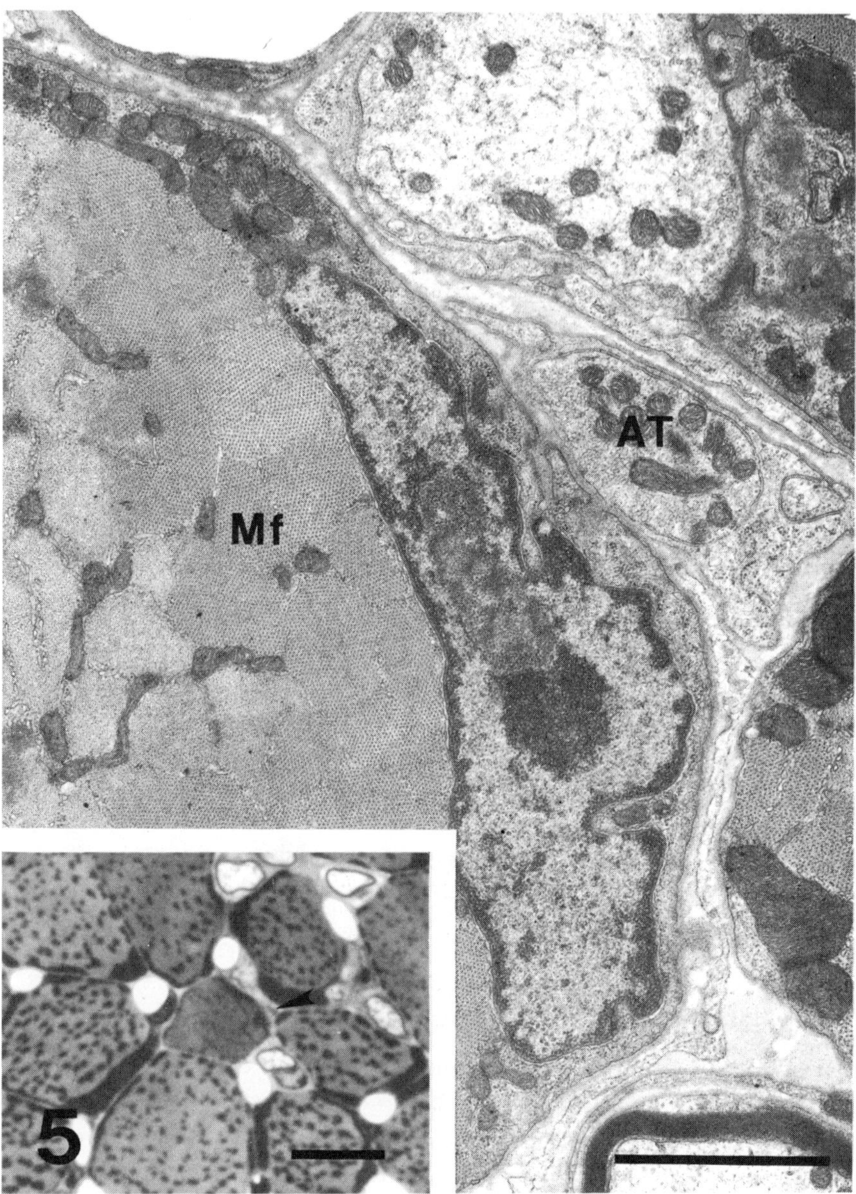

Figure 2.5. An electron micrograph of a fine fiber (Mf) from the adult mouse lateral rectus muscle. The axon terminal (AT) of the neuromuscular junction does not lie in a primary synaptic gutter. The secondary postjunctional folds are shallow and very infrequent. The neuromuscular junction is not easy to distinguish in the light micrograph of the adjacent semithin plastic section (insert). (Insert bar = 10 microns, bar = 2 microns).

three fiber types. The folds are spaced further apart than those of the white fibers, and are also straight and unbranched. The axon terminals of the white fibers contain the greatest number of synaptic vesicles.[97]

Despite the differences in metabolic and physiologic properties and in endplate structure, there is no difference in the distribution of the intramembranous particles in the endplate region membranes of the fiber types.[40] Unlike the diaphragm, which has three distinct fiber types, the rat EDL muscle contains only white (fast twitch) fibers. The neuromuscular junctions of the EDL white fiber type are reported to have a structure more similar to the red fibers of the diaphragm, with a larger area of "sole plate" sarcoplasm than the red (slow twitch) fibers of the soleus muscle.[40]

Mouse EOM displays variation in motor endplate structure when compared with limb muscle. Both of the presumed twitch fiber types with focal innervation, termed coarse and granular muscle fibers,[25] have sparse and shallow postjunctional folds (Fig. 2.4) when compared with limb twitch fibers (Fig. 2.3). Additionally, the EOMs contain a fiber type which has a multi-terminal innervation. This is the same fiber type which displays multiple cholinesterase positive sites, and is assumed to be slow or tonic[61] in its contractile properties, and may[60] or may not[62] be capable of propagating an action potential. In the chicken ALD similar fibers with multi-terminal innervation respond to a prolonged depolarization with a prolonged contraction, and the fibers are capable of propagating an action potential. These fibers may also have a polyneuronal innervation.[50]

The EOM fibers with multi-terminal innervation do not have a well-developed postsynaptic apparatus. The axon terminal does not lie within a primary synaptic gutter and has few, if any, secondary postjunctional folds (Fig. 2.5). Rather, the axon terminal sits on the surface of the myofiber, which does not have the large area of sarcoplasm, aggregation of mitochondria or multiple nuclei forming a "sole plate." An exception is the fiber type with multi-terminal innervation in human EOM. The fine fibers have neuromuscular junctions with well-developed secondary postjunctional folds. Although the fibers have multiple sites of innervation, they may not be tonic in their contractile properties as are comparable fiber types in other vertebrates, and this may account for the difference in the structure of their neuromuscular junction.

In addition to tonic or slow fibers, amphibian muscle has twitch fibers with neuromuscular junctions (T-terminals) intermediate in structure between the multi-terminal and focal endplates. The axon terminates in a number of branches that run for a short distance parallel to the longitudinal axis of the myofiber. Adjacent sites of transmitter release, the active zones, are separated by Schwann cell processes that protrude between the axon terminal and the sarcolemma. Each axon terminal has a separate Schwann cell.[78] The axon terminal lies in a shallow primary gutter, and the secondary postjunctional folds are sparse and branched at their depths, forming a T-shaped fold. The active zones lie over the openings to the secondary postjunctional folds and the localization of acetylcholine receptors and basal lamina are similar to the mammalian, focal neuromuscular junction.[101]

Morphogenesis of the Neuromuscular Junction

Localization of Cholinesterase Activity

Motor endplates are easily localized in muscle utilizing a histochemical technique for cholinesterase activity. This technique has been utilized to follow the appearance and maturation of endplates in embryonic and early postnatal muscle.[4,18,24,26,71,72,81,91,94,117] With light microscopy, the histochemical reaction product for cholinesterase activity first appears as a diffuse stain in myotubes at embryonic stages. As the neuromuscular junction forms, the reaction product accumulates, forming a straight line along the surface of the myotube. In developing mouse rectus femoris muscle the appearance of reaction product coincides with the period when the basal lamina material is accumulating in the primitive synaptic gutter. With increasing maturation the shape of the endplate transforms to an oval ring and finally develops internal ramifications.[4,24,26] During the postnatal maturation of myofibers, there is a concomitant increase in fiber diameter and the area of the cholinesterase reaction product (motor endplate).

In addition to acetylcholinesterase, butyrylcholinesterase (BuChE) is located at the neuromuscular junction. The enzymatic activity and cytochemical localization of both enzymes has been studied in developing postnatal rat diaphragm.[18] Both enzymes are found at all stages examined from the newborn to adult, but the activity of BuChE drops off dramatically during the postnatal period (past seven days). The activity of AChE remains unchanged. In electron micrographs, cytochemical reaction product for both enzymes is localized to the synaptic gutter, the intercellular space between axon and Schwann cell, and the nuclear envelope and tubular reticulum of both myotubes and Schwann cells.[18]

Acetylcholine Receptors

Acetylcholine receptors (AChRs) are localized to the neuromuscular junction in adult striated muscle.[42,78] Labelled neurotoxins, in particular alpha-bungarotoxin (α-BuTx),[28] have been utilized to follow the appearance of AChRs at developing neuromuscular junctions. The shape of the developing motor endplate as visualized with labelled neurotoxin is similar to that of histochemical cholinesterase, and when used in combination, the cholinesterase activity outlines the area of neurotoxin binding.[68] A major difference between the localization of AChRs and cholinesterase is the occurrence of extrajunctional receptors in developing and denervated muscle.[12,21,83] Initially, the AChRs are localized over the entire myotube membrane with sites of increased density (hot spots). Electron microscopic observations demonstrate that these sites have an increased sarcoplasmic membrane density, and do not always coincide with the sites of axonal contact.[20,69] In tissue culture the hot spots will form on myotubes that have developed from aneurogenic limb tissue,[8] and will form at additional sites once axonal contact has occurred.[48] As the neuromuscular junction matures, the AChRs accumulate at the endplate and the density of extrajunctional receptors drops until the adult level is reached.[12,21]

Only a single study to date has examined the appearance of antigens specific to the motor endplate basal lamina at the developing neuromuscular junction.[126] Although this was a developmental study, the neuromuscular junctions were those forming at ectopic sites in adult rat soleus muscle. Acetylcholine receptors appeared first at the synapses and were followed by AChE and finally by antigens specific to the endplate basal lamina.

Fine Structure

A number of structures have been identified which play a role in synaptic transmission, the functional aspect of the neuromuscular junction. These structures are the axon terminal with its active zones and synaptic vesicles, the basal lamina with its associated acetylcholinesterase, and the primary synaptic gutter and the crests of the secondary postjunctional folds with their membrane densities and acetylcholine receptors. An ideal study of motor endplate morphogenesis would include: (1) identification of temporal stages, (2) identification of the cell types, (3) physiological recordings to determine the onset of function (spontaneous and evoked endplate activity), and

(4) morphological studies identifying the various structures or macromolecules involved in the onset of physiological activity. Such a study would require the use of specific antibodies to identify the cell types based upon their surface antigens,[49,55,125] intracellular recordings with a cell marker, and cytochemical, immunocytochemical, thin-section and freeze-fracture electron microscopy to visualize the morphogenesis of both the pre- and postsynaptic membranes with their structural specializations associated with the release and binding of acetylcholine, and the depolarization of the postsynaptic membrane. Unfortunately, such an intensive study has not been reported, but numerous studies (Table 2.2) on a variety of vertebrate muscles have utilized many of the aforementioned techniques to elucidate the morphogenesis of the neuromuscular junction.

A summary of the fine structure of the morphogenesis of motor endplates in the hindlimb of the mouse is illustrated in Fig. 2.6. This illustration is based upon observations of the embryonic and early postnatal rectus femoris and flexor hallucis brevis muscles.[24,26] In the mouse hindlimb the important events in the formation of motor endplates occur over an approximate two-week period from embryonic day 13 through postnatal day seven. By embryonic day 13 all the major nerves of the hindlimb plexus are organized.[24] At the stage when axons first enter the proximal, preaxial region of the hindlimb bud (quadriceps femoris), the pre-muscle mass is uniformly comprised of an embryonic cell type. This cell has a large nucleus in comparison with scant cytoplasm. The nucleus is euchromatic and contains multiple nucleoli. The cytoplasm, devoid of myofibrils, is rich in polyribosomes, but has few mitochondria or cisternae of granular endoplasmic reticulum compared with more differentiated cell types. The embryonic cells are most similar to those identified as myoblasts in regenerating limbs of amphibians.[54]

Axons containing microtubules, neurofilaments and cisternae of agranular endoplasmic reticulum, but devoid of ribosomes, penetrate the pre-muscle mass and course along the surface of the embryonic cells (Fig. 2.7). Occasionally axons are expanded with less opaque axoplasm and few microtubules, but with an abundance of smooth-surfaced vesicles and cisternae of agranular endoplasmic reticulum. The vesicle-containing axons are similar to descriptions of growth cones.[1,127] A second cell type is associated with the clusters of axons. This cell type is similar to the embryonic cells, but has shorter cisternae of endoplasmic reticulum and has a sparse fuzzy-coat of basal lamina on its surface. Identification of the second cell type is difficult, but its characteristics, in particular the basal lamina, are

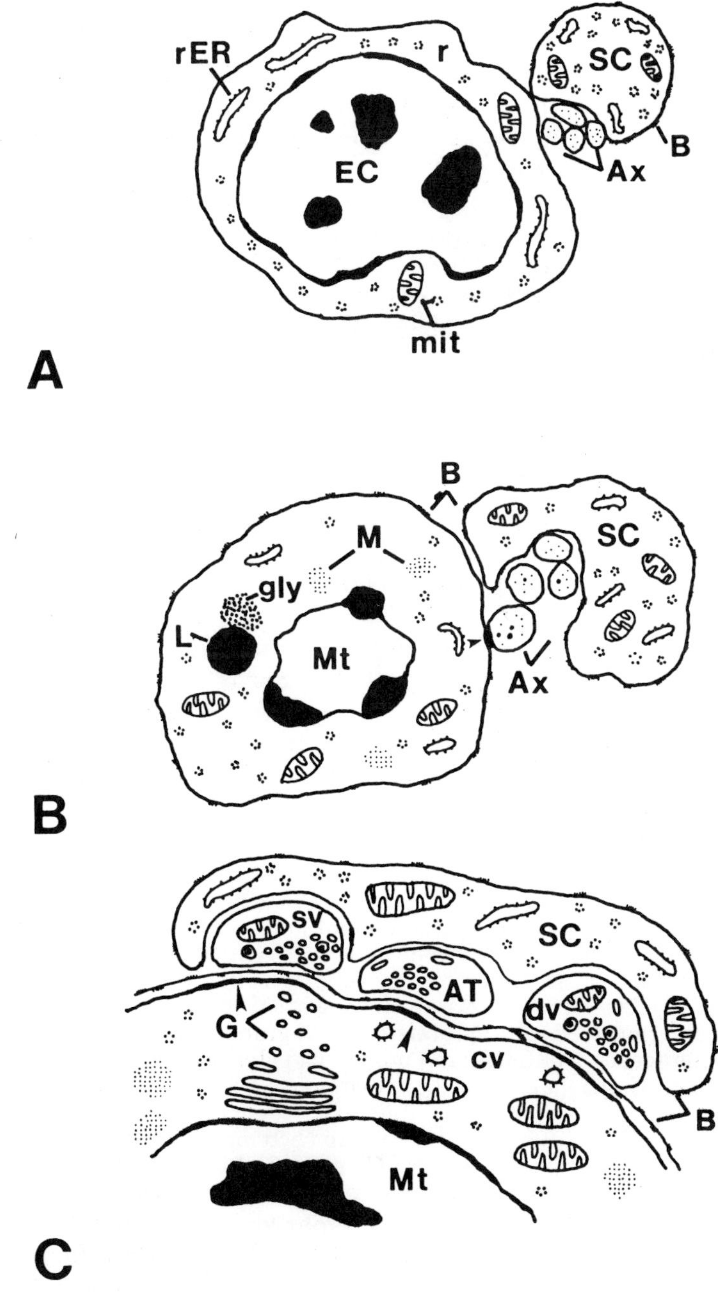

(Continued)

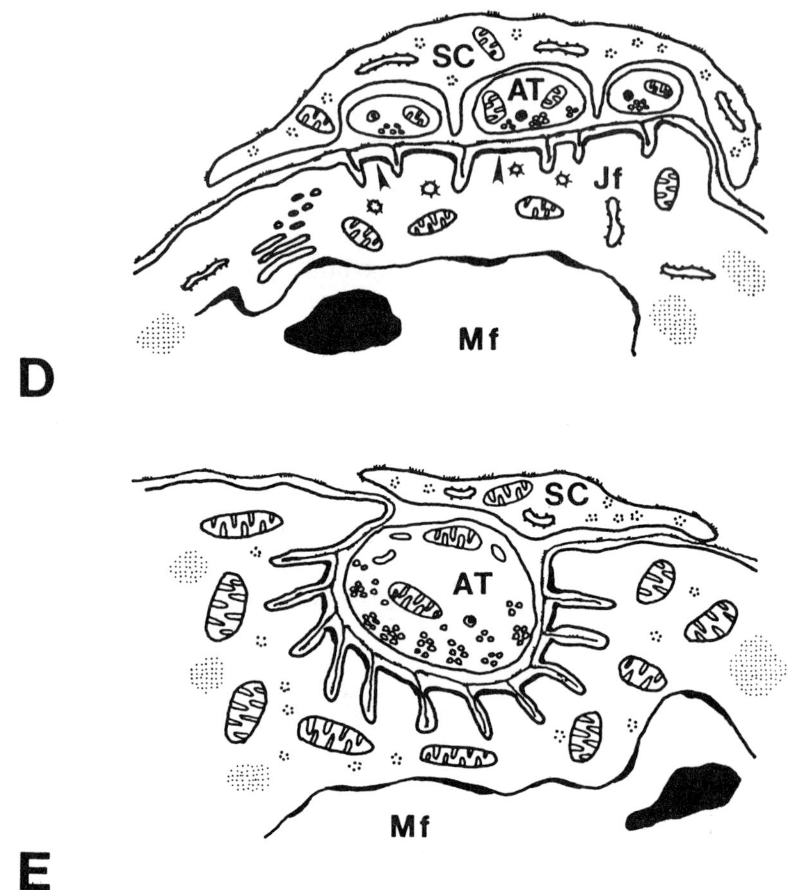

Figure 2.6. Summary of neuromuscular junction morphogenesis. **A.** Axons (Ax) and accompanying Schwann cells (SC) contact embryonic cells (EC) of the pre-muscle mass. The embryonic cells (most likely myoblasts) are characterized by a large euchromatic nucleus, sparse cytoplasm in comparison with more differentiated cell types, cisternae of granular endoplasmic reticulum (rER), mitochondria (mit), and numerous polyribosomes (r). The Schwann cells are distinguishable by their numerous polyribosomes and small cisternae of granular endoplasmic reticulum, and their sparse fuzzy-coat of basal lamina (B). **B.** Clusters of axons (Ax) and accompanying Schwann cells (SC) contact immature myotubes (Mt). The myotubes are characterized by central nuclei, accumulations of glycogen granules (gly), lipid droplets (L), and peripherally located myofibrils (M). Sites of contact between axons and myotubes display symmetrical patches of increased membrane density (arrowheads). **C.** Clusters of axon terminals (AT) sit on the surface of the myotube (Mt). The axons are covered on their external surface and partially separated from each other by a Schwann cell (SC). Synaptic (sv) and dense-

most similar to Schwann cells. Tissue culture studies demonstrate
that non-migrating Schwann cells associated with axons develop a
basal lamina.[19] At the early sites of contact between embryonic cells
(myoblasts), axons and Schwann cells, there are no signs of specialization signaling the formation of the neuromuscular junction. It is
possible that early contact specializations are present between axons
and myoblasts, but are difficult to identify. The early embryonic cells
(mesenchymal) are the substrate upon which the expanding axons
grow in their route through the limb bud.[1] Without the immunocyto-
logical markers utilized in tissue culture studies,[49,55,125] it is impossi-
ble to positively distinguish myoblasts from the embryonic cells
destined to differentiate as fibroblasts, Schwann cells or perineural
cells at the early stages of limb development.

During the following 24–48 hours myoblasts start fusing to form
myotubes. The myotubes are characterized by multiple elongated
nuclei, accumulations of glycogen granules and most importantly,
peripherally located myofibrils. Clusters of axons and associated
Schwann cells are found adjacent to myotubes and embryonic cells
(Fig. 2.8). Often the axons approach the myotubes but are separated
from them by an intervening Schwann cell process. At occasional

---

core (dv) vesicles are in the axon terminals. The subsynaptic sarcoplasm is
devoid of myofibrils, but contains numerous mitochondria, coated (cv) and
Golgi vesicles (G). The postsynaptic membrane has not formed secondary
folds, but displays patches (arrowheads) of increased sarcoplasmic density.
Both the myotube and Schwann cell have a fuzzy-coat of basal lamina (B)
which extends through the postsynaptic cleft. **D.** Axon terminals (AT) on the
surface of the immature myofiber (Mf) are separated from each other by
processes of the overlying Schwann cell (SC). Dense-core vesicles are
infrequent, but synaptic vesicles are numerous and cluster adjacent to the
presynaptic membrane. The subsynaptic sarcoplasm, devoid of myofibrils, is
rich in mitochondria, coated vesicles and Golgi vesicles, but as yet has not
accumulated to form a deep primary synaptic gutter. The postsynaptic membrane forms infrequent and shallow secondary postjunctional folds (Jf). The
crests of the folds display patches of increased density (arrowheads), and the
myofiber basal lamina extends throughout the synaptic cleft, including the
depths of the secondary folds. **E.** The mature neuromuscular junction has
axon terminals (AT) lying in deep primary synaptic gutters on the surface of
the myofiber (Mf). A Schwann cell (SC) process caps the external surface of
the axon terminal. Synaptic vesicles, cisternae of agranular endoplasmic
reticulum and mitochondria have accumulated in the terminal. The subsynaptic sarcoplasm has numerous mitochondria and nuclei. The postsynaptic sarcolemma is formed into numerous deep secondary postjunctional folds.
A prominent basal lamina extends throughout the synaptic cleft, including
the depths of the secondary postjunctional folds.

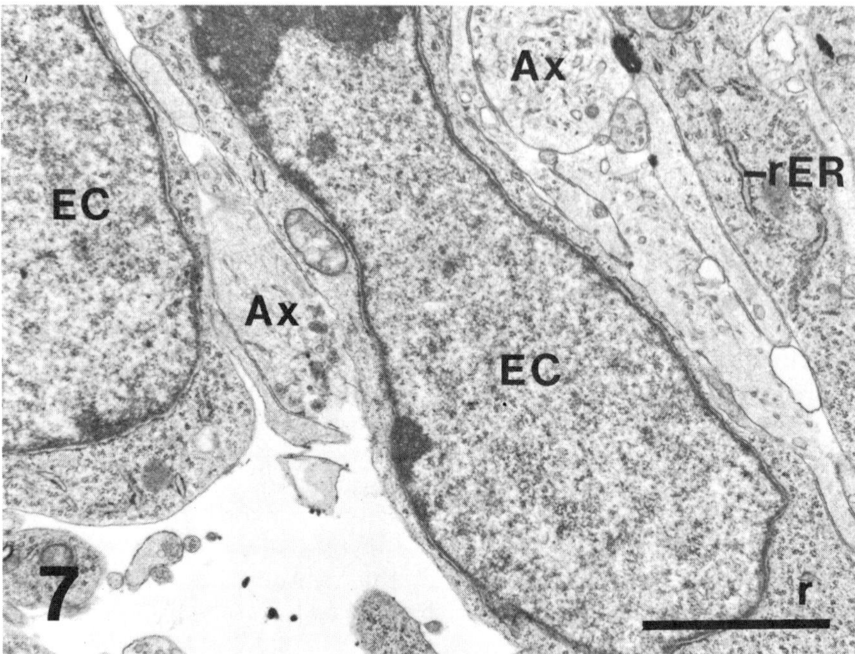

Figure 2.7. Clusters of axons (Ax) are in contact with embryonic cells (EC) in the dorsal pre-muscle mass of the embryonic day 13 mouse. The embryonic cells are characterized by a large euchromatic nucleus, scant cytoplasm in comparison with more differentiated cell types, numerous polyribosomes (r) and few cisternae of granular endoplasmic reticulum (rER). (Bar = 2 microns).

sites the axons directly contact the myotube surface. Many of the sites of contact display symmetrical patches of increased membrane density. Occasional axons contain sparse numbers of synaptic and dense-core vesicles. The myotube surface has a slight fuzzy-coat of basal lamina. The symmetrical patches of increased membrane density may be the first sign of synapse formation. Alternatively, they may be nonspecific sites of cell adhesion, since they also occur between adjacent axons, and between axons and Schwann cells.

During the following days (approximately embryonic day 18), axons and axon terminals accumulate on the surface of the myotube (Fig. 2.9). The axons are capped externally and partially separated from each other by a Schwann cell. Terminals contain clusters of synaptic vesicles and a few large (100 nm) dense-core vesicles. Regions of the axolemma display patches of increased cytoplasmic den-

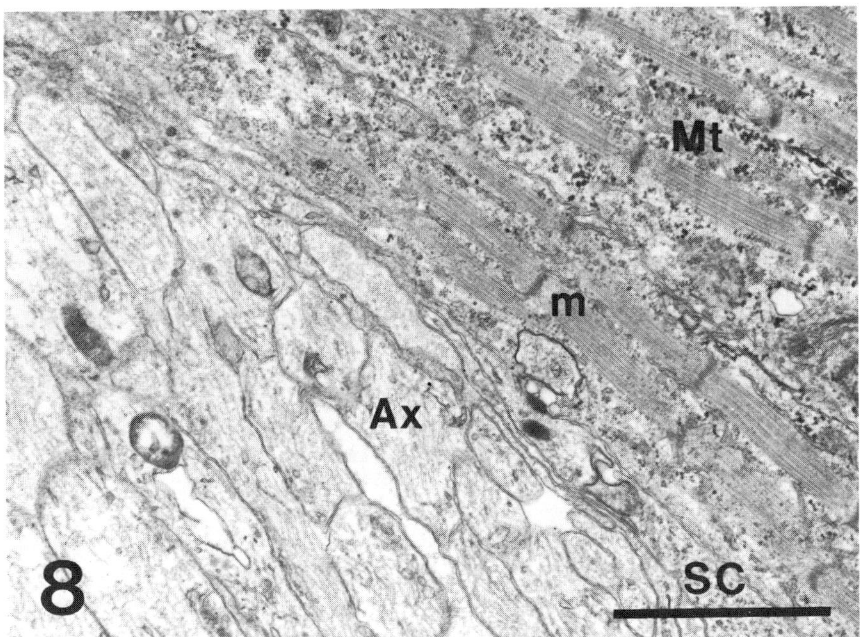

Figure 2.8. Clusters of axons (Ax) and an associated Schwann cell (SC) are adjacent to an immature myotube from the embryonic day 14 mouse rectus femoris muscle. The myotube is easily distinguishable by its numerous myofibrils (M). (Bar = 2 microns).

sity. The gap between axon terminal and myotube contains a prominent basal lamina. The postsynaptic membrane forms neither a primary gutter nor secondary postjunctional folds, but there are patches of increased membrane density. The sarcoplasm is rich in mitochondria, Golgi vesicles and coated vesicles, but the "sole plate" characteristic of many mature neuromuscular junctions has not formed. The immature neuromuscular junction appears similar to that of the EOM fibers with multi-terminal innervation.

The Golgi vesicles contain newly synthesized acetylcholine receptors.[43] The function of the coated vesicles is not known, but they may play a role in the intercellular communication between axon and myotube. Coated vesicles are capable of pinocytotically taking up extracellular materials as they form,[130] including possible substances released along with acetylcholine from synaptic vesicles.

During the following week the myotubes and their neuromuscular junctions continue to mature (Fig. 2.10). The myotube nuclei are

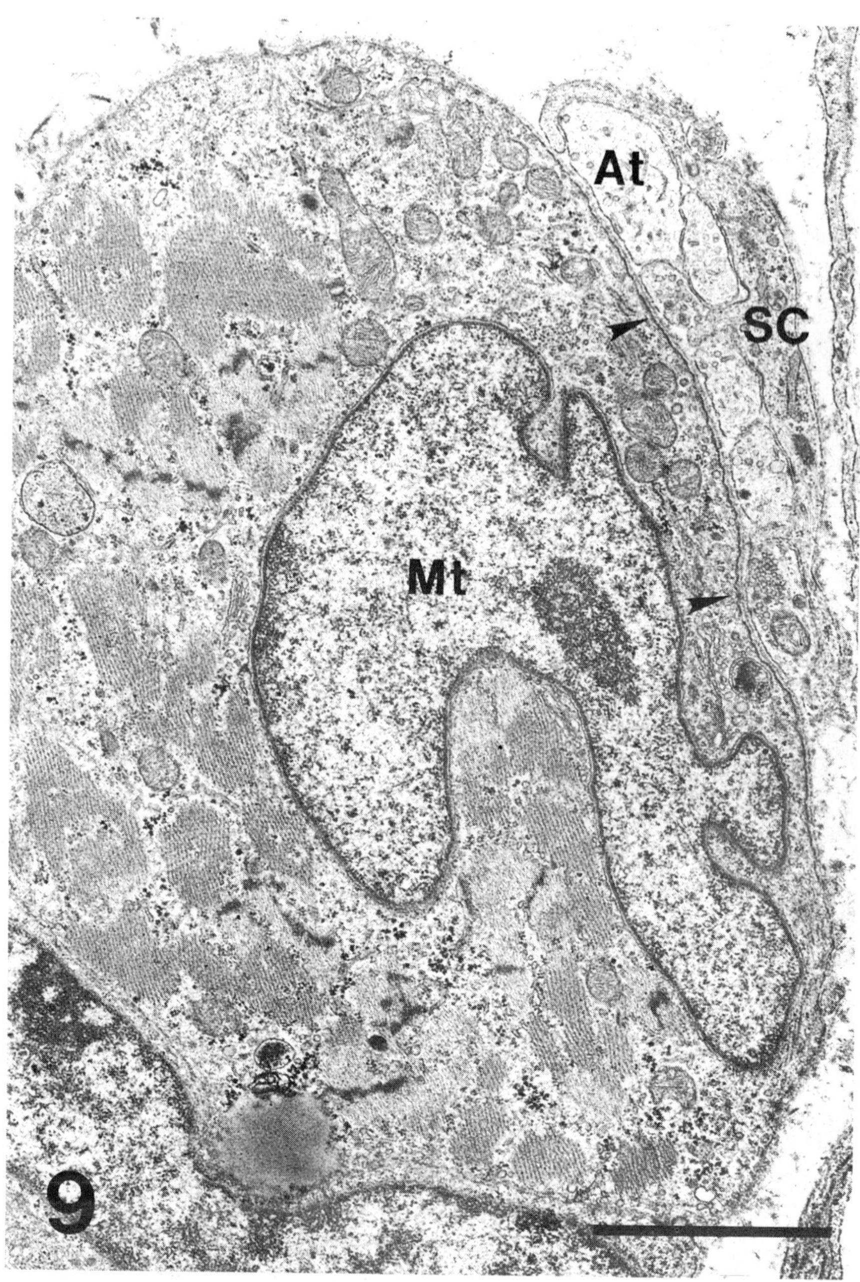

Figure 2.9. Clusters of axon terminals (AT) capped by a Schwann cell (SC) on the surface of a myotube (Mt). The axon terminals contain clusters of synaptic and dense-core vesicles (arrowheads). (Embryonic day 18 rectus femoris). (Bar = 2 microns).

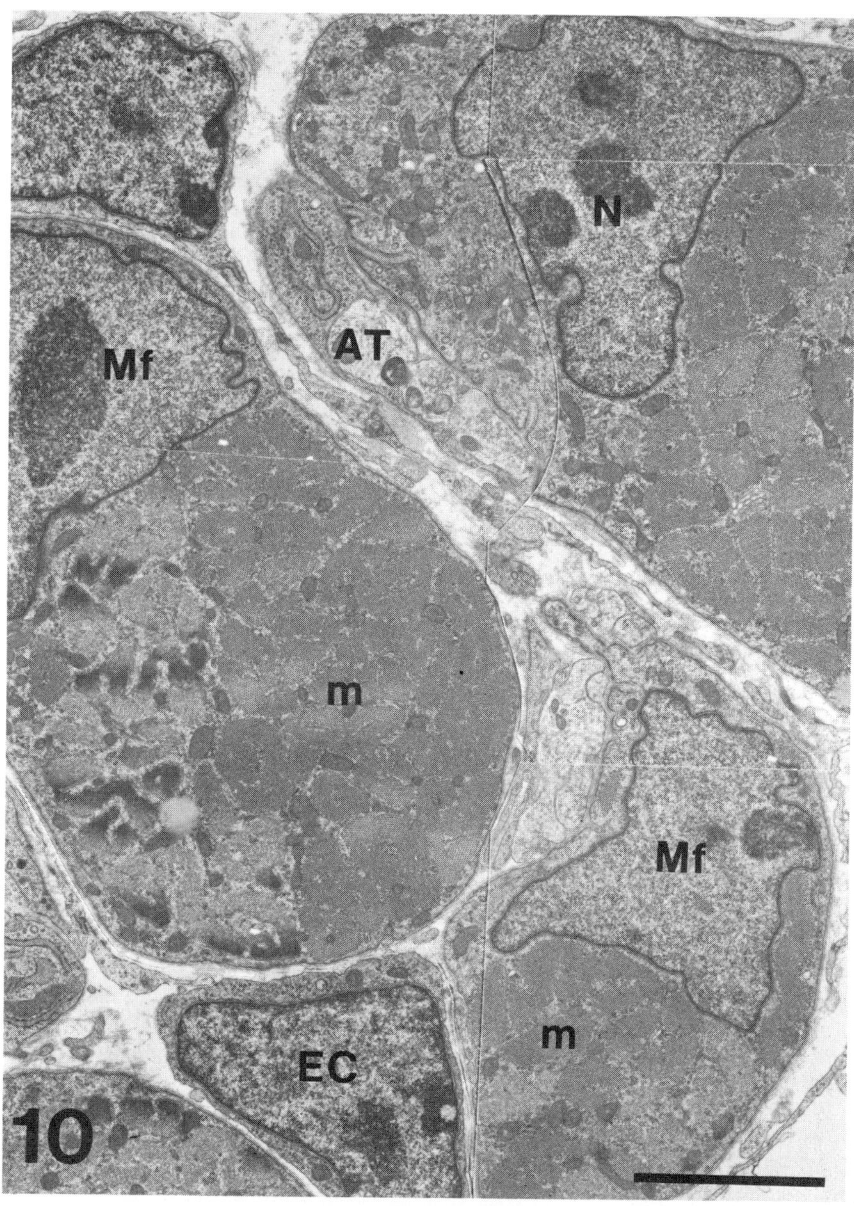

Figure 2.10. Immature myofibers (Mf) from the postnatal day seven mouse flexor hallucis brevis muscle are distinguishable by their peripherally located nuclei (N) and closely packed myofibrils (M). An embryonic cell (EC, most likely a myoblast) is associated with the myofibers. Clusters of axon terminals (AT) are localized opposite shallow postjunctional folds (arrowheads) of the immature neuromuscular junctions. (Bar = 3 microns).

displaced peripherally as myofibrils accumulate in the sarcoplasm. The primary synaptic gutter forms as sarcoplasm rich in mitochondria accumulates at the endplate, causing the axon terminals to be engulfed. The individual axon terminals are separated by Schwann cell processes which continue to cover their external surface. The crests of the secondary postjunctional folds display a prominent sarcolemmal density. A distinct basal lamina has accumulated in the synaptic cleft, including the depths of the secondary postjunctional folds. Synaptic vesicles are numerous in the axon terminals and are occasionally grouped adjacent to membrane densities (active zones). Dense-core vesicles are far less frequent than at earlier stages. The dense-core vesicles have been observed in developing and regenerating neuromuscular junctions,[24,26,66,74,92] but unlike the small catecholamine-containing dense-core vesicles,[102] their function has not been determined. The further maturation (past seven days postnatal) of the neuromuscular junction (Fig. 2.11) involves an increase in the area of the subsynaptic sarcoplasm (sole plate), and depending upon the fiber type, an increase in the number and depth of the secondary postjunctional folds.

Postnatal Maturation and Aging

With few exceptions, most adult myofibers are innervated by a single axon at a single synaptic site. During their development, limb striated myofibers pass through a transient period of polyneuronal innervation when each myofiber is innervated by one to three axons.[106] The axons innervate the same cholinesterase positive site[17] and electron microscopic observations typically detect more than one axonal profile associated with the immature endplate. By the third postnatal week the adult relationship of a single axon per motor endplate is established. While polyneuronal innervation is lost (based upon physiological recordings), one axon develops extensive terminal branches while the other axons remain immature.[95] The mechanism by which the other axons are lost is poorly understood and may relate to either the degeneration[109] or retraction[75,76,95] of axons.

Most studies of neuromuscular junction morphogenesis are confined to the embryonic and early postnatal stages. Few studies have correlated the changes in endplate structure and size with those of the myofiber in adult or aged muscle. Using histochemical cholinesterase activity to demonstrate endplates, the "mature-appearing" endplate has developed by the third postnatal week in the mouse

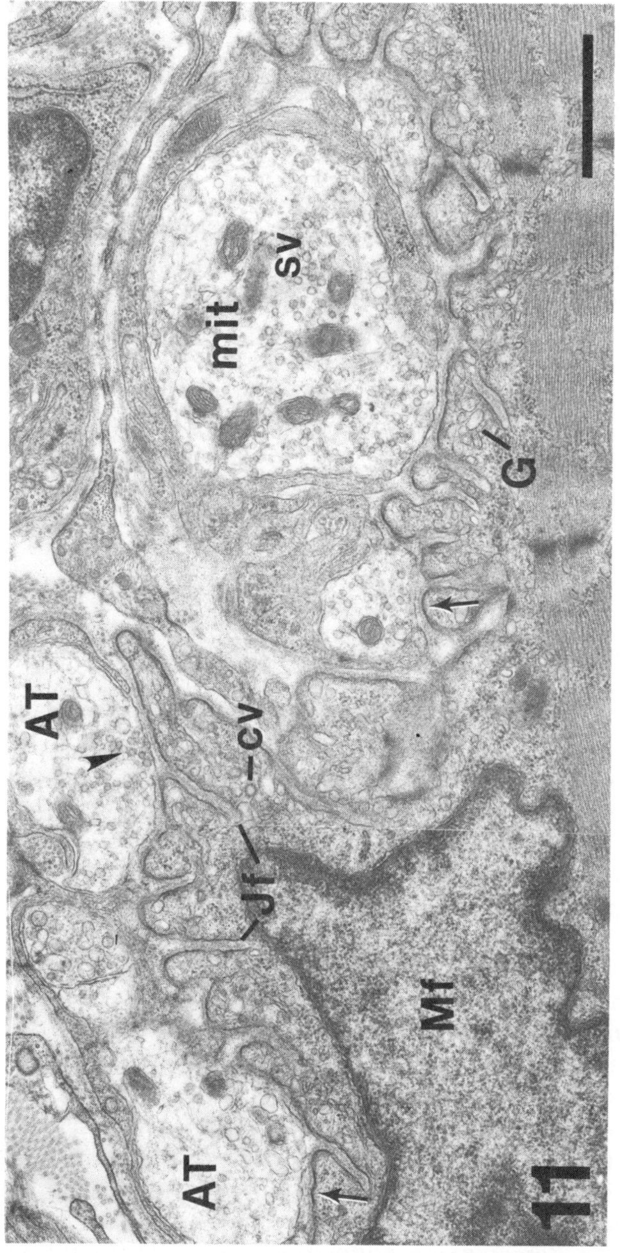

Figure 2.11. Axon terminals (AT) lie in shallow primary gutters on the surface of a myofiber (Mf) from the three-week postnatal flexor hallucis brevis muscle. The terminals contain mitochondria (mit), and numerous synaptic vesicles, including a few clusters adjacent to the presynaptic membrane (arrowhead). The axon terminals are opposite secondary postjunctional folds (Jf) which have patches of increased density at their crests (arrows). The sarcoplasm contains numerous Golgi vesicles (G) and a few coated vesicles (cv). (Bar = 1 micron).

hindlimb.[24,26,116] Although the shape and appearance of the endplates do not change, they continue to enlarge as the myofibers grow in length and diameter.

As animals grow older there is an increase in the complexity of the motor endplate associated with considerable axonal remodeling.[31,41,123,124] In rat soleus muscle the typical endplate in the young adult (3 months) is formed from one or two branches of the pre-terminal axon and is approximately 43 microns in length. Two years later (27 months) the typical endplate is considerably longer (65 microns) and is more complex, with two to three branches arising from the pre-terminal node.[41] The complex endplate may eventually separate to form smaller, adjacent endplates on the same fiber.[123] The increase in axonal complexity is matched by an increase in the number of discrete regions of high AChR density.[31] Changes in the fine structure of aged neuromuscular junctions are less well documented. Degeneration of axons is not common, but postjunctional folds without an overlying axon terminal have been observed in both rabbit diaphragm[15] and rat soleus[23] muscles. The lack of axonal profiles suggests a loss either by retraction or degeneration.

Human Studies

The studies of neuromuscular junction morphogenesis in human muscle are few and have been limited by a lack of adequately preserved specimens.[16,46,47] The descriptions that have been made are similar to those of other mammals. The period from the initial contact between axons and myotubes through the appearance of secondary postjunctional folds occurs between the 10th and 16th weeks of gestation for the upper arm.

The Relationship Between Structure and Function During Endplate Morphogenesis

Functional (electrophysiological) studies have been correlated with morphological observations in a number of neuromuscular models. The most thoroughly studied animal is the rat and an excellent summary on the intercostal muscle has been written by Dennis and his co-workers.[36] In both the diaphragm[10] and intercostal[36] muscles, axons are already present in the pre-muscle mass at the time when myoblasts first fuse to form myotubes. This is also true for the musculature of the mouse hindlimb.[24] The presence of functional neuromuscular junctions is determined by the recording of miniature endplate potentials (mepps) from the myotubes.[92] When intracellular recordings have been made it has been demonstrated that functional synapses are present as soon as myotubes can be penetrated by the microelectrode.[36] The recording of mepps occurs at the stage when cholinesterase activity is first detected[10] and synaptic vesicles may[92] or may not[80] be detected by electron microscopy. Regardless of the situation at earlier stages, synaptic vesicles are present in the axon terminals at the stage when evoked potentials can first be recorded.[80] The mepps are infrequent at early stages but become more frequent concomitantly with the structural maturation of the neuromuscular junction.[92]

Although the functional onset of activity is dependent upon structural maturation, the reverse does not appear to be the case. When neuromuscular contacts form in culture in the presence of a cholinergic blocking agent (curare), the curare does not interfere with the formation of synapses. The evoked potentials recorded immediately after the removal of the curare from the culture medium are identical to those recorded from control myotubes. Although the curare does not interfere with the establishment of neuromuscular junctions either *in vitro* or *in vivo*,[51] the lack of functional activity may interfere with the regulation of the distribution of endplates in muscle. Chick ALD muscle developing in the presence of curare has a closer spacing of adjacent synaptic contacts on the fibers with multi-terminal innervation (81 ± 3 microns compared with 133 ± 4 microns for controls).[51] Alpha-bungarotoxin will block the latter stages of motor endplate maturation in rat soleus muscle. Following α-BuTx treatment, the postnatal neuromuscular junctions fail to lose their excess axon profiles and do not develop the increased complexity of postjunctional folds, nor do the mitochondria or nuclei accumulate to form the "sole plate."[39]

Summary

The vertebrate neuromuscular junction displays structural diversity that ranges from fibers with focal innervation to fibers with multi-terminal innervation. All types of neuromuscular junctions have an axon that contacts a myofiber at one or more sites. The axon terminal may branch to form a T-shaped synapse (Endbushel), as in amphibians; a compact oval endplate with internal ramifications (en plaque), as in mammals; or may contact the myofiber at various sites along its length (en grappe). Regardless of the structural form, all neuromuscular junctions have certain features in common. The axon terminal contains mitochondria and cholinergic synaptic vesicles, and the axolemma has vesicle release sites (the active zones). A basal lamina with acetylcholinesterase is present in the synaptic cleft. The postsynaptic sarcolemma has acetylcholine receptors concentrated in high-density patches opposite the presynaptic active zones. Depending upon the fiber type, the postsynaptic sarcolemma has varying numbers of secondary postjunctional folds which may be shallow or deep in twitch fibers, or absent in "slow" fibers. The secondary postjunctional folds either extend to the myofibrils or end within a large area of sarcoplasm with aggregates of mitochondria and numerous nuclei (the sole plate).

Morphogenesis of the neuromuscular junction is initiated when axons and associated Schwann cells enter a pre-muscle mass comprised of a relatively undifferentiated cell type (myoblast). Within a few days the myoblasts fuse to form myotubes. The axons subsequently form contacts with the myotubes. The early contacts are characterized by symmetrical patches of increased membrane density, a sparse fuzzy-coat of basal lamina in the gap and a few synaptic and dense core vesicles in the axon. In subsequent days axon terminals accumulate on the surface of the myotube. Synaptic and dense core vesicles aggregate in the terminals which are partially separated from each other by processes of an overlying Schwann cell. The postsynaptic sarcolemma develops focal densities which are likely associated with the accumulation of acetylcholine receptors. As the neuromuscular junction matures, a primary gutter forms to engulf the axon terminals, secondary postjunctional folds form and the basal lamina accumulates in the synaptic cleft, including the depths of the secondary folds.

Cell-to-cell interactions must certainly play a role in determining not only the site(s) of nerve-muscle contact on a myofiber, but also the structural organization. Yet to be determined is why different fiber types have such diversely structured neuromuscular junctions. The diversity of neuromuscular junction morphology must be a reflection of the specific functions of different fiber types and their metabolic and physiologic properties. Perhaps through studies of nerve-muscle interaction during morphogenesis, insight will be gained into the relationships between structure of the neuromuscular junction and myofiber function.

References

1. Al-Ghaith LK, Lewis JH: Pioneer growth cones in virgin mesenchyme: An electron microscopic study in the developing chick wing. *J Embryol Exp Morphol* 68:149–160, 1982.
2. Alvarado J, Van Horn C: Muscle cell types of the cat inferior oblique. In Lennerstrand G, Bach-y-Rita P (eds): *Basic Mechanisms of Ocular Motility and Their Clinical Implications.* Oxford, Pergamon Press, 1975.
3. Andersson-Cedergren E: Ultrastructure of motor endplate and sarcoplasmic components of mouse skeletal muscle fiber as revealed by three-dimensional reconstructions from serial sections. *J Ultrastruct Res Suppl* 1:1–191, 1959.
4. Atsumi S: The histogenesis of motor neurons with special reference to the correlation of their endplate formation. *Acta Anat* 80:161–182, 1971.
5. Atsumi S: Development of neuromuscular junctions of fast and slow muscles of the chick embryo. *J Neurocytol* 6:691–709, 1977.
6. Bach-y-Rita P, Ito F: In vivo studies on fast and slow muscle fibers in cat extraocular muscles. *J Gen Physiol* 49:1177–1198, 1966.
7. Bach-y-Rita P, Lennerstrand G: Absence of polyneuronal innervation in cat EOM. *J Physiol* 244:613–624, 1975.
8. Bekoff A, Betz WJ: Acetylcholine hot spots: Development on myotubes cultured from aneural limb buds. *Science* 193:915–917, 1976.
9. Bennett MR, McLachlen EM, Taylor RS: The formation of synapses in reinnervated striated muscle. *J Physiol* 233:481–500, 1973.
10. Bennett MR, Pettigrew AG: The formation of synapses in striated muscle during development. *J Physiol* 241:515–545, 1974.
11. Bennett MR, Pettigrew AG: The formation of synapses in amphibian striated muscle during development. *J Physiol* 252:203–239, 1975.
12. Bevan S, Steinbach JH: The distribution of alpha-bungarotoxin binding sites on mammalian skeletal muscle developing in vivo. *J Physiol* 267:195–213, 1977.
13. Bird MM: Ultrastructural observations on rapid formation of neuromuscular junctions in vitro. *Cell Tissue Res* 217:647–659, 1981.
14. Birks RI, Huxley HE, Katz B: The fine structure of the neuromuscular junction of the frog. *J Physiol* 150:134–144, 1960.
15. Bixby JL: Ultrastructural observations on synapse elimination in neonatal rabbit skeletal muscle. *J Neurocytol* 10:81–100, 1981.
16. Blechschmidt VE, Daikoku SH: Die Entstehung der motorischen Innervation in der menschlichen Zungermuskulatur. *Acta Anat* 63:179–198, 1966.
17. Brown MC, Jansen JKS, Van Essen D: Polyneuronal innervation of skeletal muscle in newborn rats and its elimination during maturation. *J Physiol* 261:387–422, 1976.
18. Brzin M, Skatelj J, Tennyson VM, Kiauta T, Budinikas-Schoenabeck M: Activity, molecular forms and cytochemistry of cholinesterase in developing rat diaphragm. *Muscle Nerve* 4:505–513, 1981.

19. Bunge MB, Williams AK, Wood PM, Uitto J, Jeffery JJ: Comparison of nerve cell and nerve cell plus Schwann cell cultures, with particular emphasis on basal lamina and collagen formation. *J Cell Biol* 84:184–202, 1980.
20. Burrage TG, Lentz TL: Ultrastructural characterization of surface specializations containing high density acetylcholine receptors on embryonic chick myotubes in vivo and in vitro. *Devel Biol* 85:267–286, 1981.
21. Burden S: Development of the neuromuscular junction in the chick embryo: The number, distribution and stability of acetylcholine receptors. *Devel Biol* 57:317–329, 1977.
22. Burden SJ, Sargen PB, McMahan UJ: Acetylcholine receptors in regenerating muscle accumulate at original synaptic sites in absence of nerve. *J Cell Biol* 82:412–425, 1979.
23. Cardasis CA, Padykula HA: Ultrastructural evidence indicating reorganization at the neuromuscular junction in the normal rat soleus muscle. *Anat Rec* 200:41–59, 1981.
24. Carry MR: *Early Development of Nerve-Muscle System of Mouse Hindlimb*. Ph.D. dissertation, Colorado State University, 1979.
25. Carry MR, O'Keefe L, Ringel SP: Histochemistry of mouse extraocular muscle. *Anat Embryol* 164:403–412, 1982.
26. Carry MR, Morita M, Nornes HO: Morphogenesis of motor endplates along the proximodistal axis of the mouse hindlimb. *Anat Rec* 207:473–485, 1983.
27. Caujunco F: Development of the human motor endplate. Carnegie Inst Wash Publ 541 *Embryol* 30:127–152, 1942.
28. Chang CC, Lee CY: Isolation of neurotoxins from the venom of Bungarus multicinctus and their modes of neuromuscular blocking action. *Arch Int Pharmaco Ther* 144:241–257, 1963.
29. Coers C: Structure and organization of the myoneural junction. *Int Rev Cytol* 22:239–268, 1967.
30. Cole WV: Motor endings in the striated muscle of vertebrates. *J Comp Neurol* 102:671–715, 1955.
31. Courtney J, Steinbach JH: Age changes in neuromuscular junction morphology and acetylcholine receptor distribution of rat skeletal muscle fibers. *J Physiol* 320:435–447, 1981.
32. Couteaux R: Localization of cholinesterases at the neuromuscular junction. *Int Rev Cytol* 4:335–375, 1955.
33. Couteaux R: Motor endplate structure. In Bourne GH (ed): *The Structure and Function of Muscle*, Vol 2, part 2. New York, Academic Press, 1973.
34. Dale HH, Feldberg W, Vogt M: Release of acetylcholine at voluntary motor nerve endings. *J Physiol* 86:353–380, 1936.
35. Daniels MP, Vogel Z: Immunoperoxidase staining of alpha-bungarotoxin binding sites in muscle endplates shows distribution of acetylcholine receptors. *Nature* 254:339–341, 1975.
36. Dennis MJ, Ziskind-Conhaim L, Harris AJ: Development of neuromuscular junctions in rat embryos. *Devel Biol* 81:266–279, 1981.
37. Desaki J, Uchara Y: The overall morphology of neuromuscular junctions as revealed by scanning electron microscopy. *J Neurocytol* 10:101–110, 1981.

38. Droz B, Rambourg A, Koenig HL: Smooth endoplasmic reticulum: structure and role in the renewal of axonal membrane and synaptic vesicles by fast axonal transport. *Brain Res* 93:1–13, 1975.

39. Duxon MJ: The effect of postsynaptic block on development of the neuromuscular junction in postnatal rats. *J Neurocytol* 11:395–408, 1982.

40. Ellisman MH, Rash JH, Staehlin AL, Porter KR: Studies of excitable membranes. II. A comparison of specializations at neuromuscular junctions and nonjunctional sarcolemmas of mammalian fast and slow twitch muscle fibers. *J Cell Biol* 68:744–752, 1976.

41. Fagg GE, Scheff SW, Cotman CW: Axonal sprouting at neuromuscular junction of adult and aged rats. *Exp Neurol* 74:847–854, 1981.

42. Fambrough DM: Control of acetylcholine receptors in skeletal muscle. *Physiol Rev* 59:165–227, 1979.

43. Fambrough DM, Devreotes PN: Newly synthesized acetylcholine receptors are located in the Golgi apparatus. *J Cell Biol* 76:237–244, 1978.

44. Fernard VSV, Hess A: The occurrence, structure and innervation of slow and twitch fibers in the tensor tympani and stapedius of the cat. *J Physiol* 200:547–554, 1969.

45. Fertuck H, Salpeter M: Quantitation of junctional and extrajunctional acetylcholine receptors by EM autoradiography after ^{125}I-alpha-bungarotoxin binding at the neuromuscular junction. *J Cell Biol* 69:144–161, 1976.

46. Fidzianska A: Electron microscopic study of the development of human foetal muscle, motor endplate and nerve. *Acta Neuropathol* 17:234–247, 1971.

47. Fidzianska A: Human ontogenesis: II. Development of the human neuromuscular junction. *J Neuropathol Exp Neurol* 39:606–615, 1980.

48. Frank E, Fischbach G: Early events in neuromuscular junction formation in vitro. *J Cell Biol* 83:143–158, 1979.

49. Friedlander M, Fischman DA: Immunological studies of the embryonic muscle cell surface. Antiserum to the prefusion myoblast. *J Cell Biol* 81:193–214, 1981.

50. Ginsborg BL: Some properties of avian skeletal muscle fibers with multiple neuromuscular junctions. *J Physiol* 154:581–598, 1960.

51. Gorden T, Perry R, Tuffery AR, Vrbova G: Possible mechanisms determining synapse formation in developing skeletal muscle of the chick. *Cell Tissue Res* 155:13–35, 1974.

52. Gozenback HR, Wasser PG: Electron microscopic studies of degeneration and regeneration of rat neuromuscular junctions. *Brain Res* 63:167–174, 1973.

53. Gray EG: The spindle and extrafusal innervation of a frog muscle. *Proc R Soc Lond Ser* B 146:416–430, 1957.

54. Hay E: The fine structure of differentiating muscle in salamander tail. *Z Zellforsch* 59:6–34, 1963.

55. Heide UL, Kaufman SJ: Use of monoclonal antibodies in the analysis of myoblast development. *Devel Biol* 81:81–95, 1981.

56. Hess A: The structure of extrafusal muscle fibers in the frog and their innervation studied by the cholinesterase technique. *Am J Anat* 107:129–151, 1960.

57. Hess A: Structural differences of fast and slow extrafusal fibers and their nerve endings in chickens. *J Physiol* 157:221–231, 1960a.

58. Hess A: The structure of slow and fast extrafusal muscle fibers in the extraocular muscles and their nerve endings in guinea pigs. *J Cell Comp Physiol* 58:63–79, 1961b.

59. Hess A: Two kinds of extrafusal muscle fibers and their nerve endings in the garter snake. *Am J Anat* 113:347–363, 1963.

60. Hess A: The sarcoplasmic reticulum, the t-system, and the motor terminals of slow and twitch fibers in the garter snake. *J Cell Biol* 26:467–476, 1965.

61. Hess A: Vertebrate slow muscle fibers. *Physiol Rev* 50:40–62, 1970.

62. Hess A, Pilar G: Slow fibers in the extraocular muscles of the cat. *J Physiol* 169:780–798, 1963.

63. Heuser JE, Reese TS: Evidence for recycling of synaptic vesicle membrane during transmitter release at the frog neuromuscular junction. *J Cell Biol* 57:315–344, 1973.

64. Heuser JE, Reese TS: Structure of the synapse. In Brookhart JM, Mountcastle VB, Kandel ER (eds): *The Nervous System*. Bethesda, Amer Physiol Soc, 1979.

65. Hinsey JC: The innervation of skeletal muscle. *Physiol Rev* 14:514–585, 1934.

66. Hirano H: Ultrastructural study on the morphogenesis of the neuromuscular junction in the skeletal muscle of the chick. *Z Zellforsch* 79:198–208, 1967.

67. Hirokawa N, Heuser JE: Internal and external differentiations of the postsynaptic membrane at the neuromuscular junction. *J Neurocytol* 11:487–510, 1982.

68. Ishikawa Y, Shimada Y: Acetylcholine receptors and cholinesterase in developing chick skeletal muscle fibers. *Devel Brain Res* 5:187–197, 1982.

69. Jacob M, Lentz T: Localization of acetylcholine receptors by means of horseradish peroxidase-alpha-bungarotoxin during the formation and development of the neuromuscular junction in the chick embryo. *J Cell Biol* 82:195–211, 1979.

70. Jirmanova I: Ultrastructure of motor endplates during pharmacologically induced degeneration and subsequent regeneration of skeletal muscle. *J Neurocytol* 4:141–155, 1975.

71. Juntunen J: Morphogenesis of the cholinergic synapse in striated muscle. *Prog Brain Res* 49:351–358, 1979.

72. Juntunen J, Teravainen H: Structural development of myoneural junctions in the human embryo. *Histochemie* 32:107–112, 1972.

73. Karnovsky MJ, Roots L: A 'direct-coloring' thiocholine method for cholinesterases. *J Histochem Cytochem* 12:219–221, 1964.

74. Kelly AM, Zacks SI: The fine structure of motor endplate morphogenesis. *J Cell Biol* 42:154–169, 1969.

75. Korneliussen H, Jansen JKS: Morphological aspects of the elimination of polyneuronal innervation of skeletal muscle fibers in newborn rats. *J Neurocytol* 5:591–604, 1976.

76. Kuffler D, Thompson W, Jansen JKS: The elimination of synapses in

multiply innervated skeletal muscle fibers of the rat: dependence on distance between endplates. *Brain Res* 138:353–358, 1977.

77. Kuffler SW, Vaughan Williams EM: Small-nerve junctional potentials. The distribution of small motor nerves to frog skeletal muscle, and the membrane characteristics of the fibers they innervated. *J Physiol* 121:289–317, 1953.

78. Kuffler SW, Yoshikami D: The distribution of acetylcholine sensitivity at the post-synaptic membrane of vertebrate skeletal twitch muscles: iontophoretic mapping in the micron range. *J Physiol* 244:703–730, 1975.

79. Kulchitsky N: Nerve endings in muscle. *J Anat* 58:152–169, 1924.

80. Kullberg RW, Lentz TL, Cohen MW: Development of the myotomal neuromuscular junction in Xenopus laevis: An electrophysiological and fine-structural study. *Devel Biol* 60:101–129, 1977.

81. Kupfer C, Koelle GB: A histochemical study of cholinesterase during the formation of the motor endplate of the albino rat. *J Exp Zool* 116:397–407, 1951.

82. Lentz T: Development of the neuromuscular junction. I. Cytological and cytochemical studies on the neuromuscular junction differentiating muscle in the regenerating limb of the newt Triturus. *J Cell Biol* 42:431–443, 1969.

83. Lentz TL, Mazurkiewicz JE, Rosenthal J: Cytochemical localization of acetylcholine receptors at the neuromuscular junction by means of horseradish peroxidase-labelled alpha-bungarotoxin. *Brain Res* 132:423–442, 1977.

84. Letinsky MS, Morrison-Graham K: Structure of developing frog neuromuscular junctions. *J Neurocytol* 9:321–342, 1980.

85. Lewis PR, Hughes AFW: Patterns of myo-neural junctions and cholinesterase activity in muscles of tadpoles of Xenopus laevis. *Q J Microsc Sci* 101:55–67, 1960.

86. McMahan J, Sanes J, Marshall L: Cholinesterase is associated with the basal lamina at the neuromuscular junction. *Nature* 271:172–174, 1978.

87. Manlova S: Topographie et activité cholinesterasique des terminaisons nerveuses dans les muscles striés. *Acta Neuroveg* 25:428–434, 1963.

88. Marshall LM, Sanes JR, McMahan UJ: Reinnervation of original synaptic sites on muscle fiber basement membrane after disruption of the muscle cells. *Proc Nat Acad Sci USA* 74:3073–3077, 1977.

89. Mayr R, Gottschall H, Gruber H, Neuhuber W: Internal structure of the cat extraocular muscle. *Anat Embryol* 148:25–34, 1975.

90. Miledi R, Potter L: Acetylcholine receptors in muscle fibers. *Nature* 233:599–603, 1971.

91. Mumenthaler M, Engle WK: Cytological localization of cholinesterase in developing chick embryo skeletal muscle. *Acta Anat* 47:274–299, 1961.

92. Nakajima Y, Kidokoro Y, Klier G: The development of functional neuromuscular junctions in vitro: An ultrastructural and physiological study. *Devel Biol* 77:52–72, 1980.

93. Namba T, Nakamura T, Takahashi A, Grob D: Motor nerve endings in extraocular muscles. *J Comp Neurol* 134:385–396, 1968.

94. Nystrom B: Histochemical studies of endplate bound esterases in 'slow-red' and 'fast-white' cat muscles during postnatal development. *Acta Neurol Scand* 44:295–318, 1968.

95. O'Brien RAD, Ostberg AJC, Vrbova G: Observations on the elimination of polyneuronal innervation in developing mammalian skeletal muscle. *J Physiol* 282:571–582, 1978.

96. Pachter BR, Davidowitz J, Breinin GM: Light and electron microscopic serial analysis of mouse extraocular muscle: morphology, innervation and topographical organizations of component fiber populations. *Tissue Cell* 8:547–560, 1976.

97. Padykula HA, Gauthier GF: The ultrastructure of the neuromuscular junction of mammalian red, white and intermediate skeletal muscle fibers. *J Cell Biol* 46:27–41, 1970.

98. Page SG: A comparison of the fine structure of frog slow and twitch muscle fibers. *J Cell Biol* 26:477–497, 1965.

99. Palade G: Intracellular aspects of the process of protein synthesis. *Science* 189:347–358, 1975.

100. Peng HB, Nakajima Y, Bridgman PC: Development of the postsynaptic membrane in Xenopus neuromuscular cultures observed by freeze-fracture and thin-section electron microscopy. *Brain Res* 196:11–31, 1980.

101. Peper K, Dryer E, Sandri C, Akert K, Moor H: Structure and ultrastructure of frog motor endplate. A freeze-etching study. *Cell Tissue Res* 149:437–455, 1974.

102. Peters A, Palay SL, Webster HdeF: *The Fine Structure of the Nervous System.* Philadelphia, WB Saunders, 1976.

103. Pilar G: Further studies of the electrical and mechanical responses of slow fibers in cat EOM. *J Gen Physiol* 50:2289–2297, 1967.

104. Pilar G, Hess A: Differences in internal structure and nerve terminals of the slow and twitch muscle fibers in the cat superior oblique. *Anat Rec* 154:243–252, 1966.

105. Rash JE, Hudson CS, Ellisman ME: Ultrastructure of acetylcholine receptors at the mammalian neuromuscular junction. In Straub RW, Bolis L (eds): *Cell Membrane Receptors for Drugs and Hormones: A Multidisciplinary Approach.* New York, Raven Press, 1978.

106. Redfern PA: Neuromuscular transmission in new-born rats. *J Physiol* 209:701–709, 1970.

107. Reger JF: Electron microscopy of the motor endplate in rat intercostal muscle. *Anat Rec* 122:1–16, 1955.

108. Rosenberry TL: Acetylcholinesterase. In Martonosi A (ed): *The Enzymes of Biological Membranes*, Vol 4. New York, Plenum Publishing, 1976.

109. Rosenthal JL, Taraskevich PS: Reduction of multiaxonal innervation at the neuromuscular junction of the rat during development. *J Physiol* 270:299–310, 1977.

110. Rossi G, Cortesina G: Morphological study of the laryngeal muscles in man. *Acta Otolaryngol* 59:579–592, 1965.

111. Saito A, Zacks SI: Ultrastructure of Schwann and perineural sheaths at the mouse neuromuscular junction. *Anat Rec* 164:379–390, 1969.
112. Salpeter MM, McHenry FA, Feng H: Myoneural junctions in the extraocular muscles of the mouse. *Anat Rec* 179:201–224, 1974.
113. Silver A: A histochemical investigation of cholinesterases at neuromuscular junctions in mammalian and avian muscle. *J Physiol* 169:386–393, 1963.
114. Sisto-Daneo L, Filogamo G: Ultrastructure of developing myo-neural junctions. Evidence for two patterns of synaptic area differentiation. *J Submicrosc Cytol* 6:219–228, 1974.
115. Sisto-Daneo L, Filogamo G: Neurotization in muscle anlagens of chick embryo: Myoneural contacts in a period preceding synapse formation. *J Submicrosc Cytol* 8:303–318, 1976.
116. Slater CR: Postnatal maturation of nerve-muscle junctions in hindlimb muscles of the mouse. *Devel Biol* 94:11–22, 1982.
117. Teravainen H: Carboxylic esterases in developing myoneural junction of rat striated muscle. *Histochemie* 12:307–315, 1968a.
118. Teravainen H: Development of the myoneural junction in rat. *Z Zellforsch* 87:249–265, 1968b.
119. Teravainen H: Electron microscopic and histochemical observations on different types of nerve endings in the extraocular muscles of the rat. *Z Zellforsch* 90:372–388, 1968c.
120. Teravainen H: Axonal protrusions in small multiple endings in the extraocular muscles of the rat. *Z Zellforsch* 96:206–211, 1969.
121. Tiegs OW: Innervation of voluntary muscle. *Physiol Rev* 33:90–144, 1953.
122. Timus E, Timus M: The synaptoarchitecture of the muscle as a synchronizer for muscle contraction. *Z Mikrosk Anat Forsch* 94:545–555, 1980.
123. Tuffery AR: Growth and degeneration of motor endplates in normal cat hindlimb muscles. *J Anat* 110:221–247, 1971.
124. Tweedle CD, Stephens KE: Development of complexity in motor nerve endings at rat neuromuscular junction. *Neuroscience* 6:1657–1662, 1981.
125. Walsh FS, Phillips E: Specific changes in cellular glycoproteins and surface proteins during myogenesis in clonal muscle cells. *Devel Biol* 81:229–237, 1081.
126. Weinberg C, Sanes JR, Hall ZW: Formation of neuromuscular junctions in adult rats: Accumulation of acetylcholine receptors, acetylcholinesterase and components of synaptic basal lamina. *Devel Biol* 84:255–266, 1981.
127. Yamada KM, Spooner BG, Wessells NK: Ultrastructure and function of growth cones and axons of cultured nerve cells. *J Cell Biol* 49:614–635, 1971.
128. Zacks SI: *The Motor Endplate*. New York, Robert Krieger Publishing, 1973.
129. Zacks SI, Blumberg JM: Observations on the fine structure and cytochemistry of the mouse and human intercostal neuromuscular junctions. *J Biophys Biochem Cytol* 10:517–527, 1961.

130. Zacks SI, Saito A: Uptake of exogenous horseradish peroxidase by coated vesicles in mouse neuromuscular junctions. *J Histochem Cytochem* 17:161–170, 1969.
131. Zenker W, Anzenbacher H: On different forms of myo-neural junctions in two types of muscle fibers from the external ocular muscles of the Rhesus monkey. *J Cell Comp Physiol* 63:273–285, 1964.
132. Ziskind-Conhaim L, Dennis MJ: Development of rat neuromuscular junctions in organ culture. *Devel Biol* 85:243–251, 1981.

Chapter 3

Overview of the Physiology of the Neuromuscular Junction

Joseph J. McArdle, Ph.D.

It is essential to develop a fundamental understanding of the physiology of neuromuscular transmission in order to arrive at a working appreciation of the vast amount of information concerning the development, pathology and pharmacology of the neuromuscular junction (NMJ) as well as to gain insights into the molecular bases of as yet unexplained abnormalities of chemical synaptic transmission in general. With this in mind, the goal of the present chapter is to briefly review the information regarding the molecular bases for the function of the NMJ. To do this, the specialized systems of the muscle endplate and the motor nerve terminal which subserve their role in transmission across the NMJ will be discussed. In particular, attention will be focused upon the postsynaptic receptor and the presynaptic secretory systems. The latter is designed to release a sufficient quantity of the neuromediator, acetylcholine (ACh), to activate the focalized endplate conductance which in turn depolarizes the nonjunctional sarcolemma to the threshold of the initiation of an action potential. Classically, much of what we know of the secretory mechanism derives from studies of the postsynaptic events which the transmitter initiates. Therefore, the receptor system of the muscle endplate is discussed first. The greater part of this discussion focuses upon studies of the intact NMJ of amphibia and mammals, although references must be made to other synapses.

Acknowledgement: Data from my laboratory presented in this chapter were obtained with the financial assistance of the NINCDS (Grant NS 11055).

The Acetylcholine Receptor System (AChRS)

A useful image of the acetylcholine receptor system (AChRS) is that of a transmembrane channel which is open or closed to ion movement according to the position of a gating molecule. The latter is regulated by a third component of the system, referred to as the "trigger device,"[63] which specifically interacts with cholinergic ligands. Although the major focus of physiologic studies is upon the channel and its gate,[83,202,217,239] it is appropriate to first briefly consider the "trigger device," which is at least functionally and pharmacologically distinct from the other components.[231]

The "Trigger Device"

Two "gifts of nature" have greatly facilitated study of the "trigger device." First of all, Chang and Lee[43,44] discovered that the venom of various snakes, such as the krait *Bungarus multicinctus*, contains a protein which binds specifically and irreversibly to the receptor. Thus, binding of radioactively or fluorescently labelled α-bungarotoxin (α-BuTx) has enabled the isolation, quantitation and visualization of the receptor on the surface of cholinoceptive membranes. Secondly, the electroplaque of the sea ray *Torpedo* provides a uniquely rich source of the α-BuTx binding site. Much of what is known about the physical structure of the receptor derives from studies of this binding site.[54,104,120] For example, the receptor exists in dimeric and monomeric forms with sedimentation coefficients of 13S and 9S[118] and corresponding molecular weights of approximately 500,000 and 250,000,[136,223] respectively. The dimeric state of the receptor predominates in the intact membrane.[45] Since reducing agents stabilize the monomeric form of the receptor[45] while oxidizing agents favor the dimer,[99] Karlin et al[120] and Barrantes[18] have suggested that dimers result from sulfhydryl interactions between the peptides making up the monomeric unit. Four peptides, separated when the isolated monomer is subjected to polyacrylamide gel electrophoresis, have molecular weights of approximately 38,000, 47,000, 57,000 and 68,000[118,261] and are referred to as the α, β, γ and δ chains.

Karlin et al[118] demonstrated one ACh or α-BuTx binding site per 125,000 daltons of receptor protein. Two binding sites are associated with the monomer and its formula is presumed to be $\alpha_2 \beta \gamma \delta$.[31,120,209] Kinetic studies of the receptor in the electroplaque of *Electrophorus*[235] and frog[63] and lizard[148] skeletal muscle have indicated that two molecules of ACh are required to open a single channel. The function of one receptive unit involves the binding of ACh to two identifiable monomeric sites. These two sites are known to interact cooperatively,[65,101,147] which may explain the sigmoidal nature of the dose-response curve of the endplate to ACh.[121]

Additional studies have shed further light on the structure of the functional receptor unit in the intact membrane. For example, the ion channel itself seems to be at least 10 nm long,[155] spanning the membrane thickness and perhaps extending beyond the inner and outer membrane surfaces[107,119,136,227] to connect the extracellular and intracellular compartments. As viewed from the outer surface, the annulus of the receptor appears to have a diameter of 1.5–2.5 nm,[54] while at about three-quarters of the distance from the outer surface[110] the channel narrows to a cross-sectional area of 0.3–0.4 nm^2.[67,155,161] This narrow region of the channel is postulated to be the selectivity filter which quantitatively and qualitatively regulates ion flux. The size of the selectivity filter, which may not be fixed,[67] as well as its open time, determines the number and size of ions moving in response to activation of the receptor. The filter also selects ions on the basis of charge since it is permeable only to cations. In particular, Na^+, K^+ and Ca^{++} move down their concentration gradients through the open channel.[3,145,150,248,250] This cation selectivity may be due to negatively charged ends of dipolar molecules lining the channel wall.[19,20]

Quantitative studies of the binding of α-BuTx to the endplate of muscle from several species[8,148] have indicated that there are approximately 18,000 binding sites, equivalent to 9,000 functional units or monomers (see above) per square micrometer (μm^2), at the tops of the postsynaptic folds.[79] Because of this dense packing, the receptor apparently exists in the postsynaptic membrane as a semicrystalline mosaic[42,207] which is maintained by a fine cytoskeletal structure.[107] Two proteins have been proposed as the structural material. The first is actin, which is known to be associated with synaptic structures.[255] Hall et al[97] employed an antibody specific for cytoplasmic actin[159] and showed a close association of actin and high densities of the receptor. Further evidence for a close association of actin and the receptor comes from the observation that actin is a contaminant of receptor protein synthesized in a cell-free system.[193] Although several groups have found actin to be isolated in association with the receptor of electric organ, it is not yet established which peptide represents actin. In the absence of alkaline pretreatment, Hamilton et al[99] found that actin comigrated with a 43,000 molecular weight peptide on electrophoretic gels of receptor from *Torpedo californica*. The finding that alkaline extraction of this peptide[46,73,206] enhanced the receptor mobility in membrane fragments from *Torpedo marmorata*[157] further suggested its role in the maintainence of a high density of receptor. However, Sobel et al[237] did not confirm the electrophoretic similarity of actin and the 43,000 molecular weight (mol wt) peptide from *Torpedo marmorata* electric organ. Strader et al[243] demonstrated that an additional 47,000 mol wt peptide with properties similar to actin could be isolated from the receptor of *Torpedo californica* on electrophoretic gels containing 12.5% acrylamide. It is not known if alkaline treatment extracts this peptide from receptor-containing membranes to account for the reported elevation of receptor mobility.[157]

The second candidate for the material maintaining high densities of receptor is collagen. Kalcheim et al[117] found in cultured myotubes that collagen and receptor synthesis were coupled. Furthermore, collagenase prevented the formation of receptor aggregates on the sarcolemma. A high density of receptor at the motor endplate assures the high safety factor of neuromuscular transmission since the number of receptors normally activated by the neurally released ACh is several times the minimal needed to depolarize the sarcolemma to threshold.[8] Thus, it is essential to understand the process underlying the formation of such clusters.

The Gate and the Channel

Our present understanding of the function of the channel component of the acetylcholine receptor system depends greatly upon techniques to record the endplate currents accompanying receptor-mediated ionic fluxes. Briefly, these techniques involve either direct or indirect recordings of the currents. The former approach utilizes an extracellular microelectrode which is positioned above the receptor-rich endplate surface. Because this electrode has a relatively low resistance and high-frequency response it can detect the localized ionic currents flowing through channels whose gates are opened by ACh. Such recordings are readily made at neuromuscular junctions viewed with Nomarski optics (Fig. 3.1). However, with the exception of the patch-voltage clamp technique, extracellular recordings are limited to the analysis of the time characteristics of the endplate currents since amplitude measurements are critically dependent upon electrode position. Even the former analysis is inaccurate when large and diffuse activation of the endplate occurs. Indirect meas-

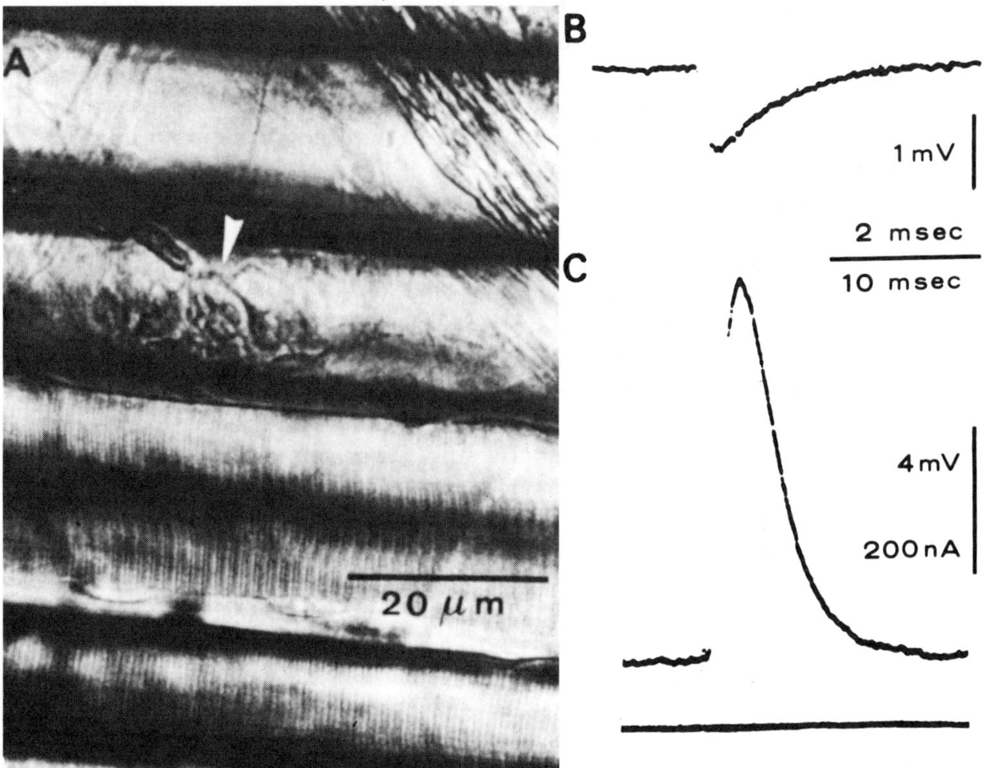

Figure 3.1. A typical endplate (arrow in A) in the triangularis sterni muscle of the mouse as it appears under Nomarski optics. B represents a miniature endplate current recorded with an extracellular recording electrode. C represents the membrane response (upper trace) to a brief current pulse (lower trace) passed through an extracellular pipette containing acetylcholine. This technique was used to obtain the ACh sensitivities presented in Table 3.3. Reproduced from McArdle et al[190] by permission.

urements of the currents obviate these difficulties. Such measurements depend upon the voltage clamp technique which is based on the following relationship:

$$I_m = C_m \, dV/dt + I_i \qquad [1]$$

This equation indicates that the total current across the endplate membrane (I_m) is equal to the sum of a capacitative ($C_m \, dV/dt$) and an ionic element (I_i). In practice, two opposite ends of the endplate membrane are impaled with microelectrodes. To reduce membrane damage these electrodes must have a relatively small tip diameter. Unfortunately, this causes an elevation of the overall time constant of the recording circuit and limits the resolution of high frequencies. However, the frequency response can be markedly increased by reducing the capacitative leakage of current across the electrode wall. This is accomplished by maintaining a minimal depth of bathing fluid over the endplate, shielding one of the clamping electrodes as close as possible to its tip and connecting this shield to a driven ground, as well as electronically introducing capacity neutralization. With these precautions, one of the intracellular microelectrodes is then used to sense the actual membrane potential which is electronically compared to a preset holding potential. Sufficient feedback is then passed through the second intracellular microelectrode to hold the membrane potential at the desired level. When the receptor is activated the feedback current changes to counter the effect of the subsequent ionic flux and the membrane potential does not change. Thus, dV/dt is 0 and the feedback current is the negative value of the true receptor-mediated current. However, the degree that this current truly reflects the endplate current is limited by the size of the activated surface since the current-passing electrode acts as a point source which can influence a length of membrane only a fraction of the space constant. Therefore, the larger the endplate the more difficult it is to approximate ideal voltage clamp conditions. Nevertheless, analysis of the time course and amplitude of such feedback currents has provided important information concerning the function of the channel and gate of the acetylcholine receptor.

The Takeuchis[247,248] were the first to make a detailed analysis of the ionic basis and voltage dependence of currents at the endplate of frog sartorius muscle fibers occurring in response to stimulation of the sciatic nerve. They treated the isolated preparations with curare in order to avoid mechanical activity. This treatment had no effect on the current properties which they investigated. Takeuchi and Takeuchi[247] did note, however, that these currents were prolonged when the endplate was clamped at more negative holding potentials. Kordaš[137] demonstrated quantitatively that the half-time of decay of neurally evoked endplate currents increased at negative holding potentials. Magleby and Stevens[165] expanded on this observation. They noted that endplate currents decayed according to a first-order exponential and that the rate constant of this decay decreased at more negative holding potentials (Fig. 3.2). The former observation led them to suggest that the decay of the endplate current was due solely to closing of the receptor's channel. Magleby and Stevens[166] then applied the general equations of rate processes to their data of the voltage sensitivity of current decay. This analysis provided theoretical support to their hypothesis that the decay of endplate current was due solely to the closing of the receptor's channel. The reciprocal of the decay rate constant thus provided an important indication of receptor function; namely, channel open time (τ). In addition, Magleby and Stevens were able to estimate the change in dipole moment associated with the movement of the gating component of the receptor from its open to its closed state as well as the associated free energy change.

Katz and Miledi explored a different approach to evaluating receptor function when they directed their attention to the increase in baseline noise produced by the diffuse application of cholinergic agonists to the endplate of frog muscle. Their initial report presented a molecular model to explain the voltage noise seen with an intracellular microelectrode.[129] They attributed this noise to the "statistical fluctuation in reaction rate, and in the frequency of elementary current pulses ('shot effects') produced by the action of ACh molecules." Therefore, equations of a random noise theory[224] were utilized to quantitatively evaluate the amplitude and the time course of the elementary events. In practice, noise is produced by exposing the endplate to a cholinergic agonist contained in the bathing medium or diffusing from a nearby micropipette. An intracellular electrode is used to record the voltage noise. However, for the reasons mentioned earlier more pertinent information is obtained by analysis of the current noise obtained with a focally positioned extracellular electrode or a conventional two-electrode intracellular voltage clamp. In their initial studies, Katz and Miledi were concerned only with recordings of ACh-evoked noise potentials (Fig. 3.3). Briefly, the ACh produced a steady level of depolarization clearly visible on a low-gain DC-coupled recording. With high-gain AC-coupled recording, the associated voltage noise was clearly apparent. Katz and Miledi analyzed this noise with the assumption that the underlying shot effect involved ". . . a minute 'blip' of instantaneous rise to amplitude a and exponential decay with a time constant τ characteristic of the min. epps (miniature endplate potentials)." Thus, the variance of the voltage noise ($\overline{E}^2$) should be

$$\overline{E}^2 = \frac{Va}{2}, \qquad [2]$$

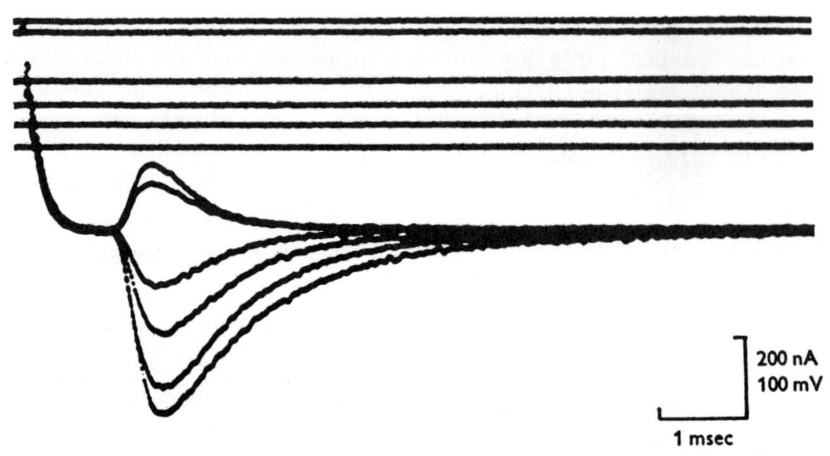

200 nA
100 mV
1 msec

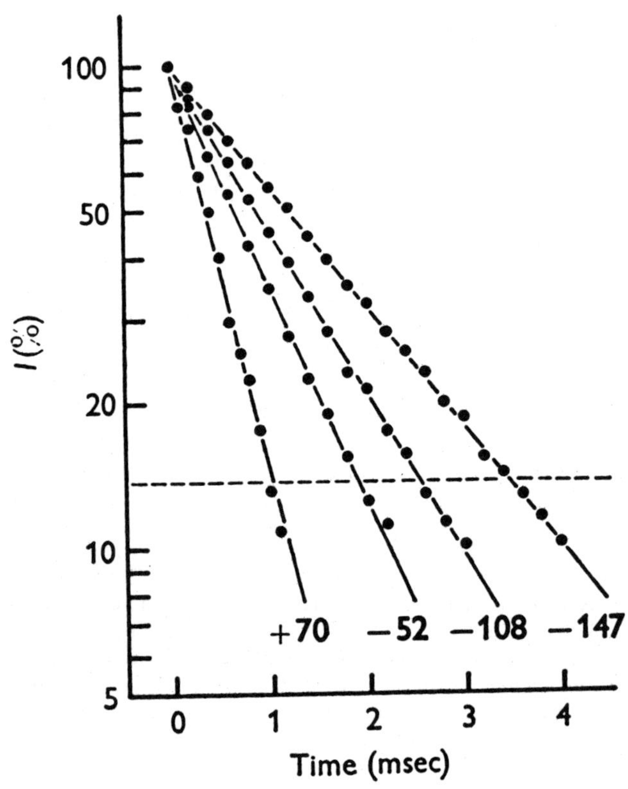

100
50
20
10
5
I (%)
+70
−52
−108
−147
0
1
2
3
4
Time (msec)

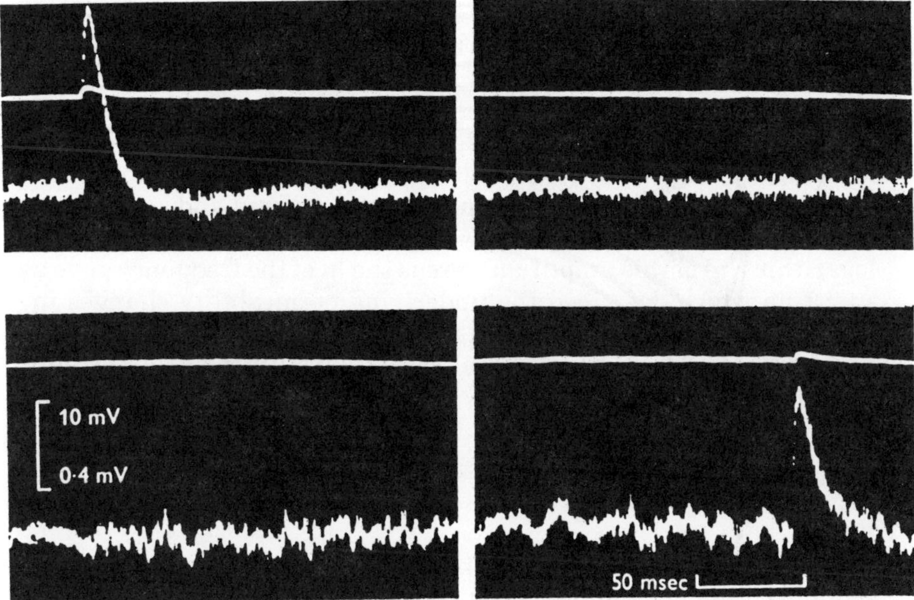

Figure 3.3. This figure is taken from Katz and Miledi[130] by permission. It depicts the voltage response of the frog motor endplate to diffusely applied acetylcholine. The two upper panels are controls while the lower two panels show the effect of acetylcholine. The upper trace in each panel shows a low-gain DC recording of resting potential while the lower trace is a high-gain AC recording in which increased membrane noise is detected after acetylcholine. Depolarization following acetylcholine is evidenced by the increased distance between the AC and DC tracings in the lower panels. Two spontaneously occurring mepps are shown.

Figure 3.2. This is a composite figure taken from the paper of Magleby and Stevens[165] by permission. The recordings represent the membrane potential (upper trace) and current (lower trace) of a voltage-clamped frog endplate in response to indirect stimulation. The effectiveness of the two-electrode voltage clamp is indicated by the fact that the membrane potential does not change during the current flow. The lower graph depicts the decay of the endplate currents at different holding potentials. To do this, the logarithm of the amplitude of the current, as a percentage of the peak current, is plotted as a function of time. At all holding potentials, the currents decay as first-order exponentials. Note the decay rate constant is greater at positive holding potentials.

where V is the mean steady-state depolarization. By measuring $\bar{E}^2$ and V, Katz and Miledi were able to calculate a to equal $0.18-0.5\ \mu V$. In order to gain insights into the time characteristics of the shot effect Katz and Miledi[130] subjected the high-gain noise to computerized spectral analysis. Briefly, a Fourier routine decomposed the digitized noise into its underlying sine and cosine components. The amplitude of these components at each frequency was squared and summed to give the corresponding spectral amplitude. A plot of the natural logarithm (ln) of this amplitude versus the ln of the frequency gave a spectrum which described the underlying permeability changes in terms of their frequencies. By taking the frequency at which the power spectrum was half maximal (f_c) and substituting its value into the following expression

$$\tau = \frac{1}{2\pi f_c} \qquad [3]$$

Katz and Miledi were able to estimate the duration of the underlying shot effect. For the voltage noise expression, this calculation gave a value equal to the time constant of the sarcolemma; for the frog sartorius muscle this value was about 10 msec. Such a value was obtained because the cable properties of the sarcolemmal membrane only passed those frequencies that were equal to or less than its own time constant. When Katz and Miledi applied the same analysis to current noise detected with an extracellular microelectrode they found τ to be approximately 1 msec $(21-25°C)$. On the basis of this information and an estimate of 10^{-10} mhos for the conductance of a single channel, Katz and Miledi calculated that 5×10^4 cations flow through the postsynaptic membrane in response to the activation of one receptor unit.

Anderson and Stevens[11] obtained comparable (10°C) results when they analyzed the endplate current noise visualized with a conventional two-electrode intracellular voltage clamp (Figs. 3.4 and 3.5). They were also able to demonstrate that the value of τ derived from such analysis exhibited the same voltage dependence as did the time constant of decay of neurally evoked endplate currents. This added further support to the hypothesis of Magleby and Stevens[165,166] that the decay of the latter was due to the closure of the receptor's channel. The energy barrier to this closure was calculated to be greater at negative holding potentials and this caused a prolongation of the mean channel open time, τ. Furthermore, Anderson and Stevens

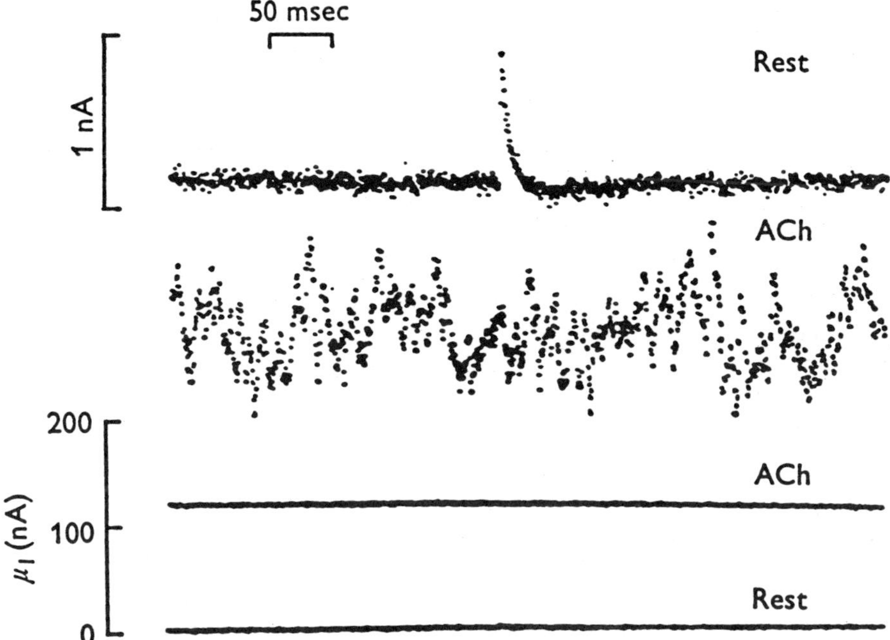

Figure 3.4. This figure is taken from Anderson and Stevens[11] by permission. It presents digitized endplate currents recorded with a conventional two-electrode voltage clamp. The upper tracings are at a high gain and show the increase in membrane current noise in the presence of acetylcholine. The low-gain traces shown below represent the steady increase of endplate current flow in the presence of acetylcholine.

were able to estimate the conductance (γ) of a single channel with their intracellular technique. To do this they used the same equations as did Katz and Miledi to evaluate the voltage fluctuations due to a single shot effect. However, Anderson and Stevens assumed that the underlying blips had the form of a square wave. For this reason, their equation [4] which relates γ to the noise variance (σ_g^2) was slightly different than the equation of Katz and Miledi for $\bar{E}^2$ (equation 2):

$$\sigma_g^2 = \mu_g\gamma \quad ; \tag{4}$$

μ_g is the mean increase of endplate conductance with which the noise is associated. Anderson and Stevens calculated a value of $2 - 3 \times 10^{-11}$ mhos for the conductance of a single channel at $8-10°C$. This would

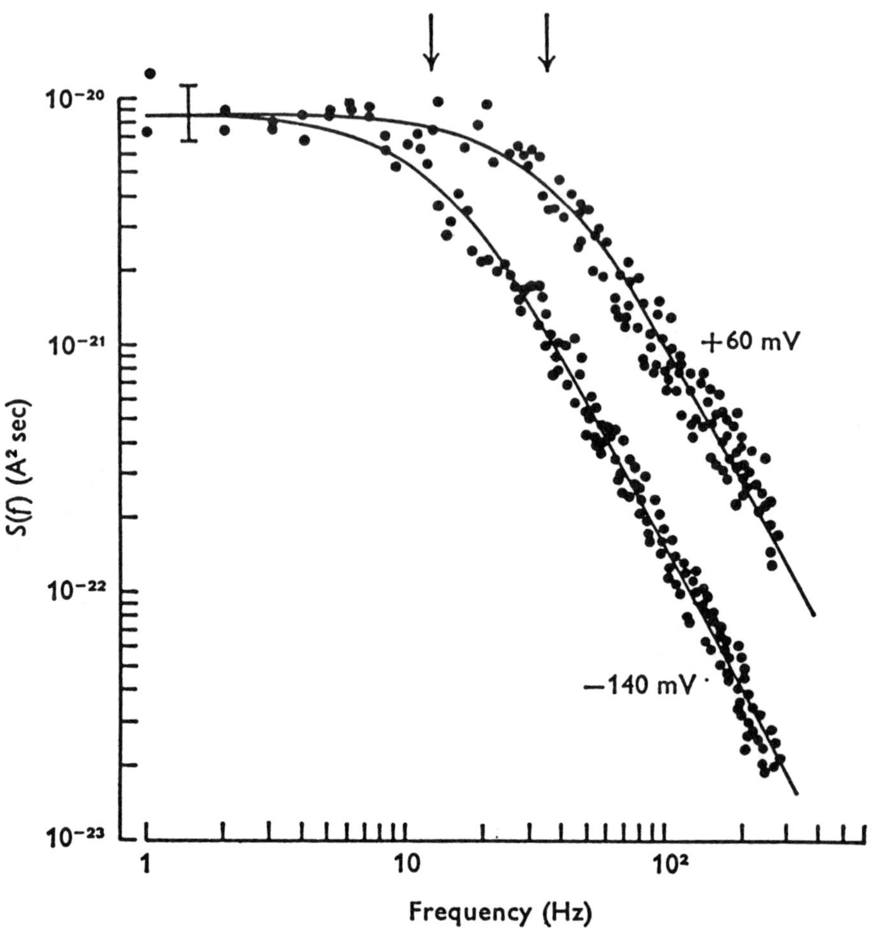

Figure 3.5. This figure is taken from Anderson and Stevens[11] by permission. It depicts the logarithm of the spectral amplitude of the acetylcholine noise signals displayed in Fig. 3.4 plotted as a function of the logarithm of frequency. Data are shown for two holding potentials ($+60\,\mathrm{mV}$ and $-140\,\mathrm{mV}$). The half-power frequency (f_c) for each spectrum is indicated by the arrows. With this value and the expression

$$\tau = \frac{1}{2\,\pi\,f_c}$$

the mean channel open time can be estimated. In agreement with the work of Magleby and Stevens, τ is greater at the more negative holding potential.[165,166]

correspond to a flow of approximately 2×10^5 cations through a channel open for 11 msec.

Clearly, the technique of noise analysis has provided important insights into the properties of the AChRS. However, the depth of the insights is limited for several reasons. In particular, the statistical nature of the analysis gives information about the average properties of a large population of receptors.

The actual shape of the elementary conductance event cannot be revealed by the noise analysis technique. As noted above, at least two shapes have been assumed. Neher and Sakmann[203] removed the necessity of such assumptions when they introduced the patch-voltage clamp technique to record the conductance change occurring when a single receptor is activated. Briefly, this technique involves pressing an extracellular pipette containing a dilute solution of a cholinergic agonist against the surface of a cholinoceptive membrane (Fig. 3.6). The patch of membrane under the tip of the pipette, as well as the inside of the pipette itself, is electronically clamped to ground. At the same time, the current required to maintain the patch at ground level is displayed on an oscilloscope. This enables visualization of the actual conductance change occurring when agonist molecules randomly activate receptor units. The resolution of these single-channel currents is greatly increased when the leakage of current across the junction of the patch and the pipette to the extracellular fluid is lowered. Such leakage is reduced when patch pipettes are properly fabricated[205] to increase the electrical resistance to current flow across this junction. Furthermore, if the patch of membrane is gently sucked into the tip of the pipette the resistance to leakage increases to the gigohm range and the resolution of single-channel events is significantly facilitated.[98] The results obtained with the patch-voltage clamp technique qualitatively confirm the voltage and pharmacologic sensitivity of the receptor as determined from analysis of noise or neurally evoked endplate currents. In addition, the patch-voltage clamp technique has revealed the shape of the elementary conductance to be that of a square wave. However, quantitative analysis of the square waves representing single-channel conductance reveals differences between the value of τ estimated from endplate currents. To a certain degree, these differences may be attributed to the variety of cholinergic agonists, temperatures and receptor types (e.g., junctional vs extrajunctional) used in patch experiments. Nevertheless, exact agreement cannot be expected since the values from patch experiments are derived directly from the underlying single events,

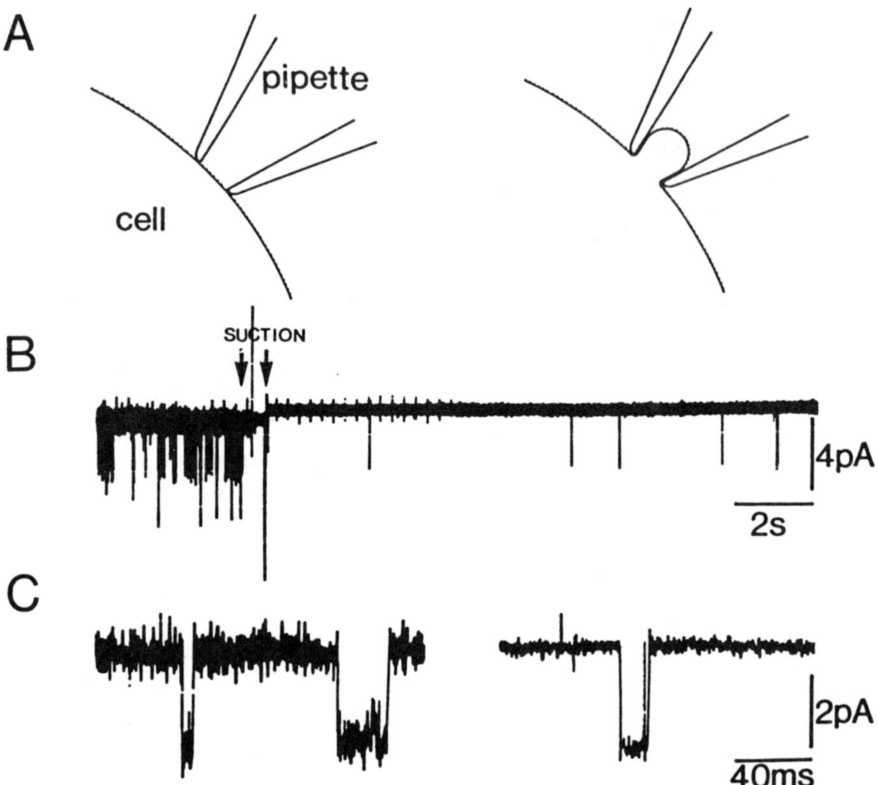

Figure 3.6. This figure, taken from Hamill et al[98] by permission, briefly depicts the patch-voltage clamp technique (see text for additional information). A pipette containing a dilute solution of a cholinergic agonist is gently pressed against a cholinoceptive membrane. As a result, the membrane activity depicted in the left of B and C is recorded through this pipette. Though single-channel events are apparent, they are obscured by the noise of the recording system. The latter is greatly reduced when the patch of membrane is gently sucked into the tip of the pipette, allowing a greater resolution of single-channel events (right of B and C).

whereas all other techniques give an average estimate of τ representing a diverse population of receptors.

Molecular Aspects of Drug Action on the AChRS

Although it is not the objective of this chapter to discuss the pharmacology of the NMJ, there are a few drug actions which should be briefly discussed at this point.

As mentioned at the end of the preceding section, different cholinergic agonists are associated with different values of τ. Katz and Miledi[131] demonstrated this phenomenon when they found that the amplitude of the shot effect, a, varied with the cholinergic agonists. For suberyldicholine (Sub), ACh and carbamylcholine or carbachol (Carb) the sequence was $a_{Sub} > a_{ACh} > a_{Carb}$. Katz and Miledi attributed this sequence to the fact that Sub produced a longer duration of channel open time, the sequence of τ being Sub > ACh > Carb. Neher and Sakmann[203] confirmed this sequence of τ using patch electrodes containing dilute solutions of Sub, ACh and Carb. The more efficacious an agonist is in maintaining the receptor in the open state the greater its intrinsic ability to produce a flux of ions. The molecular basis for such differences remains to be determined.

The preceding information suggests that drugs other than cholinergic agonists might also alter channel open time and in so doing reduce the sensitivity of the cholinoceptive membrane. Available data does suggest that such drugs exist and that their effect is due to either a direct or indirect action on the channel. With regard to the former action, Adams[2] attributed the postsynaptic depressant effects of amobarbital, thiopental and methohexital to a physical blockade of the channel once it opens (Fig. 3.7). On the other hand, Gage and his colleagues have provided extensive data suggesting that drugs may indirectly alter the channel open time. For example, in one study[86] they found that ethanol increased the endplate response to spontaneously released ACh in association with an increase of the value of τ estimated from endplate currents. Conversely, they[85,87] observed that octanol simultaneously decreased the postsynaptic sensitivity to ACh and τ. They attributed these effects of the alcohols to an action on the membrane environment of the receptor. Ethanol and octanol were proposed to increase and decrease, respectively, the stability of the open channel. This may be secondary to an action of the alcohol to increase or to decrease the energy barrier that the open channel must overcome to close. Variations of these direct and indirect actions have been hypothesized[23,24,229] to account for the complex decay of endplate currents occurring in the presence of molecules with a local anesthetic action (see Fig. 3.7). However, in a study using the patch-voltage clamp, Neher and Steinbach[204] provided direct measurements which strongly suggested that local anesthetics do block the open channel.

In 1955 Thesleff[251] demonstrated that exposure of frog muscle to blocking agents proposed to act via endplate depolarization[40,266] caused a paralysis which outlasted this action. He attributed the prolonged effect to a reduction of the endplate response to ACh. In a

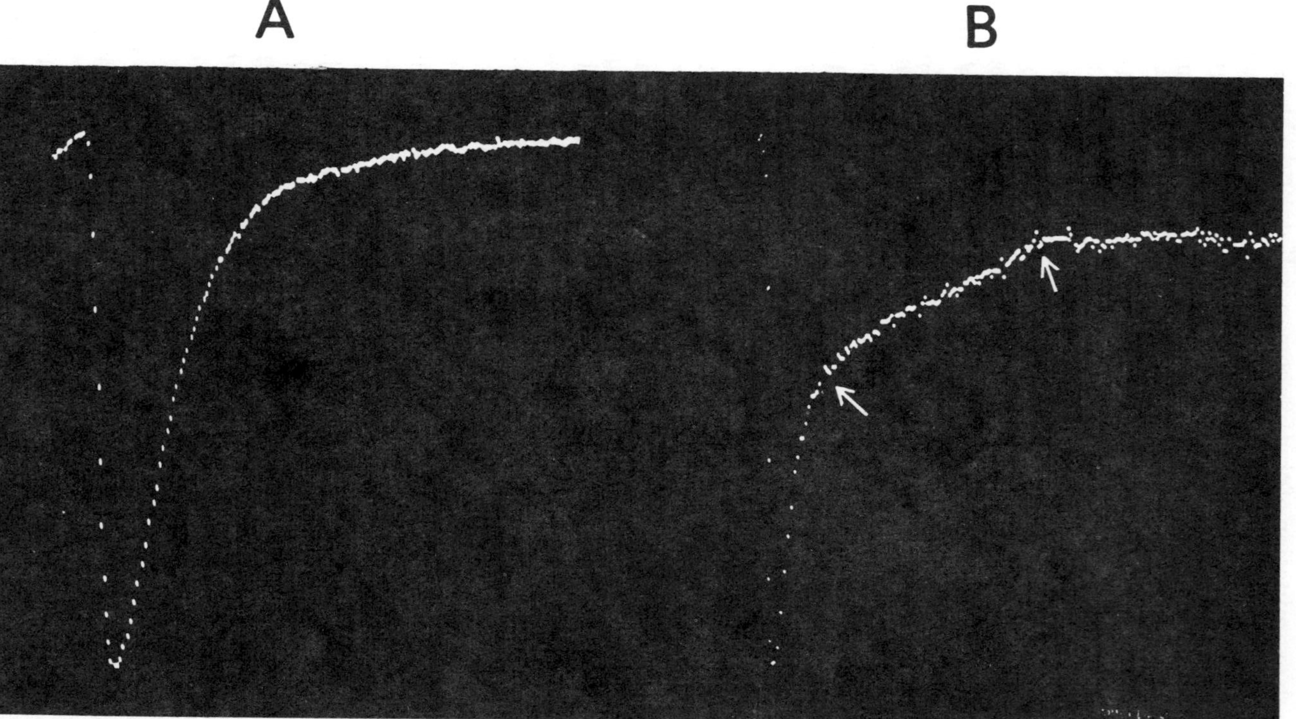

Figure 3.7. Digitized images of endplate currents recorded in a cut-fiber preparation (22°C) of the rat extensor digitorum longus muscle before (A) and after (B) exposure to the peripherally acting opiate antagonist naltrexone methyl bromide (160 μM). Note the multiple phases of current decay in B (arrows). This was interpreted as due to drug blockade of the open channel. From Argentieri and McArdle[13] by permission.

more thorough examination of this phenomenon Katz and Thesleff[121] formulated their classic model of receptor desensitization. Briefly, they suggested that a steady state normally exists at the resting endplate between nondesensitized (R) and desensitized (R') receptor. The latter is normally present at a low level.[260] When agonist molecules (A) are introduced, the AR complex rapidly forms, causing the associated channels to open. The majority of these complexes quickly dissociate, while a proportion slowly convert to a nonconducting state, AR'. In turn, some of this complex dissociates to the desensitized receptor, R'. The continued presence of A will favor R' because the desensitized receptor is presumed to have a higher affinity for ligands relative to R. The model implies that the binding and conductile properties of the receptor system change in a cyclic manner. This hypothesis underlies some current biochemical concepts concerning the receptor. In particular, one argument for isolation of a functional receptor protein is its conversion from a low- to a high-affinity state for ligands in the continued presence of agonist molecules.[245,260]

Available data suggest that the reduction of the endplate response to agonists during desensitization is due to the progressive conversion of the R population to R' and AR' rather than to gradual alteration of γ or τ of individual receptor units.[11,80] Furthermore, preliminary patch-clamp analyses suggest an all-or-none blockade of receptors during desensitization.[94,230] Adams[1] (see also references 49, 78, 158, 230) did present data that implied that desensitization involved several steps, one of which he postulated to be agonist blockade of the open channel. However, Scubon-Mulieri and Parsons[232] did not find evidence for such multiplicity of steps, and Sakmann et al,[230] as well as Magleby and Pallotta,[175] argued against blockade of channels. Kuba and Koketsu[141] also suggested a change in channel properties during desensitization since they observed a shift in the level of the extrapolated value of the membrane polarity at which endplate potentials reversed sign. Katz and Miledi,[132] as well as Lambert et al,[146] did not find such an effect of desensitization when they actually measured the reversal potential of endplate currents.

There are a number of factors which control the desensitization process. For example, an increase of temperature increases both the rate of onset and recovery from desensitization.[164] In another study, hyperpolarization increased the rate of onset without effecting recovery from desensitization.[162] Subsequently, Scubon-Mulieri and Parsons[232] did find an effect of voltage on recovery when they employed a wider range of holding potentials. Fiekers et al[80] suggested that the voltage sensitivity of the onset of desensitization was only slightly due to that of channel kinetics. They attributed this to an energy barrier to the conversion of the AR complex to the desensitized state, AR', which exceeded the energy barrier for conversion of channels to the open state.

Information from biochemical as well as biophysical studies indicate that various chemicals influence desensitization. For example, neutral detergents,[244] anesthetics,[52,95,96,267-269] and histrionicotoxin[39] stabilize the isolated receptor in its high-affinity state. SKF-525 A,[257] chlorpromazine,[164] and histrionicotoxin[7] significantly facilitate the functional desensitization of the endplate of frog muscle. On the other hand, Mathers and Usherwood[184] demonstrated that concanavalin A was effective in protecting the glutamate receptor of locust muscle from desensitization. Akasu and Karczmar[4] reported that NaF also protects the frog endplate from desensitization.

In 1966, Manthey pointed out that Ca^{++} facilitated the process of desensitization.[179] His observation has been confirmed in subsequent biophysical[80,162,201] and biochemical[53] studies of the receptor. The action of Ca^{++} is apparently on the internal surface of the receptor-containing membrane.[59] Possible physiologic sources of Ca^{++} include the extracellular medium,[3,145,150,250] as well as a pool of the cation tightly bound to the receptor molecule.[70,71,228] The work of Andreason and McNamee[12] suggests that desensitization may involve a Ca-dependent uncoupling of the recognition site of the receptor from the channel. This is based on their observation that phospholipase A, in the presence of Ca^{++}, reduced the agonist-induced efflux of Na^+ from vesicles isolated from the electroplaque of *Torpedo*. Perhaps continued exposure to agonist also brings about such uncoupling by changing the biochemical state of key membrane molecules.[5,109] However, speculations from such biochemical observations must be made cautiously. For example, the results of Andreason and McNamee may be attributed to a generalized increase of membrane leakiness after phospholipase A. This would reduce the driving force for Na^+, and therefore net efflux, through the agonist-activated receptor.[6] It is also necessary to point out that the effect of Ca^{++} on desensitization does not extend to all species. For example, Ca^{++} had relatively little effect on the ACh-induced desensitization of molluscan neurons,[35] and Pallotta and Webb[215] noted that elevation of extracellular Ca^{++} decreased desensitization of the electroplaque of *Electrophorus*. The latter finding is in obvious disagreement with the increase of desensitization which one would predict on the basis of the biochemical data.[53,245] This stresses the need to correlate biochemical with biophysical studies.[200,219]

A consideration of fundamental importance in a discussion of desensitization is whether this phenomenon has an influence upon synaptic transmission. Pagala and his colleagues[213,214] have presented data suggesting that desensitization may contribute to the failure of neuromuscular transmission in patients with myasthenia gravis.[208] This may be related to an apparent increase in affinity of the receptor for cholinergic ligands during myasthenia[72] or to the lowered number of receptors in this condition,[76] since α-BuTx, which decreases the number of functional receptors, facilitates the process of desensitization.[163] Nevertheless, the fact that τ and γ do not change during myasthenia[9,56,108] provides further evidence that the desensitization process is independent of channel conductance and gating kinetics.

Early workers did not exclude the possibility that desensitization might contribute to Wedensky inhibition occurring at the normal neuromuscular junction.[16,121,253] Thesleff reported that neural stimulation at pulse intervals of less than 25 msec caused a reduction of the endplate sensitivity to iontophoretically applied acetylcholine.[252] More recently Magleby and Pallotta demonstrated that the acetylcholine released in response to nerve stimulation was able to reduce the response of the frog endplate to acetylcholine released spontaneously from nerves.[175] They attributed this to the persistence of an AR' complex for approximately 25 msec after an endplate potential. Thus, desensitization may normally function to regulate the frequency response of synapses.[4] This may have little impact on normal neuromuscular transmission and the subsequent muscular activity because of the high safety factor insuring that endplate potentials reach the threshold for muscle action potentials. However, the process of desensitization may in some subtle way influence the properties of individual receptors during their life span.[187]

The Presynaptic Release Process

Quantal

In 1954 Del Castillo and Katz presented the quantal theory of neuromuscular transmission.[60] This was based on three fundamental observations made at the frog neuromuscular junction. First of

all, Fatt and Katz had described the spontaneously occurring miniature endplate potentials (mepps) at this synapse.[77] Secondly, Del
Castillo and Katz observed that the minimal amplitude of the endplate potentials (epps) recorded in muscle fibers whose nerves were
stimulated in the presence of an elevated concentration of extracellular Mg^{++} was equal to the mean mepp amplitude ($\overline{mepp}$).[60] Thirdly,
Del Castillo and Katz[60] also observed that the peaks in the distribution of the amplitude of epps (Fig. 3.8) in Mg^{++}-treated neuromuscular junctions could be closely predicted by multiplying the $\overline{mepp}$ by
whole numbers (m); i.e.,

$$epp = m \times \overline{mepp} \ . \tag{5}$$

On the basis of these findings, Del Castillo and Katz proposed that
mepps represented the endplate response to elementary units, or
quanta, which underlie functional neuromuscular transmission.[60]
For a given synapse, $\overline{mepp}$ provided a measure of quantal size (q).
Thus, the ratio of the mean epp amplitude ($\overline{epp}$) produced by a series
of nerve stimuli, to q ($\overline{mepp}$), provided a direct estimate of the mean
number of quantal units ($\bar{m}$) released per stimulus; i.e.,

$$\bar{m} = \frac{\overline{epp}}{\overline{mepp}} \ . \tag{6}$$

In their classic paper, Del Castillo and Katz[60] simultaneously formulated a mathematical model which provided considerable support to
their quantal hypothesis. According to this model, the average quantal content of a series of epps, $\bar{m}$, was proposed to equal the product of
the total number of quanta available for release (n) and the mean
probability ($\bar{p}$) of release; i.e.,

$$\bar{m} = n \times \bar{p} \ . \tag{7}$$

During normal function the value of $\bar{p}$ was presumed to be large.
However, under their conditions of Mg^{++} depression of neuromuscular transmission most nerve stimuli actually failed to release quanta
($m = 0$), although a stimulus occasionally released one or more quanta. Thus, they assumed that Mg^{++} greatly reduced $\bar{p}$ so that the
actual distribution of the quantal contents of a large series of epps
should be predictable according to Poisson's law; that is, the relative
frequency (f) of epps having a quantal content of x should be

$$f_x = (e^{-\bar{m}}) \left(\frac{\bar{m}^x}{x!} \right) \ . \tag{8}$$

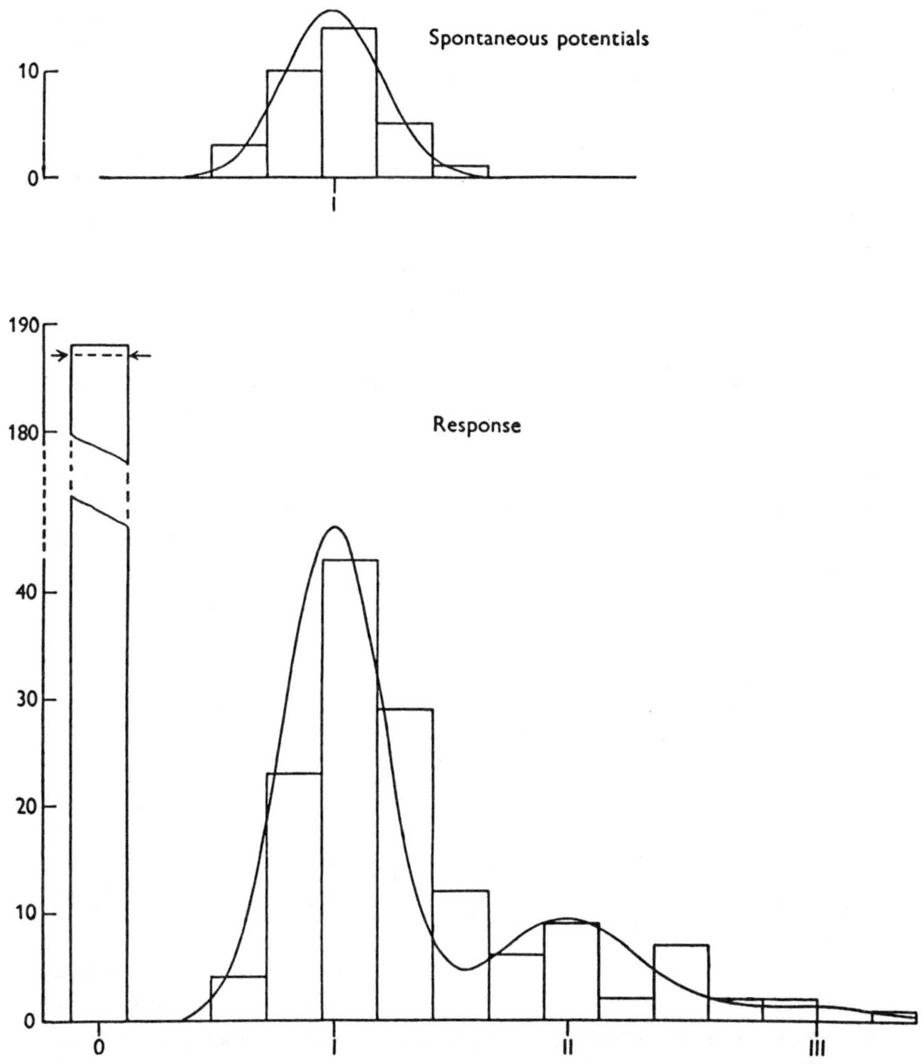

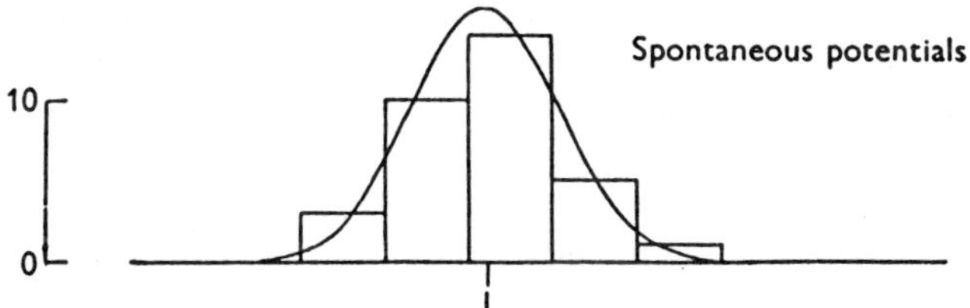

Figure 3.8. This figure is taken from Del Castillo and Katz[60] by permission. The bars in each histogram depict the amplitude distribution of miniature endplate potentials (mepps, upper) and endplate potentials (epps, lower; Mg^{++} blockade) relative to $\overline{mepp}$. The curve in the lower histogram depicts the predicted distribution if epps were due to the release of one or more units whose amplitude was equal to $\overline{mepp}$. The arrows on the lower histogram indicate the predicted number of failures assuming Poisson statistics (equation 8).

In fact, Del Castillo and Katz were able to accurately predict the distribution of the values of m with this expression when they inserted $\bar{m}$ calculated from equation 6 into equation 8. Furthermore, they were able to use equation 8 to obtain an independent estimate of $\bar{m}$ which was in complete agreement with that derived from the ratio $\overline{epp}{:}\overline{mepp}$. To do this, they set x in equation 8 equal to 0 and solved for $\bar{m}$ to obtain

$$\bar{m} = \ln \left(\frac{N}{n_o} \right) . \tag{9}$$

Del Castillo and Katz then counted the number of failures of quantal release (n_o) associated with a total number (N) of supramaximal nerve stimuli and inserted these values into equation 9 to arrive at a value of $\bar{m}$ which agreed with that obtained from equation 6. Since the coefficient of variation (C.V., the ratio standard deviation:mean) for a Poisson distribution is the square root of the reciprocal of the mean, that is,

$$\text{C.V.} = \bar{m}^{-0.5} , \tag{10}$$

$\bar{m}$ can also be derived from the following expression:

$$\bar{m} = \left(\frac{\overline{epp}}{\text{S.D.}} \right)^2 \tag{11}$$

where S.D. is the standard deviation of the epps making up a large series. The amplitude of epps can be used in this expression rather than the actual values of quantal content because C.V. is independent of the units of measurement. Therefore, C.V. would be essentially the same for the measured amplitudes and quantal contents. In summary, the work of Del Castillo and Katz precisely defined the quantal nature of synaptic transmission and provided three expressions (equations 6, 9 and 11) to calculate $\bar{m}$ in the special case where $\bar{p}$ is very low (< 0.1). Subsequent studies confirmed the quantal hypothesis and used these expressions to determine $\bar{m}$ at the neuromuscular junction of crayfish,[66] spider,[36] rat,[152] cat,[33] and man,[74] as well as at nerve-nerve synapses in the cat spinal cord[143] and ganglia of frog,[30] chick,[182] and *Aplysia*.[236]

Del Castillo and Katz made the observation that the directly measured value of $\bar{m}$ (equation 6) was less than that predicted from

Poisson statistics when $\bar{m}$ was large $(\bar{m} > 8)$.[60] They postulated several causes for this discrepancy. For example, the potential change produced by individual quanta may not summate linearly when their net amplitude of depolarization is 5% or more of the overall resting potential of a muscle fiber. In this case $\overline{epp}$ would be underestimated and as a consequence so would the directly determined value of $\bar{m}$. In addition, Del Castillo and Katz suggested that at high levels of release $\bar{p}$ may be too great $(\bar{p} > 0.1)$ for Poisson statistics to be applicable. In this case, Poisson analysis (equations 9 and 11) would overestimate $\bar{m}$. Later work evaluated the contribution of these two factors to the discrepancy which Del Castillo and Katz reported. For example, Martin showed that when the amplitude of individual epps was corrected for the effect of non-linear summation, the values of $\bar{m}$ determined from direct measurement (equation 6) and Poisson statistics (equation 11) were in agreement.[180] Furthermore, he also demonstrated that the effect of non-linear summation was greatly reduced when nerve-muscle preparations were treated with curare to reduce the net conductance increase during an epp. Thus, subsequent investigators induced subthreshold epps $(\overline{epp} < 7 \text{ mV})$ in isolated nerve muscle preparations with curare and assumed that the underlying quantal effects summed linearly. They then employed the Poisson model of quantal release to study nerve terminal function.[74] With this approach, $\bar{m}$ could be easily estimated at a wide variety of neuromuscular junctions. A study of the original literature reveals that this value varied considerably. For example, Boyd and Martin[33] found $\bar{m}$ to be 310 for the cat tenuissimus muscle and Wilson[263] obtained a value of 148 for the rat diaphragm. Such variability can be attributed to differences in experimental protocol, especially temperature and frequency of stimulation, as well as intrinsic species differences. However, the validity of information derived from the application of Poisson statistics to data obtained from curarized preparations can be questioned. This is due to the fact that numerous investigators[25,88,90,114] have found that curare acts presynaptically to depress the secretory process. This is especially apparent when epps are generated at high frequencies. Furthermore, epps do not fail intermittently in the presence of curare,[90,114] which suggests that release may be too high $(\bar{p} > 0.1)$ for Poisson statistics to be applicable. However, when $\bar{p}$ was calculated in curare-treated preparations using the fractional release method,[74,263] a value of less than 0.1 was always obtained. Briefly, this method involved eliciting epps at a frequency high enough to bring about an initial rundown in their amplitude to some steady mean value in the latter part of the train of stimuli (Fig. 3.9). The value of $\bar{m}$ was calculated for the epps in the tail of the train using equation 11. Since

$$\bar{m} = \frac{\overline{epp}}{q}, \qquad [12]$$

then

$$q = \frac{\overline{epp}}{\bar{m}} = \frac{\mathrm{SD}^2}{\overline{epp}}. \qquad [13]$$

Once this estimate of q was calculated, the quantal content of the first few epps (m_1, m_2, etc.) making up the early rundown phase of the train was plotted as a function of the total number of quanta released in the preceding epps of the train. The resulting straight line was then extrapolated to obtain the x intercept which was presumed to equal n, the number of quanta immediately available for release. The value of n was usually quite large so that the ratio $m_1{:}n$, defining fractional release, was less than 0.1. In order to avoid the pharmacologic complications associated with the depression of neuromuscular

---

Figure 3.9. The two tracings show endplate potentials (epps) recorded from cut-fiber preparations of control and reinnervating (14 days after nerve crush or 5 days after the start of reinnervation[186]) extensor digitorum longus muscles (32°C) in response to 40 stimuli delivered to the nerve at a frequency of 160 Hz. Note the initial facilitation of epp amplitude in the control which precedes the depression characteristic of the tail of the train. Intermittent failure is striking at the reinnervating endplate, which may be due to failure of the nerve action potential. The graph depicts the standard analysis of the rundown of control epp amplitude early in the train enabling an estimate of the size of the readily releaseable pool ("n") and the fractional release ("p"). To do this, Poisson statistics were assumed (see text for the questions associated with such an assumption), and the mean quantal content of the last twenty epps ($\bar{m}_{ss}$) in the train was calculated from the following expression:

$$\bar{m}_{ss} = \frac{\overline{epp}^2}{\mathrm{S.D.}}.$$

This value was found to be 128 for the control fiber. The value of q was then calculated from the following expression:

$$q = \frac{\overline{epps}}{\bar{m}_{ss}}.$$

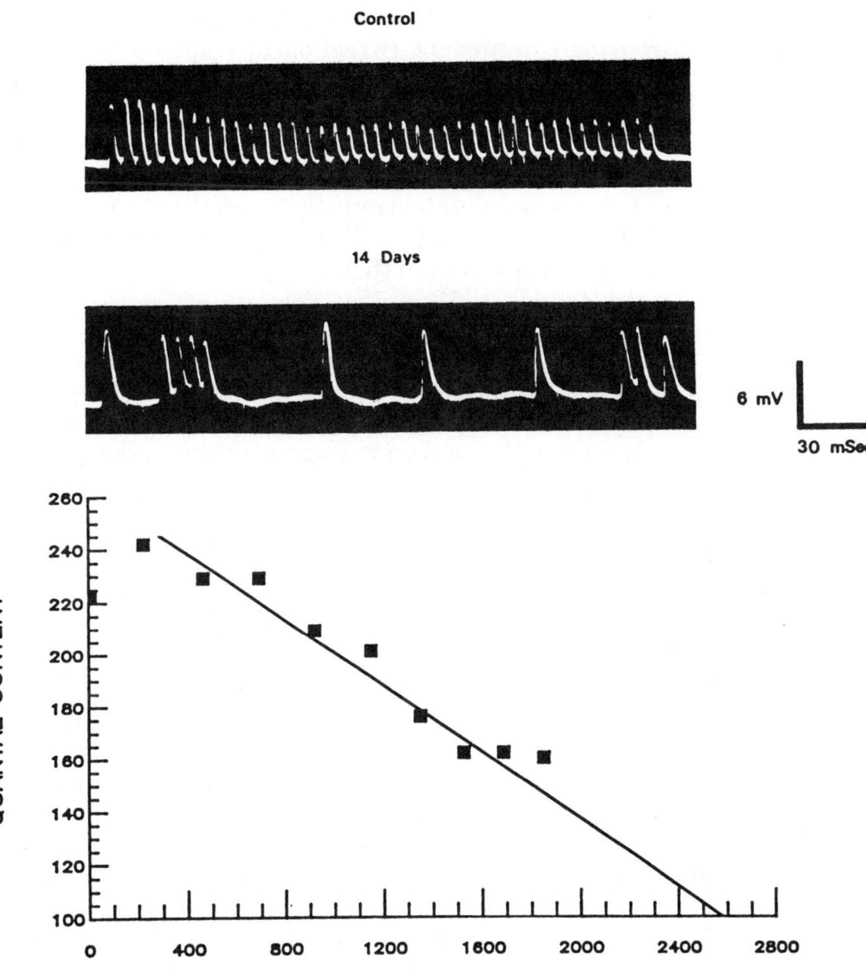

This value was found to be 0.0225 mV (a value much less than $\overline{mepp}$ actually recorded in such preparations). Knowing q, the quantal content of the first 10 epps in the train was calculated ($m_1 = \dfrac{epp_1}{q}$, etc.) and plotted as a function of the total quanta released by preceding stimuli. Two features of this rundown curve are worth noting. Firstly, the value of m_2 was greater than m_1, indicating early facilitation of quantal release. Secondly, after the 7th epp, the amplitude began to level off. Extrapolation of this curve to the x axis gave 2680 as an estimate of "n." By dividing "n" into m_1 a value of 0.083 was obtained for "p."

transmission by curare, Glavinović[91] determined $\bar{m}$ for rat dia-phragms that were cut to prevent twitching in response to nerve stimulation.[21] This enabled him to make a direct estimate of $\bar{m}$ since quantal responses could be easily recorded in this preparation. Glavinović also voltage-clamped the endplate to reduce the impact of non-linear summation.[192,241] In this way, Glavinović calculated $\bar{m}$ from the ratio of mean endplate current $\overline{(epc)}$ amplitude to mean miniature endplate current amplitude.[91] As a result, he found $\bar{m}$ to be about 40, which is much less than that obtained in earlier studies employing curare-blockade and indirect (Poisson) estimates of $\bar{m}$. Since the amplitude distribution of the epps in Glavinović's study followed a binomial distribution,[27,116,199,264,274] Poisson statis-tics clearly give an overestimate of $\bar{m}$ during normal levels of trans-mitter release. This is due to the fact that at normal levels of release the binomial estimate of $\bar{p}$ is actually about 0.9,[90,264] too large for the Poisson expressions to be applicable. In fact, Glavinović[92] dem-onstrated that kinetic estimates of $\bar{p}$ obtained from the fractional release method are wrong. Therefore, the analysis of epps in cut fiber preparations is a good way to determine the binomial parameters defining the quantal release process at undepressed neuromuscular junctions.[264] However, quantitatively similar estimates are obtained for epps recorded in glycerol-shocked preparations[233] or cut fiber preparations[14] after correction for the effects of membrane capaci-tance.[181]

Upon completing an experiment to determine $\bar{m}$, one can also obtain a value for q as well as n and $\bar{p}$, using the equations referred to above. A fundamental problem is to define the physical correlate of the latter three theoretical parameters. The greatest degree of suc-cess in solving this problem has been achieved with regard to q since considerable data exist that indicate that the presynaptic vesicle is the quantum. For example, Whittaker et al[262] showed that the synaptic vesicles from electric organs were rich in ACh. Also, Heuser and Reese[106] found that vesicle number declined during repetitive indirect stimulation of frog muscle. Furthermore, the massive re-lease of ACh in the presence of elevated K^+,[112] La^{+++},[105] or black widow spider venom[93] is associated with a depletion of synaptic vesicles. Biophysical[142] and biochemical[197] studies indicate that the quantum consists of 6,000 to 11,000 molecules of ACh, which should easily[41] fit into vesicles having a mean diameter of approxi-mately 52 nm.[106] Variation in the number of molecules per quantum probably accounts for the bell-shaped distribution of mepp ampli-tudes at a given neuromuscular junction.[60,77] In addition, there are extremes of such amplitude distributions which raise questions about the equivalence of $\overline{mepp}$ and the value of q which underlies functional transmission. On the one hand, mepps having an amplitude several times $\overline{mepp}$ occur at a low frequency. However, Liley[154] provided evidence suggesting that such "giant" mepps were due to the multiple release of quanta whose individual size was accurately represented by $\overline{mepp}$. On the other hand, Kriebel and his associates[138,139] found evidence for a population of sub-mepps whose mean amplitude was some fraction of $\overline{mepp}$. These sub-mepps hypothetically corresponded to sub-populations of vesicles that are synchronously released to produce some average value, $\overline{mepp}$. In essence, these data indicate that $\overline{mepp}$ and q are non-equivalent. However, sub-mepps were most apparent in the studies of Kriebel et al[138,139] when preparations were specially treated to induce them. Furthermore, Magleby and Miller provided compelling evidence that the sub-unit hypothesis is incorrect.[174]

The significance of n and $\bar{p}$ is much more controversial[22,100] and difficult to determine.[38] In their classic presentation, Del Castillo and Katz referred to n as the number of quanta contained in the readily releasable pool.[60] According to the functional model of Elmqvist and Quastel only a small fraction of n is released to produce each epp.[74] At high frequencies of stimulation n would be depleted so that the epp amplitude declined (see below). This depletion of n was proposed to activate the mobilization of quanta to replenish the releasable pool so that transmission does not fail. Thus, after the initial rundown of epp amplitude in response to a train of stimuli, a steady-state (ss) level of release is achieved due to the process of mobilization. At this time a value of $\bar{m}_{ss}$ can be calculated. The magnitude of $\bar{m}_{ss}$ depends upon the balance between the mobilization-input to, and the release-output from, n. Elmqvist and Quastel defined the rate of transmitter mobilization (dm/dt) as the product of $\bar{m}_{ss}$ and the frequency of stimulation.[74] Since they analyzed their data primarily with Poisson statistics the absolute values for n, $\bar{p}$, $\bar{m}$, dm/dt and q are questionable. Nevertheless, the functional model of Elmqvist and Quastel remains valid.[74] Table 3.1 summarizes some of our own results from studies of this model. Both mepps and epps were recorded in glycerol-shocked[84,233] or cut-fiber preparations[186] of rat hindlimb muscles. The direct method was thus used to estimate $\bar{m}$, while $\bar{p}$ and n were calculated from binomial expressions. Values of $\bar{m}$, n and $\bar{p}$ were first determined when the nerve was stimulated at a frequency of 1 Hz. The frequency was then increased to 160 Hz and a brief train of 40 epps was analyzed to determine $\bar{m}_{ss}$ and dm/dt.

Table 3.1

Binomial Parameters[a] Describing Transmitter Release at Neuromuscular Junctions of the Rat Extensor Digitorum Longus and Soleus Muscles

Muscle	1 Hz			160 Hz				
	$\bar{m}$	n	$\bar{p}$	m_1	"n"	"p"	$\bar{m}_{ss}$	dm/dt
Extensor[b]	48.8 ± 3.4 (18)	54.3 ± 3.6	0.99 ± 0.06	54.4 ± 2.5	1355 ± 223	0.06 ± 0.003	31.8 ± 2.6	5082 ± 410
Soleus	60.9 ± 6.2 (5)	55.5 ± 6.6	1.11 ± 0.003	59.6 ± 4.5	591 ± 43	0.10 ± 0.005	33.7 ± 4.5	5392 ± 720

a. Twitches were blocked by osmotically shocking the preparations with glycerol. 32°C. Values are presented as mean $\pm$ SEM. Numbers in parentheses indicate the number of fibers examined. $\bar{m}$, m_1, and $\bar{m}_{ss}$ are, respectively, mean quantal content of epps at a frequency of 1 Hz, quantal content of the first epp in the train of 40 epps at 160 Hz and mean quantal content of the epps in the tail of this train. These are direct estimates of m; i.e., $epp:\overline{mepp}$. $\bar{p}$ is the binomial estimate of the probability of transmitter release and n is the ratio $\bar{m}$ to $\bar{p}$. "n" is the size of the readily releasable pool as estimated from the initial rundown of epp amplitude in the 160 Hz train (see Figure 9). "p" is the fractional release and is defined as m_1: "n". dm/dt is the mobilization rate of quanta and is defined as the product of m_{ss} and 160 Hz.
b. Sellin reported very similar values.[233]

In addition, a value of "n" was estimated from the initial rundown of epp amplitudes and a value of "p" from the fractional release method. As expected from the work of Glavinović[92] the binomial estimate of $\bar{p}$ was much greater than that obtained from the fractional release procedure. Furthermore, we found that the binomial estimate of n was also much less than that derived from the rundown of epp amplitudes ("n"). Such a difference between n and "n" could be explained if they represent different functional entities in the nerve terminal. Zucker formulated a model in which he suggested that the binomial estimate of n was a reflection of the number of presynaptic release sites.[274] On the other hand, "n" may actually represent the number of quanta available to these releasing sites. As a consequence, the probability of release, $\bar{p}$, would be dependent upon membrane events, such as the activity of releasing sites, as well as the availability of quanta.

Although the precise definition of n and $\bar{p}$ remains unsettled, these parameters have been used to explain a wide variety of phenomena at the neuromuscular junction. For example, Bennett and Florin reported that the binomial value of $\bar{p}$ is normal soon after the beginning of transmission across regenerating neuromuscular junctions, while $\bar{m}$ and n recover at a relatively slower rate.[27] Since the release of transmitter is dependent upon the size of the nerve terminal,[144] Bennett and Florin suggested that the binomial estimate of n might reflect this morphological parameter.[27] However, this correlation can be questioned for at least two reasons. Firstly, n may be low at the regenerating neuromuscular junction because of some subtle defect in the release process since 3,4-diaminopyridine restores n and $\bar{p}$ to normal even at early times during the regeneration process.[14] Secondly, the motor nerves to the fast-twitch extensor digitorum longus muscle of the rat spontaneously release quanta at a greater frequency than the nerves to the slow-twitch soleus muscle,[188] even though the latter are apparently larger.[189] Quite interestingly, Gertler and Robbins presented Poisson data suggesting that $\bar{m}$ was also greater for the fast-twitch extensor muscle.[89] However, in our own comparison of these two muscles (Table 3.1) we found that the direct estimate of $\bar{m}$ was the same when the nerves were stimulated at either low (1 Hz) or high (160 Hz) frequencies. Nevertheless, the latter studies indicated that "n" was greater for the fast-twitch muscle. This may be related to the data of Padykula and Gauthier which suggest that vesicles occur at a higher density in the terminals of fast-twitch motor nerves.[212] Thus, it is likely that subtle differences between the quantal release process from different types of motor nerves remain to be discovered.

Since the postsynaptic sensitivity to acetylcholine apparently (see above discussion of desensitization) does not vary during repetitive stimulation,[115,211] alterations in n and $\bar{p}$ have also been suggested to account for the effects of such stimulation on neuromuscular transmission. The magnitude and time course of these effects are quantitated by comparing the amplitude of a test epp with a control epp. The test measurement is made at known times after a conditioning stimulus or train of stimuli of controlled frequency. When such an analysis is performed at neuromuscular junctions with a normal level of release, continuous stimulation brings about a decline in the amplitude of subsequent epps (see Fig. 3.9). Del Castillo and Katz[61] found that this depression was associated with a decline of n, while q remained unchanged. They also noted that depression was absent from frog preparations treated with elevated Mg^{++}. Similar treatment of mammalian preparations also precludes depression.[111,254] This effect of Mg^{++}, as well as the lack of significant changes of $\bar{p}$ during depression,[92,265] supports the suggestion of Liley and North[151] that depression is due to a depletion of quanta from the readily releasable pool.[26] At low levels of $\bar{m}$, mobilization of quanta[68,74] would be at least sufficient to maintain n at the preconditioning level. After repetitive stimulation, the mobilization process seems to restore n at the depressed neuromuscular junction with a time constant of about 5 sec.[246] A distinctly different cause of depression during repetitive stimulation is blockade of presynaptic action potentials. This is not associated with a depletion of n but may be due to anoxia[140] or presynaptic depolarization.[102,185]

Prior to the appearance of the depression described above, there is a brief elevation of epp amplitude.* Classically, this facilitatory phenomenon has been quantitated as the increase in amplitude or m of a test epp following a single conditioning stimulus to a Mg^{++}-treated preparation.[61] Nevertheless, such facilitation precedes depression in preparations having a high output of transmitter (curare-treated,[69,111] cut fiber preparation; see Fig. 3.9). Quite importantly, the test epp at Mg^{++}-treated amphibian,[61] crustacean,[66] and mammalian[111] neuromuscular junctions was facilitated even when the conditioning stimulus failed to release any quanta. This implies that the process responsible for facilitation is independent of transmitter secretion. In their investigation, Mallart and Martin[177] presented data suggesting that two separate processes underlie facilitation (see

---

*At very short intervals of stimulation the release process is refractory so that transmission across the synapse fails.[125]

Charlton and Bittner[47] for a similar observation in the giant synapse of squid). The first of these decayed with a time constant of 35 msec following a conditioning stimulus. They attributed this phase of potentiation to an elevation of $\bar{p}$. The time constant of decay of the second component was 250 msec and was suggested to be due to a transient increase of n secondary to mobilization brought about by transmitter release.[265]

Mallart and Martin went on to formulate a model in which each stimulus added a component to facilitation.[177] These components were proposed to sum linearly during repeated stimulation. Hubbard[111] reported similar initial effects of repetitive stimulation, although he referred to this phenomenon as primary potentiation in order to distinguish it from the later enhancement of epp amplitude after a conditioning tetanus.[167] The latter effect is classically known as post-tetanic potentiation and is observed in Mg^{++} as well as curare-blocked preparations. In the latter case, a phase of depression precedes the potentiation.[111] Nevertheless, Magleby[168] presented data suggesting that potentiation and depression can be operative at the same time after a conditioning tetanus. This would imply that distinct processes are involved.[171] In a series of kinetic studies Magleby and Zengel carefully explored the phenomen of potentiation. When they followed its time course in Mg^{++}-blocked frog muscle or rabbit superior cervical ganglion,[272] they uncovered an enhancement of the amplitude of the excitatory postsynaptic potential which occurred between facilitation and potentiation.[169,273] They called this phenomenon augmentation and showed that like potentiation it was due to the increase of $\bar{m}$.[172] These two effects of repetitive stimulation were found to have quite different time courses: augmentation decayed with a time constant of about 7 sec after a conditioning tetanus, while the time constant of potentiation could be as much as 60 sec.[172] Thus, the processes enhancing transmitter release could be studied separately. In this way, Magleby and Zengel[170] found that each stimulus of the conditioning train, regardless of its frequency, causes transmitter release to be increased by about 1% of control during potentiation. In addition, they found that the various phenomena enhancing transmitter release were differentially affected by prolonged stimulation,[171] temperature,[172] and ions,[271] which further supports the hypothesis that distinct mechanisms are involved.[149,173,176] Nevertheless, considerable data suggest that these mechanisms to enhance transmitter release result in an increase of $\bar{p}$[74,113,168,177,178,226] and/or n[92,220] due, at least in part, to mobilization of transmitter.[160] In addition, Birks[29] has discovered that repetitive stimulation of the cat superior cervical ganglion dramatically increases its store of acetylcholine. However, this elevation lasts for several hours after termination of the conditioning stimulus. Thus, it cannot account for the relatively short-term enhancement of transmitter release.

In order to gain insight into possible mechanisms underlying activity-induced enhancement of transmitter release, it is necessary to consider the sequence of events involved. For convenience these are summarized diagrammatically in Fig. 3.10. The amplitude of the nerve action potential would certainly influence the amplitude of the subsequent nerve terminal depolarization. If the latter were increased for some time after a conditioning stimulus, a test epp might be expected to be associated with enhanced transmitter release.[62,153]

Takeuchi and Takeuchi[249] presented data suggesting that facilitation at the squid giant synapse was due to a change in the size of presynaptic potential. However, Charlton and Bittner were unable to confirm this observation.[48] Likewise, Martin and Pilar found no change of the presynaptic action potential during facilitation of transmitter release at the avian ciliary ganglion.[183] Similar findings have been obtained at the crayfish neuromuscular junction.[210,275] Furthermore, repetitive activity is known to increase transmitter release even in the absence of a test stimulus. This is indicated by an enhancement of mepp frequency[34,111] which occurs over a time course similar to the augmentation and potentiation of stimulus-evoked release.[221] Thus, steps 1 and 2 (see Fig. 3.10) can be eliminated as primary contributors to the enhancing effects of repetitive activity. Since extracellular Ca^{++} markedly influences facilitation[126] and potentiation,[226] steps 4 to 8 as well as 12 and 13 are likely to be involved.

In their classic studies of stimulus-evoked transmitter release, Katz and Miledi[124,125,128] established that depolarization of the motor nerve terminal alone was not able to activate release. The latter occurred only when Ca^{++} was present during the terminal depolarization. In this condition, inward Ca^{++} current is activated (steps 4 to 6)[156] to increase the concentration of Ca^{++} within the nerve terminal ($[Ca]_t$, step 7). This then raises the probability of quantal release (step 8)[75,194,195] leading to exocytosis (step 9). Thus, the inward movement, accumulation and action of Ca^{++} would make a significant contribution to the overall delay in transmitter release (steps 4 to 9).[123] Miledi and Parker have reported that approximately 4×10^{-16} mole of Ca^{++} enter the nerve terminal (t) of the squid's giant synapse during a single impulse.[196] Quite importantly, their data indicated that the resultant increase of $[Ca]_t$ out-

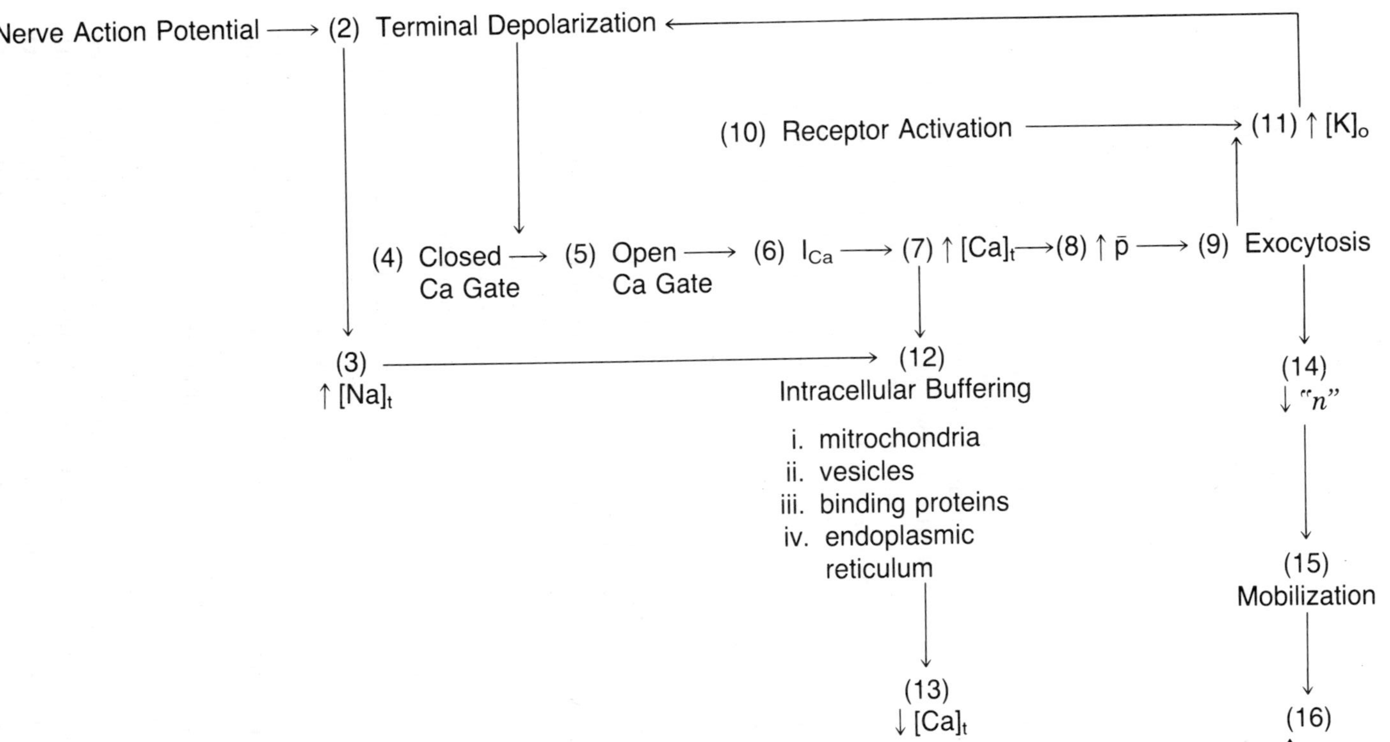

Figure 3.10. Schematic summarizing the processes which contribute to stimulus enhancement of transmitter release. I_{ca} indicates inward Ca^{++} current across the nerve terminal membrane, "n" the size of the readily available pool of transmitter, $[\ ]_t$ and $[\ ]_o$ the intraterminal and synaptic cleft concentrations of ions, respectively. See text for discussion.

lasts the stimulus-evoked release. Therefore, more of the Ca^{++} brought into the nerve terminal by a closely following test impulse would be available to the release process since the Ca^{++} buffering mechanisms (step $12^{10,221}$) would still be occupied with the conditioning Ca^{++} load. Following a conditioning tetanic stimulus, the buffering mechanisms may be swamped, allowing for the slow decline of $[Ca]_t$, or some related intermediate, to cause facilitation as well as augmentation and potentiation.[26,126,170] Since Dodge and Rahamimoff[64] have suggested that four Ca^{++} are necessary for the release of a single quantum, it is also conceivable that residual $[Ca]_t$ would further enhance the release process by cooperating with the Ca^{++} brought in by the test pulse. This possibility requires the assumption that four Ca^{++} are also involved in enhanced release. Younkin has presented data suggesting that three or four Ca^{++} are involved in facilitated transmitter release.[270] This is not so for potentiation,[170] which further suggests that normally evoked, facilitated and potentiated release do not involve the same Ca^{++} action.[55] Clarification is required with regard to the role of the four Ca^{++} during normally evoked release[216,221] in order to precisely define the role of Ca^{++} in enhanced release.

Figure 3.10 also indicates other factors which may act to enhance transmitter release. For example, an elevation of $[Na]_t$ (step 3) could occur if the extrusion mechanism for this cation were saturated as a result of the action potentials associated with repetitive activity. The Na^+ could then increase $[Ca]_t$, as well as transmitter release,[28,222,240] by competing with the Ca^{++} buffering mechanisms for energy stores needed to extrude Na^+, or by actually releasing intracellularly bound Ca^{++}.[221] Repetitive stimulation might also increase I_{Ca} (step 5)[242] or bring about a prolonged activation of mobilization (steps 14 and 15) which causes n to overshoot its normal level. Such stimulation of mobilization may actually require Ca^{++}. Finally, repeated receptor activation is likely to cause a change in the local concentration of K^+ (steps 10 and 11) in the space surrounding the neuromuscular junction. The K^+ may then influence the polarity of the nerve terminal to enhance or depress transmitter release.[185]

Before concluding this section, it is appropriate to briefly describe the conductance changes of the nerve terminal which activate I_{Ca} and, as a result, transmitter release. When Katz and Miledi locally applied the specific blocker of the Na^+ channel tetrodotoxin (TTX) onto the unmyelinated terminals of frog motor nerves they observed that transmitter release did not occur from those portions of the ending distal to the site of toxin application.[127] Therefore, they concluded that action potentials must propagate to the very ends of motor nerves to ensure maximal release of transmitter from the terminal arborizations. This implies that the Na^+ and K^+ channels underlying the action potential as well as the Ca^{++} channels must all be inserted along the entire length of the terminal membrane which contains the vesicle releasing sites. Katz and Miledi attributed the necessity of action potential propagation throughout the terminal to the fact that the actual length (L) of the unmyelinated terminal is much greater than the length constant (λ) of the membrane. Thus, electronic spread of current would be unable to thoroughly activate the nerve ending. Katz and Miledi[127] pointed out that this would not be true for a short nerve ending in which L was less than or equal to λ. Brigant and Mallart[37] have presented convincing evidence that indicates that the short motor nerve endings in mouse muscle rely upon electrotonic spread of current to activate transmitter release. This derives from their hypothesis that the different waveforms of the extracellular currents recorded from precisely localized regions of mouse motor nerve endings were due to the segregation of Na^+, K^+ and Ca^{++} channels along the length of the terminal membrane. To demonstrate this, Brigant and Mallart applied established channel blockers and looked for alterations in the currents.[37] For example, when they iontophoresed tetrodotoxin onto the region of the motor nerve ending closest to the last internode they found a marked suppression of an inward current, which is likely to be due to Na^+ because of the specificity of the toxin. In contrast, similar treatment of the extreme distal ends of the axon had no effect on the current recorded at that site. Therefore, action potentials cannot propagate to the ends of mouse motor nerves since Na^+ channels are not there. However, Brigant and Mallart showed that the local spread of current from the last node of Ranvier was sufficient to boost the depolarization of distal nerve endings and thus enhance transmitter release.[37] Brigant and Mallart found that the K^+ channel blockers tetraethylammonium (TEA) and 3,4-diaminopyridine (DAP) had no effect when applied to the proximal portion of the nerve ending. On the other hand, distal application of these chemicals produced blockade of an outward current, leaving behind a prolonged inward Ca^{++} current which was blocked by cobalt. The former effect indicated that K^+ channels are located only on the distal portions of the terminals. Thus, the proximal and distal portions of mouse motor nerve endings resemble the nodal and internodal regions of myelinated mammalian nerves, respectively, where Na^+ and K^+ channels are distinctly localized.[32,50,51,225] This is another example of the heterogeneity of excitable membranes.

Molecular

In addition to spontaneous and stimulus-evoked quantal release of acetylcholine from motor nerves, there is also molecular release from isolated nerve-muscle preparations. Mitchell and Silver[198] pointed out that this may account for most of the acetylcholine released from muscle.[81,93,218] Katz and Miledi noted that local application of curare to the frog endplate caused a resting muscle fiber to be hyperpolarized.[133] Thus, they concluded that molecular release of acetylcholine caused a steady depolarization of about 40 μV. Vyskočil and Illés presented data which suggested that a ouabain-sensitive Na-K ATPase activity regulated molecular release.[258,259] In addition, Vizi and Vyskočil found that molecular release was independent of the Ca^{++} concentration of the bathing medium.[256] At present, the origin of the molecularly released acetylcholine remains obscure.[134]

Factors Influencing the Postsynaptic Sensitivity to Acetylcholine

Katz and Thesleff demonstrated that the sensitivity of the endplate to acetylcholine is directly proportional to the passive electrical resistance of the sarcolemma.[122] This relationship suggests a way in which organisms may modulate cholinergic pathways as well as an additional means of experimentally enhancing this process. In order to test the latter possibility we[191] took advantage of the ability of 20,25-diazacholesterol (20,25-DC) to increase membrane resistance due to a significant reduction of the chloride permeability of the sarcolemma.[57] However, it is appropriate to note here that Furman and Barchi did not find that 20,25-DC had the latter effects.[82] D'Alonzo and McArdle have already discussed possible causes for this discrepancy.[57]

The experiments to assay the endplate sensitivity to acetylcholine were performed upon the triangularis sterni muscle of the mouse because of the distinct advantages it offers to the study of synaptic phenomena.[190] Mice were given subcutaneous injections of 20,25-DC (50 mg/Kg) at intervals of four days and sacrificed at four days after the sixth injection. At that time, the fibers of the triangularis sterni exhibited the expected myotonic-like activity (Fig. 3.11) as well as a reduction of total cholesterol content[57] (Table 3.2). These two findings would suggest that the resistance of the triangularis sterni muscle, like that of the more thoroughly studied extensor digitorum longus and soleus muscles of the rat, would be increased. I have not yet made this measurement. Nevertheless, both the average and maximal sensitivity of the endplate to acetylcholine was enhanced (Table 3.3). Since most of the cholesterol of muscle is in the sarcolemma,[17,103,238] these preliminary data suggest that the composi-

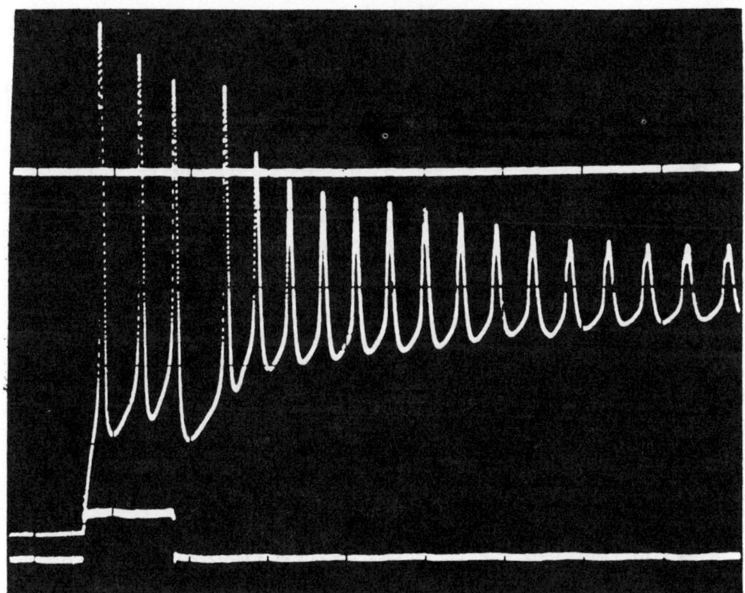

Figure 3.11. Trains of action potentials (22°C) recorded from a single fiber of the triangularis sterni muscle of a mouse treated with 20,25-diazacholesterol as described in the text. Upper trace is O mV potential and the middle trace is the membrane response to a 20 msec stimulus (lower trace) delivered through a second intracellular electrode.

Table 3.2
Mean Cholesterol Content (μg/g Muscle) of Extensor, Soleus and Triangularis Sterni Muscles from Control and Animals Treated with 20,25-Diazacholesterol (20,25-DC).

	Control	*20,25-DC*
Extensor	248	137
Soleus	365	102
Triangularis	422	227

Table 3.3
Average and Maximum Endplate Sensitivity to Acetylcholine (mV/nCoul) of Fibers in the Triangularis Sterni Muscle from Control and 20,25-Diazacholesterol (20,25-DC) Treated Mice.

	Average	*Maximum*
Control	2062	3395
20,25-DC	3553	5901

tion of this membrane regulates its response to cholinergic agonists. We have also obtained preliminary data indicating that the cholesterol content of the muscle increases after denervation or poisoning with botulinum toxin. If this proves to be due to a change in sarcolemmal composition it may contribute to the changes in receptor properties during denervation[13] and botulinum poisoning.[234] (For more information regarding the influence of milieu on the behavior of the acetylcholine receptor see articles by D'Alonzo and McArdle[58] and McArdle[187]).

Concluding Comments

Historically, the neuromuscular junction has provided stimulating and lasting hypotheses facilitating our understanding of synaptic function. It is certain that this increasingly accessible synapse will continue to provide us with insights into the subtle relationships between synaptic function and biochemistry.[135] Thus, our understanding of the plasticity, which underlies such complex phenomena as memory and learning, trophism, development, pathology and chemical action, will be advanced.

References

1. Adams PR: A study of desensitization using voltage clamp. *Pfluegers Arch* 360:135–144, 1975.
2. Adams PR: Drug blockade of open endplate channels. *J Physiol* 260:531–552, 1976.
3. Adams DJ, Dwyer TM, Hille B: The permeability of endplate channels to monovalent and divalent metal cations. *J Gen Physiol* 75:493–510, 1980.
4. Akasu T, Karczmar AG: Effects of anticholinesterases and sodium fluoride on neuromyal desensitization. *Neuropharm* 19:393–403, 1980.
5. Akhtar RA, Abdel-Latif AA: Calcium ion requirement for acetylcholine-stimulated breakdown of triphosphoinositide in rabbit iris smooth muscle. *J Pharmacol Exp Therap* 204:655–668, 1978.
6. Albuquerque EX, Thesleff S: Influence of phospholipase C on some electrical properties of the skeletal muscle membrane. *J Physiol* 190:123–127, 1967.
7. Albuquerque EX, Kuba K, Lapa AJ, Daly JW, Witkop B: Acetylcholine receptor and ionic conductance modulator of innervated and denervated muscle membranes. Effect of histrioniocotoxins. In Milhorat AT (ed): *Exploratory Concepts in Muscular Dystrophy II*, Amsterdam, Excerpta Medica, 1973, pp 585–597.
8. Albuquerque EX, Barnard EA, Porter CW, Warnick JE: The density of acetylcholine receptors and their sensitivity in the postsynaptic membrane of muscle endplates. *Proc Nat Acad Sci* 71:2818–2822, 1974.
9. Alemà S, Cull-Candy SG, Miledi R, Trautmann A: Properties of endplate channels in rats immunized against acetylcholine receptors. *J Physiol* 311:251–266, 1981.
10. Alnaes E, Rahamimoff R: On the role of mitochondria in transmitter release from motor nerve terminals. *J Physiol* 248:285–306, 1975.
11. Anderson CR, Stevens CF: Voltage clamp analysis of acetylcholine produced endplate current fluctuations at frog neuromuscular junction. *J Physiol* 235:655–691, 1973.
12. Andreason TJ, McNamee MG: Phospholipase A inhibition of acetylcholine receptor function in Torpedo californica membrane vesicles. *Biochem Biophys Res Comm* 79:958–965, 1977.
13. Argentieri TM, McArdle JJ: Endplate currents are prolonged at reinnervating neuromuscular junctions. *Soc Neurosci Abs* 7:2266, 1981.
14. Argentieri TM, McArdle JJ, Laxminarayan S, Michelson L: The sensitivity of regenerating nerve endings to calcium and 3,4 diaminopyridine. *Soc Neurosci Abs* 8:862, 1982.
15. Argentieri TM, McArdle JJ: Interaction of the opiate antagonist, naltrexone methyl bromide, with the acetylcholine receptor system of the motor endplate. *Brain Res* (in press).
16. Axelsson J, Thesleff S: The "desensitizing" effect of acetylcholine on the mammalian motor endplate. *Acta Physiol Scand* 43:15–26, 1958.
17. Barchi RL, Weigle JB, Chalikian DM, Murphy LE: Muscle surface membranes. Preparative methods affect apparent chemical properties and neurotoxin binding. *Biochem Biophys Acta* 550:59–76, 1979.

18. Barrantes FJ: Oligomeric forms of the membrane-bound acetylcholine receptor disclosed upon extraction of the M_r 43,000 nonreceptor peptide. *J Cell Biol* 92:60–68, 1982.
19. Barry PH, Gage PW, Van Helden DF: Cation permeation at the amphibian motor endplate. *J Memb Biol* 45:245–276, 1979.
20. Barry PH, Gage PW, Van Helden DF: Endplate channels behave as neutral site channels. *Neurosci Lett* 11:233–237, 1979.
21. Barstad JAB: Presynaptic effect of the neuromuscular transmitter. *Experientia* 18:579–580, 1962.
22. Barton SB, Cohen IS: Are transmitter release statistics meaningful? *Nature* 268:267–268, 1977.
23. Beam KG: A voltage clamp study of the effect of two lidocaine derivatives on the time course of endplate currents. *J Physiol* 258:279–300, 1976.
24. Beam KG: A quantitative description of endplate currents in the presence of two lidocaine derivatives. *J Physiol* 258:301–322, 1976.
25. Beani L, Bianchi C, Ledda F: The effect of tubocurarine on acetylcholine release from motor nerve terminals. *J Physiol* 174:172–183, 1964.
26. Bennett MR, Fisher C: The effect of calcium ions on the binomial parameters that control acetylcholine release during trains of nerve impulses at amphibian neuromuscular synapses. *J Physiol* 271:673–698, 1977.
27. Bennett MR, Florin T: A statistical analysis of the release of acetylcholine at newly formed synapses in striated muscle. *J Physiol* 238:93–107, 1974.
28. Birks RI, Cohen MW: The influence of internal sodium on the behavior of motor nerve endings. *Proc R Soc Lond Ser B* 170:401–421, 1968.
29. Birks RI: A long-lasting potentiation of transmitter release related to an increase in transmitter stores in a sympathetic ganglion. *J Physiol* 271:847–862, 1977.
30. Blackman JG, Ginsborg BL, Ray C: On the quantal release of the transmitter at a sympathetic synapse. *J Physiol* 167:402–415, 1963.
31. Boheim G, Hanke HW, Barrantes FJ, Eibl H, Sakmann B, Fels G, Maelicke A: Agonist-activated ionic channels in acetylcholine receptor reconstituted into planar lipid bilayers. *Proc Nat Acad Sci USA* 78:3586–3590, 1981.
32. Bostock H, Sears TA, Sherratt RM: The effects of 4-aminopyridine and tetraethylammonium ions on normal and demyelinated mammalian nerve fibres. *J Physiol* 313:301–315, 1981.
33. Boyd IA, Martin AR: The endplate potential in mammalian muscle. *J Physiol* 132:74–91, 1956.
34. Braun M, Schmidt RF, Zimmermann M: Facilitation at the frog neuromuscular junction during and after repetitive stimulation. *Pfluegers Archiv* 287:41–55, 1966.
35. Bregestovski PD, Bukharaeva EA, Iljin VI: Voltage clamp analysis of acetylcholine receptor desensitization in isolated mollusc neurones. *J Physiol* 297:581–595, 1979.
36. Brenner HR, Rathmayer W: The quantal nature of synaptic transmission at the neuromuscular junction of a spider. *J Gen Physiol* 62:224–236, 1973.

37. Brigant JL, Mallart A: Presynaptic currents in mouse motor endings. *J Physiol* 333:619−636, 1982.
38. Brown HT, Perkel DH, Feldman MW: Evoked neurotransmitter release: Statistical effects of nonuniformity and nonstationarity. *Proc Nat Acad Sci USA* 73:2913−2917, 1976.
39. Burgermeister W, Klein WL, Nirenberg M, Witkop B: Comparative binding studies with cholinergic ligands and histrionicotoxin at muscarinic receptors of neural cell lines. *Molec Pharmacol* 14:751−767, 1978.
40. Burns BD, Paton WDM: Depolarization of the motor endplate by decamethonium and acetylcholine. *J Physiol* 115:41−73, 1954.
41. Canepa FG: Acetylcholine Quanta. *Nature* 201:184−185, 1964.
42. Cartaud J, Benedetti L, Cohen JB, Meunier JC, Changeux JP: Presence of a lattice structure in membrane fragments rich in nicotinic receptor protein from the electric organ of Torpedo marmorata. *FEBS Lett* 33:109−113, 1973.
43. Chang CC, Lee CY: Isolation of neurotoxins from the venom of Bungarus multicinctus and their modes of neuromuscular blocking action. *Arch Int Pharmacodyn* 144:241−257, 1963.
44. Chang CC, Lee CY: Electrophysiological study of neuromuscular blocking action of cobra neurotoxin. *Brit J Pharmacol Chemother*. 28:172−181, 1966.
45. Chang HW, Bock E: Molecular forms of acetylcholine receptor. Effects of calcium ions and sulfhydryl reagent on the occurrence of oligomers. *Biochem* 16:4513−4520, 1977.
46. Changeux JP, Heidmann T, Popot JL, Sobel A: Reconstitution of a functional acetylcholine regulator under defined conditions. *FEBS Lett* 105:181−187, 1979.
47. Charlton MP, Bittner GD: Facilitation of transmitter release at squid synapses. *J Gen Physiol* 72:471−486, 1978.
48. Charlton MP, Bittner GD: Presynaptic potentials and facilitation of transmitter release in the squid giant synapse. *J Gen Physiol* 72:487−511, 1978.
49. Chesnut TJ: Components of desensitization of the frog neuromuscular junction and the effect of metabolic inhibitors. *Cell Molec Neurobiol* 2:59−63, 1982.
50. Chin SY, Ritchie JM, Rogart RB, Stagg D: A quantitative description of membrane currents in rabbit myelinated nerve. *J Physiol* 292:149−166, 1979.
51. Chiu SY, Ritchie JM: Evidence for the presence of potassium channels in the paranodal region of acutely demyelinated mammalian single nerve fibres. *J Physiol* 313:415−437, 1981.
52. Cohen JB, Changeux JP: Interaction of a fluorescent ligand with membrane-bound cholinergic receptor from Torpedo marmorata. *Biochem* 12:4855−4864, 1973.
53. Cohen JB, Weber M, Changeux JP: Effects of local anesthetics and calcium on the interaction of cholinergic ligands with the nicotinic receptor protein from Torpedo marmorata. *Molec Pharmacol* 10:904−932, 1975.
54. Conti-Tronconi BM, Raftery MA: The nicotinic cholinergic receptor:

correlation of molecular structure with functional properties. *Ann Rev Biochem* 51:491–530, 1982.

55. Cooke JD, Quastel DMJ: Cumulative and persistent effects of nerve terminal depolarization on transmitter release. *J Physiol* 228:407–434, 1973.

56. Cull-Candy SG, Miledi R, Trautmann A: Endplate currents and acetylcholine noise at normal and myasthenic human endplates. *J Physiol* 287:247–265, 1979.

57. D'Alonzo AJ, McArdle JJ: An evaluation of fast- and slow-twitch muscle from rats treated with 20,25-diazacholesterol. *Exp Neurol* 78:46–66, 1982.

58. D'Alonzo AJ, McArdle JJ: Effects of 20,25-diazacholesterol treatment on the decay of endplate currents. *Exp Neurol* 76:681–683, 1982.

59. DeBassio WA, Parsons RL, Schnitzler RM: Effect of ionophore X-537A on desensitization rate and tension development in potassium-depolarized muscle fibres. *Br J Pharmacol* 57:565–571, 1976.

60. Del Castillo J, Katz B: Quantal components of the endplate potential. *J Physiol* 124:560–573, 1954.

61. Del Castillo J, Katz B: Statistical factors involved in neuromuscular facilitation and depression. *J Physiol* 124:574–585, 1954.

62. Del Castillo J, Katz B: Changes in endplate activity produced by presynaptic polarization. *J Physiol* 124:586–604, 1954.

63. Dionne VE, Steinbach JH, Stevens CF: An analysis of the dose-response relationship at voltage-clamped frog neuromuscular junctions. *J Physiol* 281:421–444, 1978.

64. Dodge FA, Rahamimoff R: Co-operative action of calcium ions in transmitter release at the neuromuscular junction. *J Physiol* 193:419–432, 1967.

65. Dreyer F, Peper K: Density and dose-response curve of acetylcholine receptors in frog neuromuscular junctions. *Nature* 253:641–643, 1975.

66. Dudel J, Kuffler SW: The quantal nature of transmission and spontaneous miniature potentials at the crayfish neuromuscular junction. *J Physiol* 155:514–529, 1961.

67. Dwyer TM, Adams DJ, Hille B: The permeability of the endplate channel to organic cations in frog muscle. *J Gen Physiol* 75:469–492, 1980.

68. Eccles JC: *The Physiology of Nerve Cells.* Baltimore, Johns Hopkins Press, 1957.

69. Eccles JC, Katz B, Kuffler SW: Nature of the 'endplate potential' in curarized muscle. *J Neurophysiol* 4:362–387, 1941.

70. Eldefrawi ME, Eldefrawi AT, Shamoo AE: Molecular and functional properties of the acetylcholine-receptor. *Ann NY Acad Sci* 264:183–202, 1975.

71. Eldefrawi ME, Eldefrawi AT, Penfield AL, O'Brien RD, Van Campen V: Binding of calcium and zinc to the acetylcholine receptor purified from *Torpedo californica*. *Life Sci* 16:925–936, 1975.

72. Elias SB, Appel SH: Acetylcholine receptor in myasthenia gravis: increased affinity for alpha-bungarotoxin. *Ann Neurol* 4:250–252, 1978.

73. Elliot J, Dunn SMJ, Blanchard SG, Raftery MA: Specific binding of perhydrohistrionicotoxin to torpedo acetylcholine receptor. *Proc Nat Acad Sci USA* 76:2576–2579, 1979.

74. Elmqvist D, Quastel DMJ: A quantitative study of endplate potentials in isolated human muscle. *J Physiol* 178:505–529, 1965.

75. Erulkar SD, Rahamimoff R, Rotshenker S: Quelling of spontaneous transmitter release by nerve impulses in low extra-cellular calcium solutions. *J Physiol* 278:491–500, 1978.

76. Fambrough DM, Drachman DB, Satyamurti S: Neuromuscular junction in myasthenia gravis: Decreased acetylcholine receptors. *Science* 182:293–295, 1973.

77. Fatt P, Katz B: Spontaneous subthreshold activity at motor nerve endings. *J Physiol* 117:109–128, 1952.

78. Feltz A, Trautmann A: Desensitization at the frog neuromuscular junction: A biphasic process. *J Physiol* 322:257–272, 1982.

79. Fertuck HC, Salpeter MM: Quantitation of junctional and extrajunctional acetylcholine receptors by electron microscope autoradiography after ^{125}I-alpha-bungarotoxin binding at mouse neuromuscular junctions. *J Cell Biol* 69:144–158, 1976.

80. Fiekers JF, Spannbauer PM, Scubon-Mulieri B, Parsons RL: Voltage dependence of desensitization. Influence of calcium and activation kinetics. *J Gen Physiol* 75:511–529, 1980.

81. Fletcher P, Forrester T: The effect of curare on the release of acetylcholine from mammalian motor nerve terminals and an estimate of quantum content. *J Physiol* 251:131–144, 1975.

82. Furman RE, Barchi RL: 20,25-diazacholesterol myotonia. An electrophysical study. *Ann Neurol* 10:251–260, 1981.

83. Gage PW: Generation of endplate potentials. *Physiol Rev* 56:177–247, 1976.

84. Gage PW, Eisenberg RS: Action potentials without contraction in frog skeletal muscle fibers with disrupted transverse tubules. *Science* 158:1702–1703, 1967.

85. Gage PW, McBurney RN, Van Helden D: Endplate currents are shortened by octanol: Possible role of membrane lipid. *Life Sci* 14:2277–2283, 1974.

86. Gage PW, McBurney RN, Schneider GT: Effects of some aliphatic alcohols on the conductance change caused by a quantum of acetylcholine at the toad endplate. *J Physiol* 244:409–429, 1975.

87. Gage PW, McBurney RN, Van Helden D: Octanol reduces endplate channel lifetime. *J Physiol* 274:279–298, 1978.

88. Galindo A: Prejunctional effect of curare: its relative importance. *J Neurophys* 34:289–301, 1971.

89. Gertler RA, Robbins N: Differences in neuromuscular transmission in red and white muscles. *Brain Res* 142:160–164, 1978.

90. Glavinović MI: Presynaptic action of curare. *J Physiol* 290:499–506, 1979.

91. Glavinović MI: Voltage clamping of unparalysed cut rat diaphragm for study of transmitter release. *J Physiol* 290:467–480, 1979.

92. Glavinović MI: Change of statistical parameters of transmitter release during various kinetic tests in unparalysed voltage-clamped rat diaphragm. *J Physiol* 290:481–497, 1979.

93. Gorio A, Hurlbut WP, Ceccarelli B: Acetylcholine compartments in mouse diaphragm: A comparison of the effects of black widow spider venom, electrical stimulation and high concentrations of potassium. *J Cell Biol* 78:716–733, 1978.

94. Gration KAF, Lambert JJ, Usherwood PNR: A comparison of glutamate single-channel activity at desensitizing and nondesensitizing sites. *J Physiol* 310:49P, 1981.

95. Grünhagen HH, Changeux JP: Studies on the electrogenic action of acetylcholine with *Torpedo marmorata* electric organ. IV: Quinacrine: a fluorescent probe for the conformational transitions of the cholinergic receptor protein in its membrane-bound state. *J Mol Biol* 106:497–516, 1976.

96. Grünhagen HH, Changeux JP: Studies on the electrogenic action of acetylcholine with *Torpedo marmorata* electric organ. V. Qualitative correlation between pharmacological effects and equilibration processes of the cholinergic receptor protein as revealed by the structural probe quinacrine. *J Mol Biol* 106:517–535, 1976.

97. Hall ZW, Lubit BW, Schwartz JH: Cytoplasmic actin in postsynaptic structures at the neuromuscular junction. *J Cell Biol* 90:789–792, 1982.

98. Hamill OP, Marty A, Weber E, Sakmann B, Sigworth FJ: Improved patch-clamp techniques for high-resolution current recording from cells and cell-free membrane patches. *Pfluegers Arch* 391:85–100, 1981.

99. Hamilton SL, McLaughlin M, Karlin A: Formation of disulfide-linked oligomers of acetylcholine receptor in membrane from *Torpedo* electric tissue. *Biochem* 18:155–163, 1979.

100. Hansert E, Wernig A, Carmody JJ: Transmitter release statistics are meaningful. *Nature* 271:688, 1978.

101. Hartzell HC, Kuffler SW, Yoshikami D: Post-synaptic potentiation: Interaction between quanta of acetylcholine at the skeletal neuromuscular synapse. *J Physiol* 251:427–463, 1975.

102. Hatt H, Smith DO: Synaptic depression related to presynaptic axon conduction block. *J Physiol* 259:367–393, 1976.

103. Headon D, Barrett F, Joyce N, O'Flaherty J: Cholesterol in muscle membranes. *Mol Cell Biochem* 17:117–123, 1977.

104. Heidmann T, Changeux JP: Structural and functional properties of the acetylcholine receptor protein in its purified and membrane-bound states. *Ann Rev Biochem* 47:317–357, 1978.

105. Heuser J, Miledi R: Effect of lanthanum ions on function and structure of frog neuromuscular junctions. *Proc R Soc Lond Ser B* 179:247–260, 1971.

106. Heuser JE, Reese TS: Evidence for recycling of synaptic vesicle membrane during transmitter release at the frog neuromuscular junction. *J Cell Biol* 57:315–344, 1973.
107. Heuser JE, Salpeter SR: Organization of acetylcholine receptors in quick frozen, deep-etched, and rotary-replicated *Torpedo* postsynaptic membrane. *J Cell Biol* 82:150–173, 1979.
108. Hohlfeld R, Sterz R, Kalies I, Peper K, Wekerle H: Neuromuscular transmission in experimental autoimmune myasthenia gravis (EAMG). Quantitative ionophoresis and current fluctuation analysis at normal and myasthenic rat endplates. *Pfluegers Arch* 390:156–160, 1981.
109. Hokin LE, Hokin MR: Acetylcholine and the exchange of inositol and phosphate in brain phosphoinositide. *J Biol Chem* 233:818–821, 1958.
110. Horn R, Brodwick MS, Dickey WD: Asymmetry of the acetylcholine channel revealed by quaternary anesthetics. *Science* 210:205–207, 1980.
111. Hubbard JI: Repetitive stimulation at the mammalian neuromuscular junction, and the mobilization of transmitter. *J Physiol* 169:641–662, 1963.
112. Hubbard JI, Kwanbunbumpen S: Evidence for the vesicle hypothesis. *J Physiol* 194:407–420, 1968.
113. Hubbard JI, Jones SF, Landau EM: The effect of temperature change upon transmitter release, facilitation and post-tetanic potentiation. *J Physiol* 216:591–609, 1971.
114. Hubbard JI, Wilson DF: Neuromuscular transmission in a mammalian preparation in the absence of blocking drugs and the effect of D-tubocurarine. *J Physiol* 228:307–325, 1973.
115. Hutter OF: Post-tetanic restoration of neuromuscular transmission blocked by D-tubocurarine. *J Physiol* 118:216–227, 1952.
116. Johnson EW, Wernig A: The binomial nature of transmitter release at the crayfish neuromuscular junction. *J Physiol* 218:757–767, 1971.
117. Kalcheim C, Vogel Z, Duksin D: Embryonic brain extract induces collagen biosynthesis in cultured muscle cells: Involvement in acetylcholine receptor aggregation. *Proc Nat Acad Sci USA* 79:3077–3081, 1982.
118. Karlin A, Weill CL, McNamee MG, Valderamma R: Facets of the structures of acetylcholine receptors from *Electrophorus* and *Torpedo*. *Cold Spring Harbor Symp Quant Biol* 40:203–210, 1975.
119. Karlin A, Holtzman E, Valderamma R, Damle V, Hsu K, Reyes F: Binding of antibodies to acetylcholine receptors in *Electrophorus* and *Torpedo* electroplax membranes. *J Cell Biol* 76:577–592, 1978.
120. Karlin A, Damle V, Hamilton S, McLaughlin M, Valderamma R, Wise P: Acetylcholine receptors in and out of membranes. In Ceccarelli B, Clementi F (eds): *Advanced Cytopharmacology*, Vol 3. New York, Raven Press, 1979, pp 183–189.
121. Katz B, Thesleff S: A study of the 'desensitization' produced by acetylcholine at the motor endplate. *J Physiol* 138:63–80, 1957.

122. Katz B, Thesleff S: On the factors which determine the amplitude of the 'miniature endplate potential'. *J Physiol* 137:267–278, 1957.

123. Katz B, Miledi R: The measurement of synaptic delay, and the time course of acetylcholine release at the neuromuscular junction. *Proc R Soc London Ser B* 161:483–495, 1965.

124. Katz B, Miledi R: The timing of calcium action during neuromuscular transmission. *J Physiol* 189:535–544, 1967.

125. Katz B, Miledi R: A study of synaptic transmission in the absence of nerve impulses. *J Physiol* 192:407–436, 1967.

126. Katz B, Miledi R: The role of calcium in neuromuscular facilitation. *J Physiol* 195:481–492, 1968.

127. Katz B, Miledi R: The effect of local blockage of motor nerve terminals. *J Physiol* 199:729–741, 1968.

128. Katz B, Miledi R: Tetrodotoxin-resistant electric activity in presynaptic terminals. *J Physiol* 203:459–487, 1969.

129. Katz B, Miledi R: Membrane noise produced by acetylcholine. *Nature* 226:962–963, 1970.

130. Katz B, Miledi R: The statistical nature of the acetylcholine potential and its molecular components. *J Physiol* 224:665–669, 1972.

131. Katz B, Miledi R: The characteristics of endplate noise produced by different depolarizing drugs. *J Physiol* 230:707–717, 1973.

132. Katz B, Miledi R: The reversal potential at the desensitized endplate. *Proc R Soc London Ser B* 199:329–334, 1977.

133. Katz B, Miledi R: Transmitter leakage from motor nerve endings. *Proc R Soc London* 196:59–72, 1977.

134. Katz B, Miledi R: Does the motor nerve evoke nonquantal transmitter release? *Proc R Soc London Ser B* 212:131–137, 1981.

135. Kelly RB, Deutsch JW, Carlson SS, Wagner JA: Biochemistry of neurotransmitter release. *Ann Rev Neurosci* 2:399–446, 1979.

136. Klymkowski MW, Stroud RM: Immunospecific identification and three-dimensional structure of a membrane-bound acetylcholine receptor from *Torpedo californica*. *J Mol Biol* 128:319–334, 1979.

137. Kordaš M: The effect of membrane polarization on the time course of the endplate current in frog sartorius muscle. *J Physiol* 204:493–502, 1969.

138. Kriebel ME, Stolper DR: Non-poisson distribution in time of small- and large-mode miniature and endplate potentials. *Am J. Physiol* 229:1321–1329, 1975.

139. Kriebel ME, Llados F, Matteson DR: Spontaneous subminiature endplate potentials in mouse diaphragm muscle: Evidence for synchronous release. *J Physiol* 262:553–581, 1976.

140. Krnjević K, Miledi R: Failure of neuromuscular propagation in rats. *J Physiol* 140:440–461, 1958.

141. Kuba K, Koketsu K: Decrease of Na^+ conductance during desensitization of the frog endplate. *Nature* 262:504–505, 1976.

142. Kuffler SW, Yoshikami D: The number of transmitter molecules in a quantum: an estimate from iontophoretic application of acetylcholine at the neuromuscular synapse. *J Physiol* 251:465−482, 1975.
143. Kuno M: Quantal components of excitatory postsynaptic potentials in spinal motoneurones. *J Physiol* 175:81−99, 1964.
144. Kuno M, Turkanis SA, Weakly JN: Correlation between nerve terminal size and transmitter release at the neuromuscular junction of the frog. *J Physiol* 213:545−556, 1971.
145. Kusano K, Miledi R, Stinnakre J: Postsynaptic entry of calcium induced by transmitter action. *Proc R Soc London Ser B* 189:49−56, 1975.
146. Lambert DH, Spannbauer PM, Parsons RL: Desensitization does not selectively alter sodium channels. *Nature* 268:553−555, 1977.
147. Land BR, Podleski TR, Salpeter EE, Salpeter MM: Acetylcholine receptor distribution on myotubes in culture correlated to acetylcholine sensitivity. *J Physiol* 269:155−176, 1977.
148. Land BR, Salpeter EE, Salpeter MM: Acetylcholine receptor site density affects the rising phase of miniature endplate currents. *Proc Nat Acad Sci USA* 77:3736−3740, 1980.
149. Landau EM, Smolinsky A, Lass Y: Post-tetanic potentiation and facilitation do not share a common calcium-dependent mechanism. *Nature New Biol* 244:155−157, 1973.
150. Lassignal NL, Martin AR: Effect of acetylcholine on postjunctional membrane permeability in eel electroplaque. *J Gen Physiol* 70:23−36, 1977.
151. Liley AW, North KAK: An electrical investigation of effects of repetitive stimulation on mammalian neuromuscular junction. *J Neurophysiol* 16:509−527, 1953.
152. Liley WW: The quantal components of the mammalian endplate potential. *J Physiol* 133:571−587, 1956.
153. Liley AW: The effects of presynaptic polarization on the spontaneous activity at the mammalian neuromuscular junction. *J Physiol* 134:427−443, 1956.
154. Liley AW: Spontaneous release of transmitter substance in multiquantal units. *J Physiol* 136:595−605, 1957.
155. Linder TM, Quastel DMJ: A voltage clamp study of the permeability change induced by quanta of transmitter at the mouse endplate. *J Physiol* 281:535−556, 1978.
156. Llinás R, Steinberg IZ, Walton K: Presynaptic calcium currents and their relation to synaptic transmission: Voltage clamp study in squid giant synapse and theoretical model for the calcium gate. *Proc Nat Acad Sci USA* 73:2918−2922, 1976.
157. Lo MMS, Garland PB, Lamprecht J, Barnard EA: Rotational mobility of the membrane-bound acetylcholine receptor of *Torpedo* electric organ measured by phosphorescence depolarization. *FEBS Lett* 111:407−412, 1980.

158. Lorković H: Desensitization in denervated mouse muscles. *Pfluegers Arch* 391:171–177, 1981.

159. Lubit BW, Schwartz JH: An antiactin antibody that distinguishes between cytoplasmic and skeletal muscle actins. *J Cell Biol* 86:891–897, 1980.

160. Maeno T, Edwards C: Neuromuscular facilitation with low-frequency stimulation and effects of some drugs. *J Neurophysiol* 32:785–792, 1969.

161. Maeno T, Edwards C, Anraku M: Permeability of the endplate membrane activated by acetylcholine to some organic cations. *J Neurobiol* 8:173–184, 1977.

162. Magazanik LG, Vyskočil F: Dependence of acetylcholine desensitization on the membrane potential of frog muscle fiber and on the ionic changes in the medium. *J Physiol* 210:507–518, 1970.

163. Magazanik LG, Vyskočil F: Desensitization at the motor endplate. In Rang HP (ed): *Drug Receptors*. Baltimore, University Park Press, 1973, pp 105–119.

164. Magazanik LG, Vyskočil F: The effect of temperature on desensitization kinetics at the postsynaptic membrane of the frog muscle fiber. *J Physiol* 249:285–300, 1975.

165. Magleby KL, Stevens CF: The effect of voltage on the time course of endplate currents. *J Physiol* 223:151–171, 1972.

166. Magleby KL, Stevens CF: A quantitative description of endplate currents. *J Physiol* 223:173–197, 1972.

167. Magleby KL: The effect of repetitive stimulation on facilitation of transmitter release at the frog neuromuscular junction. *J Physiol* 234:327–352, 1973.

168. Magleby KL: The effect of tetanic and post-tetanic potentiation on facilitation of transmitter release at the frog neuromuscular junction. *J Physiol* 234:353–371, 1973.

169. Magleby KL, Zengel JE: A dual effect of repetitive stimulation on post-tetanic potentiation of transmitter release at the frog neuromuscular junction. *J Physiol* 245:163–182, 1975.

170. Magleby KL, Zengel JE: A quantitative description of tetanic and post-tetanic potentiation of transmitter release at the frog neuromuscular junction. *J Physiol* 245:183–208, 1975.

171. Magleby KL, Zengel JE: Long-term changes in augmentation, potentiation, and depression of transmitter release as a function of repeated synaptic activity at the frog neuromuscular junction. *J Physiol* 257:471–494, 1976.

172. Magleby KL, Zengel JE: Augmentation: A process that acts to increase transmitter release at the frog neuromuscular junction. *J Physiol* 257:449–470, 1976.

173. Magleby KL, Zengel JE: Stimulation-induced factors which affect augmentation and potentiation of transmitter release at the neuromuscular junction. *J Physiol* 260:687–717, 1976.

174. Magleby KL, Miller DC: Is the quantum of transmitter release composed of subunits? A critical analysis in the mouse and frog. *J Physiol* 311:267–287, 1981.
175. Magleby KL, Pallotta BS: A study of desensitization of acetylcholine receptors using nerve-released transmitter in the frog. *J Physiol* 316:225–250, 1981.
176. Magleby KL, Zengel JE: A quantitative description of stimulation-induced changes in transmitter release at the frog neuromuscular junction. *J Gen Physiol* 80:613–638, 1982.
177. Mallart A, Martin AR: An analysis of facilitation of transmitter release at the neuromuscular junction of the frog. *J Physiol* 193:679–694, 1967.
178. Mallart A, Martin AR: The relation between quantum content and facilitation at the neuromuscular junction of the frog. *J Physiol* 196:593–604, 1968.
179. Manthey AA: The effect of calcium on the desensitization of membrane receptors at the neuromuscular junction. *J Gen Phys* 49:963–976, 1966.
180. Martin AR: A further study of the statistical composition of the end-plate potential. *J Physiol* 130:114–122, 1955.
181. Martin AR: The effects of membrance capacitance on nonlinear summation of synaptic potentials. *J Theor Biol* 59:179–187, 1976.
182. Martin AR, Pilar G: Quantal components of the synaptic potential in the ciliary ganglion of the chick. *J Physiol* 175:1–16, 1964.
183. Martin AR, Pilar G: Presynaptic and post-synaptic events during post-tetanic potentiation and facilitation in the avian ciliary ganglion. *J Physiol* 175:17–30, 1964.
184. Mathers DA, Usherwood PN: Effects of concanavalin A on junctional and extrajunctional L-glutamate receptors on locust skeletal muscle fibers. *Comp Biochem Physiol* 59c:151–155, 1978.
185. Matyushkin DP, Shabunova IA, Sharovarova GM, Vinogradova IM: On potassium functional feedback in neuromuscular junction. *J Neurosci Res* 3:441–450, 1978.
186. McArdle JJ: Complex endplate potentials at the regenerating neuromuscular junction of the rat. *Exp Neurol* 49:629–638, 1975.
187. McArdle JJ: Molecular aspects of the trophic influence of nerve on muscle. *Prog Neurobiol* 21:135–198, 1983.
188. McArdle JJ, Albuquerque EX: A study of reinnervation of fast and slow mammalian muscles. *J Gen Physiol* 61:1–23, 1973.
189. McArdle JJ, Sansone FM: Re-innervation of fast and slow twitch muscle following nerve crush at birth. *J Physiol* 271:567–586, 1977.
190. McArdle JJ, Angaut-Petit D, Mallart A, Bournaud R, Faille L, Brigant JL: Advantages of the triangularis sterni muscle of the mouse for investigations of synaptic phenomena. *J Neurosci Meth* 4:109–115, 1981.

191. McArdle JJ, D'Alonzo AJ: Reduction of cholesterol content of muscle increases the endplate response to acetylcholine. *Neurosci Abs* 7:701, 1981.

192. McLachlin EM, Martin AR: Non-linear summation of endplate potentials in the frog and mouse. *J Physiol* 311:307−324, 1981.

193. Merlie JP, Hofler JG, Sebbane R: Acetylcholine receptor synthesis from membrane polysomes. *J Biol Chem* 256:6995−6999, 1981.

194. Meiri H, Rahamimoff R: Clumping and oscillations in evoked transmitter release at the frog neuromuscular junction. *J Physiol* 278:513−523, 1978.

195. Miledi R: Transmitter release induced by injection of calcium ions into nerve terminals. *Proc R Soc London Ser B* 183:421−425, 1973.

196. Miledi R, Parker I: Calcium transients recorded with arsenazo III in the presynaptic terminal of the squid giant synapse. *Proc R Soc London Ser B* 212:197−211, 1981.

197. Miledi R, Molenaar PC, Polak RL: Free and bound acetylcholine in frog muscle. *J Physiol* 333:189−199, 1982.

198. Mitchell JF, Silver A: The spontaneous release of acetylcholine from denervated hemidiaphragm of the rat. *J Physiol* 165:117−129, 1963.

199. Miyamoto MD: Binomial analysis of quantal transmitter release at glycerol treated frog neuromuscular junctions. *J Physiol* 250:121−142, 1975.

200. Moreau M, Changeux JP: Studies on the electrogenic action of acetylcholine with *Torpedo marmorata* electric organ. I. Pharmacologic properties of the electroplaque. *J Mol Biol* 106:457−467, 1976.

201. Nastuk WL, Parsons RL: Factors in the inactivation of postjunctional membrane receptors of frog skeletal muscle. *J Gen Physiol* 56:218−249, 1970.

202. Neher E, Stevens CF: Conductance fluctuations and ionic pores in membranes. *Ann Rev Biophys Bioeng* 6:345−381, 1977.

203. Neher E, Sakmann B: Single channel currents recorded from membrane of denervated frog muscle fibers. *Nature* 260:799−801, 1976.

204. Neher E, Steinbach JH: Local anaesthetics transiently block currents through single acetylcholine receptor channels. *J Physiol* 277:153−176, 1978.

205. Neher E, Sakmann B, Steinbach JH: The extracellular patch clamp: A method for resolving currents through individual open channels in biological membranes. *Pfluegers Arch* 375:219−228, 1978.

206. Neubig RR, Krodel EK, Boyd ND, Cohen JB: Acetylcholine and local anesthetic binding to Torpedo nicotinic postsynaptic membranes after removal of nonreceptor peptides. *Proc Nat Acad Sci USA* 76:690−694, 1979.

207. Nickel E, Potter LT: Ultrastructure of isolated membranes of Torpedo electric tissue. *Brain Res* 57:508−517, 1973.

208. Niemi WD, Nastuk WL, Chang HW, Penn AS, Rosenberry TL: Electrophysiological studies of thymectomized and nonthymectomized acetyl-

     choline receptor-immunized animal models of myasthenia gravis. *Exp Neurol* 63:1–27, 1979.

209. O'Brien RD, Gibson RE, Sumikawa K: The nicotinic acetylcholine receptor from *Torpedo* electroplax. *Prog Brain Res* 49:279–291, 1979.

210. Ortiz CL: Crayfish neuromuscular junction: Facilitation with constant nerve terminal potential. *Experientia* 28:1035–1036, 1972.

211. Otsuka M, Endo M, Nonomura Y: Presynaptic nature of neuromuscular depression. *Jpn J Physiol* 12:573–584, 1962.

212. Padykula HA, Gauthier GF: The ultrastructure of the neuromuscular junctions of mammalian red, white and intermediate skeletal muscle fibers. *J Cell Biol* 46:27–41, 1970.

213. Pagala MKD, Namba T, Grob D: Desensitization to acetylcholine at motor endplates in normal humans, patients with myasthenia gravis and experimental models of myasthenia gravis. *Ann NY Acad Sci* 377:567–582, 1981.

214. Pagala MKD, Tada S, Namba T, Grob D: Neuromuscular transmission in neonatal mice injected with serum globulin of myasthenia gravis patients. *Neurology* 32:12–17, 1982.

215. Pallotta BA, Webb GD: The effects of external Ca $(^{2+})$ and Mg $(^{2+})$ on the voltage sensitivity of desensitization in *Electrophorus electricus* electroplaques. *J Gen Physiol* 75:693–708, 1980.

216. Parnas H, Segal LA: A theoretical study of calcium entry in nerve terminals, with application to neurotransmitter release. *J Theor Biol* 91:125–169, 1981.

217. Peper K, Bradley RJ, Dreyer F: The acetylcholine receptor at the neuromuscular junction. *Physiol Rev* 62:1271–1340, 1982.

218. Polak RL, Sellin LC, Thesleff S: Acetylcholine content and release in denervated or botulinum poisoned rat skeletal muscle. *J Physiol* 319:253–359, 1981.

219. Popot JL, Sugiyama H, Changeux JP: Studies on the electrogenic action of acetylcholine with *Torpedo marmorata* electric organ. II. Permeability response of the receptor-rich membrane fragments to cholinergic agonists *in vitro*. *J Mol Biol* 106:469–483, 1976.

220. Quilliam JP, Tamarind DL: Some effects of preganglionic nerve stimulation on synaptic vesicle populations in rat superior cervical ganglion. *J Physiol* 235:317–331, 1973.

221. Rahamimoff R, Erulkar SD, Lev-Tov A, Meiri H: Intracellular and extracellular calcium ions in transmitter release at the neuromuscular synapse. *Ann NY Acad Sci* 307:583–597, 1978.

222. Rahamimoff R, Lev-Tov A, Meiri H: Primary and secondary regulation of quantal transmitter release: Calcium and sodium. *J Exp Biol* 89:5–18, 1980.

223. Reynolds JA, Karlin A: Molecular weight in detergent solution of acetylcholine receptors from *Torpedo californica*. *Biochem* 17:2035–2038, 1978.

224. Rice SO: Mathematical analysis of random noise. *Bell Syst Tech J* 23:282–332, 1944.

225. Ritchie, JM, Rogart RB: Density of sodium channels in mammalian myelinated nerve fibers and nature of the axonal membrane under the myelin sheath. *Proc Nat Acad Sci USA* 74:211–215, 1977.

226. Rosenthal J: Post-tetanic potentiation at the neuromuscular junction of the frog. *J Physiol* 203:121–133, 1969.

227. Ross MJ, Klymkowski MW, Agard DA, Stroud RM: Structural studies of a membrane bound acetylcholine receptor from *Torpedo californica*. *J Mol Biol* 116:635–659, 1977.

228. Rubsamen H, Hess GP, Eldefrawi AT, Eldefrawi ME: Interaction between calcium and ligand-binding sites of the purified acetylcholine receptor studied by use of a fluorescent lanthanide. *Biochem Biophys Res Comm* 68:56–63, 1976.

229. Ruff RL: A quantitative analysis of local anesthetic alteration of miniature endplate currents and endplate current fluctuations. *J Physiol* 264:89–124, 1977.

230. Sakmann B, Patlak J, Neher E: Single acetylcholine-activated channels show burst-kinetics in presence of desensitizing concentrations of agonist. *Nature* 286:71–73, 1980.

231. Schiebler W, Hucho F: Reconstitution of active acetylcholine receptor by hybridization of binding site blocked with ion channel-blocked acetylcholine receptor protein. *Biochem Biophys Acta* 597:626–630, 1980.

232. Scubon-Mulieri B, Parsons RL: Desensitization and recovery at the potassium-depolarized frog neuromuscular junction are voltage-sensitive. *J Gen Physiol* 71:285–299, 1978.

233. Sellin LC: Studies of neurotrophic effects on mammalian skeletal muscle during reinnervation. Ph.D. dissertation, College of Medicine and Dentistry of New Jersey, 1977.

234. Sellin LC, Thesleff S: Pre- and post-synaptic actions of botulinum toxin at the rat neuromuscular junction. *J Physiol* 317:487–495, 1981.

235. Sheridan RE, Lester HA: Rates and equilibria at the acetylcholine receptor of Electrophorus electroplaques. A study of neurally evoked post-synaptic currents and of voltage-jump relaxations. *J Gen Physiol* 70:187–219, 1977.

236. Simonneau M, Tauc L, Baux G: Quantal release of acetylcholine examined by current fluctuation analysis at an identified neuro-neuronal synapse of *Aplysia*. *Proc Nat Acad Sci USA* 77:1–5, 1980.

237. Sobel A, Weber M, Changeux JP: Large-scale purification of the acetylcholine-receptor protein in its membrane-bound and detergent-extracted forms from *Torpedo marmorata* electric organ. *Eur J Biochem* 80:215–224, 1979.

238. Sommer JR, Dolber PC, Taylor I: Filipin-cholesterol complexes in sarcoplasmic reticulum of frog skeletal muscle. *J Ultrastruct Res* 72:272–285, 1980.

239. Spivak CE, Albuquerque EX: Dynamic properties of the nicotinic receptor ionic channel complex: activation and blockade. In Hanin I,

Goldberg A (eds): *Progress in Cholinergic Biology: Models of Cholinergic Synapses.* New York, Raven Press, 1982, pp 323–357.

240. Statham HE, Duncan CJ: The effect of sodium ions on MEPP frequency at the frog neuromuscular junction. *Life Sci* 20:1839–1846, 1977.

241. Stevens CF: A comment on Martin's relation. *Biophys J* 16:891–895, 1976.

242. Stinnakre J, Tauc L: Calcium influx in active *Aplysia* neurons detected by injected aequorin. *Nature New Biol* 242:113–115, 1973.

243. Strader CD, Lazarides E, Raftery MA: The characterization of actin associated with postsynaptic membranes from *Torpedo californica.* *Biochem Biophys Res Comm* 92:365–373, 1980.

244. Sugiyama H, Changeux JP: Interconversion between different states of affinity for acetylcholine of the cholinergic receptor protein from *Torpedo marmorata. Eur J Biochem* 55:505–515, 1975.

245. Sugiyama H, Popot JL, Changeux JP: Studies on the electrogenic action of acetylcholine with *Torpedo marmorata* electric organ. III. Pharmacological desensitization *in vitro* of the receptor-rich membrane fragments by cholinergic agonists. *J Mol Biol* 106:485–496, 1976.

246. Takeuchi A: The long-lasting depression in neuromuscular transmission of frog. *Jpn J Physiol* 8:102–113, 1958.

247. Takeuchi A, Takeuchi N: Active phase of frog's endplate potential. *J Neurophysiol* 22:395–411, 1959.

248. Takeuchi A, Takeuchi N: On the permeability of endplate membrane during the action of transmitter. *J Physiol* 154:52–67, 1960.

249. Takeuchi A, Takeuchi N: Electrical changes in pre- and post-synaptic axons of the giant synapse of *Loligo. J Gen Physiol* 45:1181–1193, 1962.

250. Takeuchi N: Effects of calcium on the conductance change of endplate membrane during the action of transmitter. *J Physiol* 167:141–155, 1963.

251. Thesleff S: The mode of neuromuscular block caused by acetylcholine, nicotine decamethonium and succinylcholine. *Acta Physiol Scand* 34:218–231, 1955.

252. Thesleff S: Motor endplate 'desensitization' by repetitive nerve stimuli. *J Physiol* 148:659–664, 1959.

253. Thesleff S: Effects of motor innervation on the chemical sensitivity of skeletal muscle. *Physiol Rev* 40:734–752, 1960.

254. Thies RE: Neuromuscular depression and the apparent depletion of transmitter in mammalian muscle. *J Neurophysiol* 28:427–442, 1965.

255. Toh BH, Gallichio HA, Jeffrey PL, Livett BG, Muller HK, Cauchi MN, Clarke FM: Anti-actin stains synapses. *Nature* 64:648–650, 1976.

256. Vizi ES, Vyskočil F: Changes in total and quantal release of acetylcholine in the mouse diaphragm during activation and inhibition of membrane ATPase. *J Physiol* 286:1–14, 1979.

257. Vyskočil F, Magazanik LG: The desensitization of postjunctional muscle membrane after intracellular application of membrane stabilizers and snake venom polypeptides. *Brain Res* 48:417–419, 1972.

258. Vyskočil F, Illés P: Non-quantal release of transmitter at mouse neuromuscular junction and its dependence on the activity of $Na^+ - K^+$ ATPase. *Pfluegers Arch* 370:295–297, 1977.

259. Vyskočil F, Illés P: Electrophysiological examination of transmitter release in non-quantal form in the mouse diaphragm and the activity of membrane ATP-ase *Physiol Bohemoslav* 27:449–455, 1978.

260. Weber M, David-Pfeuty T, Changeux JP: Regulation of binding properties of the nicotinic receptor protein by cholinergic ligands in membrane fragments from *Torpedo marmorata. Proc Nat Acad Sci USA* 72:3443–3447, 1975.

261. Weill CL, McNamee MG, Karlin A: Affinity-labeling of purified acetylcholine receptor from *Torpedo californica. Biochem Biophys Res Comm* 61:997–1003, 1974.

262. Whittaker VP, Essman WB, Dowe GHC: The isolation of pure cholinergic synaptic vesicle from the electric organs of elasmobranch fish of the family torpidinidae. *Biochem J* 128:833–846, 1972.

263. Wilson DF: Effects of caffeine on neuromuscular transmission in the rat. *Am J Physiol* 225:862–865, 1973.

264. Wilson DF: Estimates of quantal-release and binomial statistical-release parameters at rat neuromuscular junction. *Am J Physiol* 233:C157–C163, 1977.

265. Wilson DF: Depression, facilitation, and mobilization of transmitter at the rat neuromuscular junction. *Am J Physiol* 237:C31–C37, 1979.

266. Wray D: Prolonged exposure to acetylcholine: Noise analysis and channel inactivation in cat tenuissimus muscle. *J Physiol* 310:37–56, 1981.

267. Young AP, Brown FF, Halsey MJ, Sigman DS: Volatile anesthetic facilitation of *in vitro* desensitization of membrane bound acetylcholine receptor from *Torpedo californica. Proc Nat Acad Sci USA* 75:4563–4567, 1978.

268. Young AP, Oshiki JR, Sigman DS: Allosteric effects of volatile anesthetics on the membrane-bound acetylcholine receptor protein. II. Alteration of alpha-bungarotoxin binding kinetics. *Molec Pharmacol* 20:506–510, 1981.

269. Young AP, Sigman DS: Allosteric effects of volatile anesthetics on the membrane-bound acetylcholine receptor protein. I. Stabilization of the high-affinity state. *Molec Pharmacol* 20:498–505, 1981.

270. Younkin SG: An analysis of the role of calcium in facilitation at the frog neuromuscular junction. *J Physiol* 237:1–14, 1974.

271. Zengel JE, Magleby KL: Differential effects of Ba^{++}, Sr^{++}, and Ca^{++} on stimulation-induced changes in transmitter release at the frog neuromuscular junction. *J Gen Physiol* 76:175–211, 1980.

272. Zengel JE, Magleby KL, Horn JP, McAfee DA, Yarowsky PJ: Facilitation, augmentation, and potentiation of synaptic transmission at the superior cervical ganglion of the rabbit. *J Gen Physiol* 76:213–231, 1980.
273. Zengel JE, Magleby KL: Augmentation and facilitation of transmitter release. A quantitative study at the frog neuromuscular junction. *J Gen Physiol* 80:583–611, 1982.
274. Zucker RS: Changes in the statistics of transmitter release during facilitation. *J Physiol* 229:787–810, 1973.
275. Zucker RS, Lara-Estrella LO: Is synaptic facilitation caused by presynaptic spike broadening? *Nature* 278:57–59, 1979.

Chapter 4

Pharmacology of the Neuromuscular Junction

Frank G. Standaert, M.D.

Introduction

The processes by which a motor nerve sends signals to a skeletal muscle are described in the preceding chapter. Simplistically stated, transmitter acetylcholine, made and stored in the motor nerve ending, is released in response to an action potential in the motor axon. The transmitter diffuses across the synaptic cleft and binds receptors. The protein of the receptor responds by forming a channel for the passage of ions into the muscle and the flow of ions creates the depolarizing endplate potential. The depolarization of the endplate, in turn, creates a potential gradient across the adjoining muscle membrane that opens voltage-dependent sodium channels and starts a wave of electrical and mechanical activity that sweeps along the muscle and causes it to contract. Meanwhile, the acetylcholine unbinds from the receptor and diffuses until it contacts the enzyme, acetylcholinesterase, which destroys it and ends its role in transmission. Simultaneously, recovery processes in the nerve and muscle are in action with the result that the neuromuscular junction is reset quickly to its starting point. Drugs can, and do, react with each of the processes involved in transmission.

Ideally, the actions of a drug on neuromuscular transmission would be tied to this process in such a way as to make the drug's effects understandable and its use rationally and scientifically based. This ideal is not with us yet. Recent advances in our understanding of receptors, the mechanism of release of transmitter and the response to it, and of the kinetic behavior of transmitters and drugs have greatly clarified critical parameters; some of these will be described in this chapter, but many drug actions remain cryptic. In these cases, use of the drug has to be based upon such deductions as can be supported by observation and the descriptions of these drugs must remain empirical.

Sites of Action

Some of the most remarkable advances in drug knowledge have come from studies of cholinergic receptors in motor endplates. The receptor surface of the postjunctional membrane appears in electro-myographs of mammalian skeletal muscle to be little different from that described in earlier studies with electroplax and frog.[91,249,482] The acetylcholine receptors (AChR) are arranged in clusters, densely packed in tidy two-by-two rows at the outermost edge of the junctional folds where this density reaches 9,000 to 10,000/μm^2 of postjunctional membrane.[226,253] The receptors appear as small, discrete 8 to 9 nm diameter rosette-shaped protrusions containing a central darkened pore. The protein extends through the membrane, protruding about 8.5 nm into the extracellular phase and 2 nm into the cytoplasm.[297] The acetylcholine receptors would seem to be positioned precisely to receive acetylcholine molecules released from the nerve terminal a scant 50 nm away and to permit the exchange of ions between extracellular fluid and cytoplasm. There appears to be an underlying cytoskeleton in the submembrane which restricts the receptors to this most efficacious location. Electron micrographs reveal an elaborate meshwork connecting the outer membrane receptor surface with underlying filaments. This interwoven lattice is thought to anchor the receptors in their dense, ordered arrangement at the tips of the outer folds.[110,226,253,419]

The endplate nicotinic acetylcholine receptor has been extracted and purified from a variety of sources, particularly, the electric organs of certain fish that are extraordinarily rich in cholinergic receptors. These have provided most of the material for study, but the endplate nicotinic receptor of other species, including humans,[385,527] has been isolated and found to be similar to that of the fish. The exact chemical composition of the receptor varies slightly from one species to another, but in most, it is a protein made up of five subunits: two of these, the alpha units, are about 40 K daltons and one each of the others is about 50, 55 and 65 K daltons molecular weight.[217,219,231,437,438]

The five subunits are arranged in a ring, or rosette.[258,286,461] The center of the ring is a potential space which, when opened, forms a channel through which cations can pass.

The alpha subunits consistently label as the ACh binding site while the functional role of the other subunits is not known with certainty. Drugs binding to other subunits[39,408] change the kinetics of the binding of drugs to the recognition sites on the alpha subunits of the receptor.[407,408] The ion channel formed by the endplate receptor is distinctive in that it is not specific for any single ion.[7,161,164] It is lined with negatively charged groups that effectively exclude negatively charged drugs and molecules, yet permit cations to enter; it is large enough to pass all biologic cations[4] and even large enough to pass certain organic cations: choline, guanidine, and triethanolamine ions.[161,164,235] The walls of the channel are irregular, so that certain organic molecules can enter the mouth of the channel without penetrating the entire channel. If this happens, the function of the system is disrupted. Other, slender drugs, such as decamethonium and carbachol, can pass entirely through the channel and enter the muscle cytoplasm.[7,113,114,115,544] They also disrupt the channel's function while they are in it and presumably disorder cytoplasmic function as well.

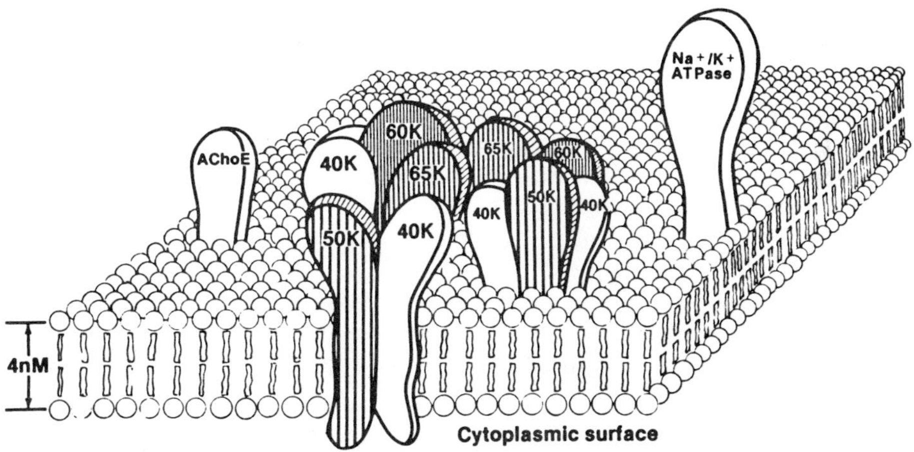

Figure 4.1. Sketch of receptor/ionophores and some proteins in postjunctional membrane. The central figure labels the five subunits of the receptor protein and is cut away to show its ion channel; another receptor approximating a dimeric organization is to the right. Acetylcholinesterase (AChoE) and sodium potassium ATPase are also sketched.

The cholinergic receptors are inserted into a lipoprotein membrane and are held in place by a cytoskeleton. The nature and function of the lipoprotein has been analyzed in electroplaque membranes,[217,344,591] yet its role is not well known. It is known that the receptor/ionophore will not function without the lipoprotein, i.e., the protein will not change conformation to produce an ion channel unless it is in a lipid environment.[330,333,361] It also is thought that lipid soluble drugs may enter the membrane and/or the boundary area where the receptor protein is inserted into the membrane, to influence the conformation of the protein, the binding characteristics of the protein, and the kinetics of the opening and closing of the ion channel.[203,283,308] Drugs that have these effects clearly have the capacity to influence the time course and strength of neuromuscular transmission.

This arrangement of receptors is true of the muscle immediately subjacent to the nerve, the sole plate of the neuromuscular junction; but the rest of normal mature mammalian muscle cells is devoid of these receptors, which means that normally only the endplate itself is sensitive to cholinergic agonists or antagonists. This makes the endplate "chemically sensitive," a property that is not shared by the rest of the membrane of the muscle cell. In contrast, the extrajunctional membrane of the muscle cell contains electrically excitable, or voltage-dependent, selective ion channels that make this membrane "electrically excitable" but not sensitive to cholinergic drugs. This juxtaposition of a chemically excitable membrane and an electrically excitable one confers on muscle the special properties that account for the endplate's response to cholinergic drugs and is the reason why cholinergic drugs do not affect normal muscle directly. It is also why drugs, such as succinylcholine, may depolarize the endplate while not causing a sustained depolarization and contraction of the muscle; this process is described below.

The concentration of cholinergic receptors in the endplate is dependent on the presence of an active nerve. When the nerve is removed or inactivated, as by injury to the nerve or spinal cord, then a new class of receptors, called extrajunctional receptors, are synthesized by the muscle and inserted everywhere in the muscle membrane.[84,169,498,588] These extrajunctional receptors are chemically excitable and are responsible for the response to cholinergic agonists of muscles without functional nerves. There is great theoretical interest in the origin and control of these receptors,[165,178,179,198,355,425,435,464,525] but there also is practical interest among anesthesiologists who may administer agonists like succinylcholine to patients with denervated muscles; if they do, they then have to deal with the adverse effect of the outpouring of potassium and the contractures the drug may produce.[27,84,228,277,533] Anesthesiologists may also have to deal with the greater difficulty in blocking neuromuscular transmission with nondepolarizing agents, a phenomenon regularly observed in people whose muscles are deprived of an input from an active nerve by stroke, spinal cord injury, or even by immobilization of the limb, as by a cast.[220,229,256,386,479,500] Immobilized,[190,340,458] paralyzed,[74,423] disused,[84,169,316,424] or denervated[169,423,526] skeletal muscle undergoes changes in the structure and receptor surface of the neuromuscular junction. Changes in the receptor population occur both at the endplate surface and across the extrajunctional sarcolemna following loss of neuronal activity. The density of the acetylcholine receptors at the tips of the endplate does not decline but undergoes a rapid transient increase [175,334,327,403,404] characterized by a heterogenous population of receptors having two metabolic lifetimes.[38,327,334] Across the nonendplate membrane surface, extrajunctional receptors appear with increased density,[165,234,423] having a single-channel open time double that of endplate receptors and a lower single-channel conductance.[68,203] Changes in the neuromuscular junction in response to denervation and disuse do not seem to be limited to the affected limb; there can also be structural changes in the endplate and a slight increase in the number of extrasynaptic receptors in contralateral or non-immobilized extremities. The dose requirements for nondepolarizing blocking drugs are raised in hemiparetic patients in both paralyzed muscles and in non-affected extremities.[479] Extrajunctional receptors and phenomena related to them are described in the next chapter.

Although muscle is not the focus of this chapter, drugs that influence the lipids and proteins of endplate membrane may also dissolve into the lipid of muscle membrane and by influencing the various ion-controlling proteins in it may influence the time course and strength of muscle contraction. While these do not change neuromuscular transmission directly, the effect on muscle performance may be just as important as that on transmission. Changes in muscle contraction strength may also be confused with changes in transmission even though the processes are different and ought to be thought about individually.

Many drugs are known to affect the prejunctional component of the neuromuscular transmission system, the motor nerve terminal. This structure contains apparatus for receiving an electrical signal from the motor axon and transducing it into a chemical signal to send across the synaptic cleft to the muscle. The motor nerve terminal contains mechanisms for synthesizing transmitter, storing it, mobilizing it from the synthesis sites to the release sites and for regulating

all of these processes. It also contains the cellular apparatus needed
to produce energy for these processes and to maintain this part of the
cell in good order. The nerve terminal membrane is known to contain
receptors that respond to nicotinic cholinergic drugs, alpha-adrenergic
drugs and other putative transmitters and opiates. It may have
muscarinic and other receptors. The reaction of drugs with these
prejunctional structures is of obvious importance to the functional
status of the nerve, and to neuromuscular transmission, but the
nerve ending is very difficult to study experimentally and full understanding of prejunctional drug action is not yet available.

Postjunctional Drug Actions

The endplate receptor/ionophore is the most studied part of the
neuromuscular junction and the best understood substrate for drug
action. The receptor offers many potential sites for drug binding, but
only a handful of these sites are known to have significant functional
consequences. The most important are the so-called recognition sites
on each of the alpha (40 K dalton) subunits. These are the receptor
points of classic pharmacology. When acetylcholine binds to both
subunits the protein changes conformation and allows cations to
pass.[400,481,545] Other agonists that bind to the recognition site
cause the same conformation change. While antagonists compete for
the recognition site, they do not activate the protein; instead, they
occlude the recognition site and prevent agonists from acting. This
competition for the recognition site is the classic agonist-antagonist
competition of neuromuscular pharmacology.

The ion channel is a more recently recognized site of action for
drugs that may impair neuromuscular transmission. Some drugs,
including some antibiotics, quinidine, histrionicotoxin, and tricyclic
antidepressants, may bind to areas around the mouth of the receptor
and physically occlude it or impede a conformation change so that
sodium, calcium and potassium ions cannot pass through the channel
as they usually do. Other drugs, notably organic cations such as the
usual neuromuscular blocking drugs, and others, such as the local
anesthetics, may enter channels opened by normal agonist activity
and either bind to some point in the passageway or merely physically
occlude the channel; in either case the channel is not as permeable as
normal to the passage of the depolarizing physiologic ions. The group
of drugs that binds to unopened channels has become known as closed
channel blocking agents; the ones that enter a channel are called

open channel blocking agents. Both produce nondepolarizing, noncompetitive blockade of transmission. The open channel group also may display use dependence, the magnitude of the effect depending upon how frequently the channel is opened by use of the system, and they may display voltage dependence; that is, the rate and degree of penetration of the open channel depends upon the electrostatic force applied to the charged organic molecule by the electrical field that exists across the endplate membrane. The closed channel drugs may act as a cap at the mouth of a channel, thus preventing ions from crossing, or they may dissolve in the protein and prevent a functional channel from forming.[180,505]

These phenomena are subjects of intense investigation. By use of an electrophysiological method called patch clamping it is possible to catch in a micropipette a piece of membrane that contains a single receptor-channel complex. By manipulating the system and applying drugs appropriately, the effects of drug-receptor/ionophore interactions on a molecular scale can be recorded. It has been shown that an ion channel, opened by reaction with two ions of acetylcholine, acts like a gate or a switch. The protein becomes almost instantly permeable to ions and remains permeable until one of the acetylcholine molecules diffuses off the protein, about 0.3 msec after it arrives.[47] The ionophore then snaps shut, ending the current. During the time that it is open about $1-3$ pA (or about 1×10^4 ions per msec) cross the membrane and depolarize the tiny segment of membrane around the protein.[240,398] This is a remarkable amplification; the current carried by just two molecules of acetylcholine is transformed into a current carried by tens of thousands as many inorganic cations.

Ion flow through an opened channel is the elemental unit of neuromuscular transmission. The current through a single channel is miniscule, but the currents through channels are additive; two simultaneously open channels permit twice as much current flow and a greater area of depolarization. Since each neuromuscular junction contains about 2×10^6 channels,[255] and many of these can be opened simultaneously, as for example, in response to a burst of transmitter from the nerve, the total current is substantial enough to create the endplate potential that triggers neuromuscular transmission.

Understanding the effects of drugs on ion channels, and appreciating the additive qualities of ion flow through many channels, provides the basis for understanding drug effects on the motor endplate. Since the total current flow establishes normal neuromuscular transmission, it follows that anything that changes total current flow will change neuromuscular transmission. For example, in neonates or in myasthenia gravis the endplate contains fewer receptors than normal. Hence, there is less current flow and a smaller margin of safety for transmission. Similarly, *d*-tubocurarine, by occluding recognition sites, prevents channels from opening and thereby reduces total current flow. This causes the familiar reduction in endplate potential and the possibility of transmission failure. In like manner, materials that otherwise deplete the pool of active channels will reduce total current and weaken transmission.

Although less obvious, drugs that interfere with the channel by changing its opening or closing characteristics, or that plug the channel and prevent ions from passing, will also modify total current, endplate potential and neuromuscular transmission. For example, carbachol reacts with the receptor in a manner similar to acetylcholine, but its binding is not as solid and the drug quickly unbinds and drifts away, allowing the channel to close. Since carbachol is not attached to an alpha unit as long as acetylcholine, and the channel is not open as long, fewer physiologic ions flow for each ion of carbachol. In other words, carbachol is not as strong an amplifier as acetylcholine and therefore appears less potent.[463] In another example, certain local anesthetics, such as the lidocaine derivative known as QX222, enter the channel opened by acetylcholine,[8,399,260,462] but do not bind there, hopping in and out a dozen or more times every time the channel opens. Since physiologic ions cannot flow while the local anesthetic is in the channel, the average number of ions that crosses an open channel is reduced, as is the total current, the endplate potential and the strength of neuromuscular transmission.

Other drugs, including certain of the usual neuromuscular blocking drugs, may enter the channel, but not leave it easily.[449,106,6,421,308] These also cause weakening of transmission, as do the closed channel blockers that alter the opening of the channel and do not permit ions to pass.[9,13,472,180,505,341] Still others, notably procaine, as well as drugs that dissolve in the membrane lipid, change the opening or closing characteristics of the channel, thus interfering with its switching function and modifying current flow and transmission.[299,180,6,242,201,202] Channel action is potentially a very important mechanism of drug action about which much is known, but even more is to be learned. As our knowledge of these phenomena increases we are certain to be able to predict the drug actions with more surety.

The resting (not bound to a drug) and the active (channel opened by an agonist) states of the receptor/ionophore are the ones of most interest in terms of the occurrence of transmission, but they are only a few of the states in which the protein can exist. The receptor is a large, flexible protein set into a fluid lipid matrix; it is capable of dynamic action and is constantly in transition from one conformation to another. Most of these conformations and their physiologic significances are not known, but this does not mean that they may not influence drugs or may not be influenced by drugs. For example, among the many conformations that can be assumed by the receptor protein are ones termed "desensitized." In these states receptors exposed to agonists are sequestered into a conformation that binds the agonist tightly—more tightly than the normal resting receptor— but does not open the ion channel and so does not let current flow to depolarize the membrane. The membrane retains its resting potential despite the presence of agonist and seems to be insensitive or desensitized to the agonist. Experimentally, signs of desensitization of the endplate can be detected within seconds of the application of agonist, and the desensitization persists for several seconds after agonist is removed.

Present theory holds that this experimentally observed shift in receptor properties is only an exaggeration of normal physiology. Receptors are large, dynamic proteins in which a number of the conformations are in equilibrium with one another. Normally, this equilibrium provides a number of receptors in the "resting" conformation that may change into the active, open ionophore conformation when agonists bind to them. However, other conformations also are in the equilibrium including ones called "desensitized." These receptors are not detected by usual physiologic methods, but may be recognized by special techniques. The usual condition of the equilibrium between normal resting and desensitized states favors the former, making receptors available to bind to acetylcholine and causing neuromuscular transmission; however, this equilibrium can be shifted by many other drugs so that desensitized receptors become more prevalent. Production of desensitization by agonists is the classic example, but antagonists also bind well to, and produce, desensitized receptors. Interestingly, many drugs not usually associated with the neuromuscular junction encourage the formation of the desensitized state; by reducing the number of available resting receptors, these drugs weaken neuromuscular transmission and add to the action of nondepolarizing agents, such as *d*-tubocurarine. Among the groups are some local anesthetics,[546,153,486] the volatile anesthetics (e.g., halothane, chloroform),[589,590] certain antibiotics (e.g., polymyxin B),[75] phenothiazines[337,339,83] and barbiturates.[65,143] Some drugs, notably meproadifen, are so effective in producing desensitized receptors that they immediately displace the equilibrium in this direction and produce a desensitized block which is not preceded by noticable depolarization.[341] The endplate is nondepolarized, but the blockade is very different from that produced by the usual nondepolarizing agents such as *d*-tubocurarine.

Several desensitized states are recognized but they all are nondepolarizing and the blockage of transmission is not a competitive blockade.[183,420,154,93] Functionally, the acceleration and/or the perpetuation of desensitized receptors by drugs effectively removes these units from the pool which is available for the normal functioning of the neuromuscular junction. In other words, an agent that increases the number of desensitized receptors reduces the reserve of the neuromuscular junction and weakens neuromuscular transmission.

The time that acetylcholine is bound to alpha units and thus the time the channel is open determines the duration of depolarization of the membrane patch. Since the acetylcholine residence time on the receptor is brief—less than 1 msec—the depolarization is also brief. In principle, the acetylcholine molecule that diffuses off a receptor may attach to another receptor and open its ionophore, thus repeatedly depolarizing the membrane. In practice, this does not happen because the muscle endplate is so rich in the enzyme acetylcholinesterase that acetylcholine is as likely to land on the enzyme and be destroyed as it is to land on a second receptor and open its channel. Because of this, the average acetylcholine molecule helps open only one channel before it is destroyed and the depolarization of the endplate caused by a single burst of neurotransmitter is very brief, not much longer than the nerve potential that caused it.

This brief depolarization caused by acetylcholine can be extended in several ways. One way is to inhibit acetylcholinesterase in order that an acetylcholine molecule may participate in several depolarizing events before it finally escapes the junctional cleft and diffuses away from receptors. Another way is to provide acetylcholine to replace molecules that are destroyed. The extreme example of this occurs *in vitro* where acetylcholine is provided continuously; in this case depolarizing events continue until other phenomena, such as desensitization, intervene. A similar, but less extreme, situation occurs *in vivo* when drugs such as 4-aminopyridine are given to prolong the release of transmitter from the nerve ending.

It is apparent that increasing the amount of acetylcholine or the time it is in the junctional cleft will increase the flow of depolarizing ions across the muscle membrane and prolong the endplate potential. This is the molecular process by which an acetylcholinesterase inhibitor, such as pyridostigmine, or a drug that prolongs the release of acetylcholine from the nerve, such as 4-aminopyridine, prolongs the endplate potential. It is less apparent how the prolonged presence of acetylcholine antagonizes the blockade produced by compounds such as *d*-tubocurarine. The explanation lies in the fact that the *d*-tubocurarine resides on the receptor for a very short time, about one millisecond.[481] Consider what would happen if it were otherwise. If tubocurarine were bound to a receptor for many milliseconds, acetylcholine released from the nerve would encounter receptors that were already occupied and would have no place to work. Inhibiting acetylcholinesterase would not help because even though the agonist were protected from destruction, it would diffuse out of the synaptic cleft before any significant number of recognition sites were freed by the departure of antagonist. In reality, the average residence time of *d*-tubocurarine on a receptor is only slightly greater than the transmission period. This gives *d*-tubocurarine a competitive advantage because the acetylcholine normally is destroyed so rapidly. If, however, acetylcholinesterase is inhibited, or if the release of acetylcholine continues for longer than usual, then acetylcholine is present longer than the antagonist is in place. This shifts the competitive advantage so that acetylcholine can occupy the recognition sites, cause the channel to open and depolarize the membrane. The blockade produced by *d*-tubocurarine is reversed, even though *d*-tubocurarine remains in the body and even though it remains in the junctional cleft. *d*-Tubocurarine can occupy receptors in the intervals when the nerve is quiet and there is no acetylcholine, but it will lose the competition when enough acetylcholine is present for a long enough time.

Such microkinetics are of great importance. They are difficult to study and are just beginning to be appreciated, but they are the true determinants of drug action at the receptors. Microkinetics determines, for instance, which blocking drugs are practical because their binding is long enough to block transmission, but short enough to be overcome by drugs that prolong the presence of transmitter. Microkinetics also determines which drugs are practical reversing agents because they prolong acetylcholine long enough for it to act on receptors that have lost antagonists, yet not so long that the agonist accumulates to dangerous levels in the synapse. Clinicians and pharmacologists generally regard acetylcholine as a short-acting drug and *d*-tubocurarine as a long-acting drug. This is true with regard to persistence in the whole organism, but with regard to binding at nicotinic receptors, the two compounds are similar, as must be true if *d*-tubocurarine is to be a useful drug.

Intuitively it would seem that compounds that depolarize the muscle endplate and maintain it in a depolarized state would cause a maintained contraction of the muscle. In fact, they do not; instead, they produce a flaccid paralysis. This anomaly is due to the special properties of the muscle endplate and to the geometric relationship of this chemically sensitive area to the much larger chemically insensitive, but electrically sensitive, area of the membrane that comprises the muscle cell membrane. The application of a cholinergic depolarizing compound such as acetylcholine, or its analogue, succinylcholine, to normal mammalian muscle activates the cholinergic receptors of the endplate and causes depolarization, but it has no action on the chemically insensitive voltage-dependent ion channels in the adjacent muscle membrane. Thus, a voltage gradient is set up across the boundary between the two areas of membrane, with the endplate relatively depolarized. This voltage gradient does what the cholinergic drug could not do directly; it opens the voltage-dependent ion channels of the muscle and may start a wave of electrical activity and contraction down the muscle. However, the muscle activity is transient. Even though the endplate remains depolarized, the muscle membrane accommodates to this depolarization by not continuously or repeatedly depolarizing. Simplistically, the sodium channels of the muscle have a triphasic cycle of activation by a voltage gradient, inactivation by intrinsic processes, and recovery in the absence of a voltage gradient. These channels must complete all three phases before they begin another cycle. If the endplate is depolarized and the depolarization is maintained, then the sodium channels in the adjacent muscle do not complete their cycle; instead, they remain in the second, inactivated, state in which they do not pass ions. Since there is no further flow of sodium across the muscle membrane, it recovers its resting potential and the muscle relaxes. At the same time, since the endplate is depolarized, additional acetylcholine from the nerve can have no effect and so nerve stimulation does not drive the muscle as it normally does. Thus, the seemingly anomalous flaccid paralysis produced by depolarizing compounds is a manifestation of an accommodation that occurs when a normally excitable membrane is exposed continuously to an adjacent, maintained depolarization. The clinical usefulness of depolarizing muscle relaxants is due entirely to the juxtaposition in a single membrane of two contiguous zones: a small one that the drug can depolarize and a much larger one that accommodates to the depolarization.

The apparent anomaly of a depolarizing compound producing a flaccid paralysis is only the first of the sequence of strange events that agonists produce at the neuromuscular junction. If the agonist is kept continuously present, as in an *in vitro* experiment or during an infusion of succinylcholine, the junctional membrane slowly regains its resting potential, even though the agonist continues to be present. Even stranger, neuromuscular transmission may return for a while, even though the drug is not changed.[274] Anticholinesterases, such as pyridostigmine, may hasten the recovery of transmission, even though they would be expected to augment the blockade of transmission produced by an agonist. Finally, if the depolarizing compound is left at the junction for a still longer time, e.g., an hour or more, neuromuscular transmission will fail again, and anticholinesterases again become ineffective, even though the membrane potential of the endplate remains unchanged and normal or near normal.[274]

The explanation of this sequence is not known. It is not even named, being referred to simply as Phase II of depolarizing drug action. (Phase I is the expected depolarizing block produced when the drug is first administered.) Some refer to it as "desensitization blockade," but this is erroneous because desensitization as noted earlier (page 129) is a term reserved for a specific state of the endplate that is produced by agonists and is thought to be due to the encouragement of specific, nonfunctional conformations of the receptor that become apparent when agonists are applied. While desensitized receptors play a role in Phase II, their appearance is only one of many phenomena that make up the series of events known as Phase II. Besides desensitization, other factors contribute, including: channel blockade by the agonist,[5] penetration of the agonist into the subendplate cytoplasm, [544,114,115] the intracellular accumulation of calcium and sodium,[410,17,372,466] the loss of intracellular potassium,[565] activation of Na-K ATPase by the increase in intracellular Na,[112] and probably much more. Desensitization *per se* occurs spontaneously and rapidly in response to agonists. It similarly clears rapidly when the agonist is removed. Phase II is a slowly developing, slowly clearing impairment of transmission that is composed of many events that change with drug, dose, time and type of muscle—fast or slow— and with the presence or absence of other drugs such as local or volatile anesthetics.

Clinically, the most practical consequence, return of neuromuscular transmission (either spontaneously or with the aid of neostigmine or pyridostigmine) after paralysis by a depolarizing compound, is equally unpredictable; the individual may recover uneventfully or he/she may suffer a prolonged paralysis that may or may not be reversible by the usual anticholinesterases. There are several indicators that may help in assessing the return of neuromuscular transmission, such as the response to a brief train ("train of four") or a tetanizing burst of stimuli applied to the nerve of the adductor policis, but they are not fully reliable and the appearance of a consequential degree of Phase II, (since some degree always occurs) is a condition that must be determined empirically in each patient given an infusion of a depolarizing compound such as succinylcholine.[319,155]

Prejunctional Drug Actions

The motor nerve ending has been noted as a potential site of drug action. The nerve ending lacks the myelin that protects the rest of the axon from ionized drugs and it has substantial exposed surface with many branch points. In addition to being surrounded by an excitable membrane and covered with membrane proteins, the nerve ending also contains all of the metabolic apparatus needed to maintain a high degree of cellular activity and the special biochemistry related to synthesis and release of transmitter. Since any signal arising in the spinal cord must traverse the proximal portion of the junction, on its way to muscle, any drug-induced change in capacity of the nerve to transmit must alter neuromuscular transmission.

Even though the nerve contains many potential sites for drug action, little is known about how drugs actually affect it. The primary impediment is size; the ending is too small and too isolated to investigate by conventional techniques. Acetylcholine, the presumed transmitter, is not detectable by electron microscopy or histochemical methods and is so labile that chemical techniques are limited. Almost every method used to study the ending is incomplete; the methods are either indirect, or utilize drugs to prevent neuromuscular transmission so that muscle contraction will not harm electrodes, or use drugs to inhibit cholinesterase from destroying the transmitter, or all of these. As a result, our currently spotty knowledge is pieced together from a variety of experiments.

The most commonly employed techniques record the endplate potentials that are assumed to be produced by acetylcholine from the nerve. An elaborate set of statistical procedures has been constructed to draw inferences from the recordings and most of what we know has been deduced from these experiments. Yet, these indirect techniques usually employ one or more drugs to control contraction and thus are subject to unknown artifacts or misinterpretation. In addition, our understanding of the most commonly recorded potential, the spontaneous miniature endplate potential (mepp), is not well connected to our analysis of stimulus-induced transmission.[572] Also, in customary electrophysiologic experiments mepps account for less than two percent of the acetylcholine released spontaneously from the nerve, while the remaining acetylcholine goes unnoticed.[292,289,561, 542,369,144]

Approaches from the neural side are more difficult and not much more direct. Superb electron micrographs have been published,[86,247, 87,252,248,222] but this approach is based on a correlation of the physiology of transmission with observed morphologic features and is not very useful for analysis of drug action. Recordings from motor axons reflect actions in the axon terminals, permitting statements about whether or not a drug acts, but not providing a detailed insight into the mechanisms involved.[454,381]

Despite the lack of any single good approach, an enormous amount of research has been done on the nerve ending and its processes. While the combined information is frustratingly incomplete, it has allowed construction of an approach to looking at drug action on the nerve ending. Customarily, those who have considered prejunctional drug action have used terms that erroneously suggest the nerve ending is an entity, and by implication, homogeneous. Morphologists have shown precise organization within the nerve ending with specialization along its course and even within the junctional surface of the membrane.[247,248,86,87,222,436] Physiologic studies are fewer, but they too suggest that different parts of the nerve ending have different biophysical properties.[69,342] The accumulated pharmacologic evidence suggests that the nerve terminals have multiple zones segregated for special functions.

With regard to drugs, the nerve ending may be regarded as having three zones of function: a proximal segment which is a continuation of the axon, but is not myelinated, and where propagation of electrical activity takes place; a distal synaptic surface from which transmitter is released; and a midzone that contains the biochemical apparatus to both maintain the system and maintain the excitation-secretion system that converts the electrical signal from an action potential signal to the chemical signal of transmission. These zones are not absolutely distinct because nerve cells by nature propagate activity from one portion to another. One zone may influence another, particularly if the drug effect is strong, yet they are distinctive enough so that they should be considered separately.

The proximal segment is the one that is easiest to investigate by electrophysiological methods. It apparently contains sodium chan-

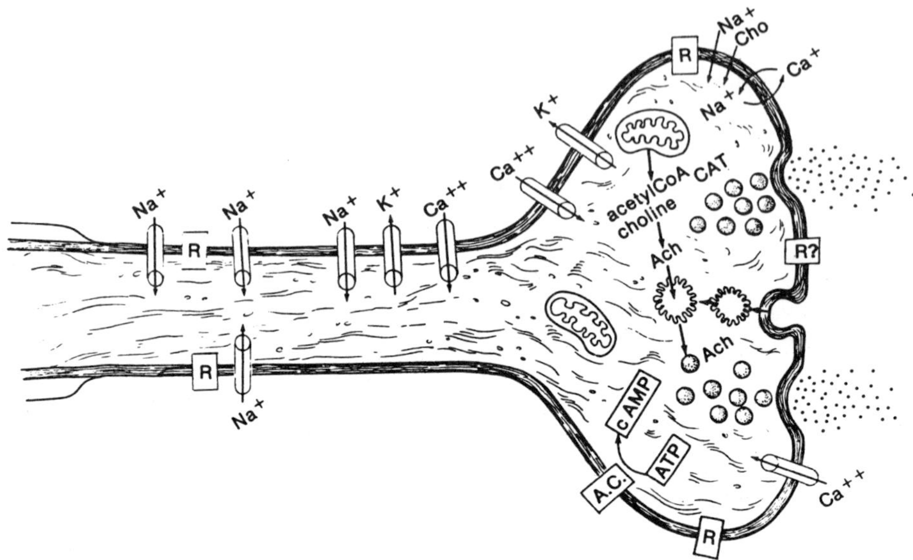

Figure 4.2.   Scheme of a motor nerve terminal. The proximal zone, immediately next to the last segment of myelin, is shown as rich in sodium channels (Na^+) that may be activated by cholinergic receptors (R). A midzone contains enzyme systems related to metabolism and transmission (CAT = choline acetyl transferase; A.C. = adenylate cyclase). Some of these are dependent on the entry of sodium and choline (Cho), processes that are linked and may be modulated by a cholinergic receptor. Between the proximal and midzone, the terminal is shown as having a variety of ion channels, but to be rich in potassium channels. The final zone, that of release, is sketched as having calcium channels and perhaps having muscarinic or nicotinic receptors (R?) that can modulate the release of transmitter (Ach).

nels that are both voltage and chemically sensitive. Clearly they respond to action potentials by propagating the potential to the more distal parts of the axon. They also respond to acetylcholine by depolarizing the membrane[261,452,455] and, if the depolarization is great enough, by initiating action potentials that are propagated antidromically (toward the cell body) and orthodromically (toward the nerve terminal) in the axon. The sharp depolarization initiated by acetylcholine is prevented by *d*-tubocurarine and by other antagonists and a variety of other neurodepressant materials.[519] The acetylcholine effect is prevented by tetrodotoxin, which indicates that sodium participates,[313,509] and distinguishes these cholinergic channels from those in the muscle endplate which are not affected by tetrodotoxin.[200,290,81] Another indicator of this difference is the observation that in the proper circumstances drugs such as *d*-tubocurarine can depolarize the membrane and even initiate action potentials[266] or repetitive activity.[417,499] Such depolarization never occurs at the neuromuscular junction, but can occur in denervated muscles when special extrajunctional receptors are produced by the muscle.[356,273,552] Like other cholinergic receptor/channel systems, those in the proximal nerve terminal desensitize in the continued presence of agonist[512] which may contribute to the neuromuscular block caused by those drugs.

In this general zone, but perhaps at the more distal part of it, are potassium channels similar to those found in other unmyelinated nerves.[69,342] The flow of current through these is impeded by potassium channel blocking drugs, such as 4-aminopyridine,[383,549,78, 216,384,300] tetraethylammonium ion,[20,53,384] phencyclidine,[50] quinidine,[581] the benzodiazepine, flurazepam,[474] and even the relaxant, gallamine.[494,495] Since impeding the potassium currents slows the recovery of neural membrane potentials, potassium blocking drugs create an abnormally long negative after-potential in the nerve ending. The broadened action potential is reflected orthodromically by an increased period of transmitter release and antidromically by repetitive action potentials. The prolongation of the release of transmitter can antagonize *d*-tubocurarine and related drugs.[383, 534,374,195]

Although drug effects at this zone can be great enough to affect more distal parts of the nerve ending, as when the drug produces repetitive nerve action potentials or prolongs the neural action potential, the effects of less intense drug actions apparently are not propagated through the nerve terminal and neither acetylcholine or similar agonists nor 4-aminopyridine or similar potassium channel blocking drugs have a significant effect on the release of vesicles from the synaptic surface; that is, they do not significantly change miniature endplate potential frequency in mammals.[55,58]

The mid-zone, or metabolic zone, of the ending is more complicated. It has been studied extensively by biochemical methods, including measurements of the enzymes, such as choline acetyltransferase, which synthesizes acetylcholine, and those that participate in the usual metabolic system.[427,553,295,232,281,282,554,571] A number of choline analogs have been tested as "false transmitters" and a substantial amount is known about how choline is taken up and acetylated, but few studies have been done with conventional neuromuscular drugs. From measurements of endplate potentials and miniature endplate potentials it is known that *d*-tubocurarine, decamethonium and related materials change the physiology of the nerve ending by decreasing the store, and presumably the synthesis and/or storage of transmitter, and the mobilization of transmitter from the synthesis sites to the release sites (see discussion of physiology in preceding chapter), but almost nothing is known about how this occurs.[265,264,207,205,381,380] Sodium seems to be important to both the uptake of choline and the synthesis, storage, and mobilization of acetylcholine.[21,31,363,439,440] Several authors have postulated that the drugs may interfere with sodium uptake,[46,555] perhaps by directly blocking sodium channels, or perhaps blocking a cholinergic receptor linked to the sodium channel.[509,510,511]

This zone also is known to contain a cyclic nucleotide system and to be modulated by drugs that interact with the system.[508,514–517,123,124] Cyclic AMP has been detected in the area by immunohistochemical methods,[515] and lipid soluble derivatives of the nucleotide increase the mobilization process.[577,284,244] In experimental situations cyclic AMP and related materials can depolarize the ending enough to generate propagated nerve action potentials and can increase the frequency of spontaneous release of transmitter, as indicated by miniature endplate potentials.[515] Although sodium obviously is involved in propagated action potentials, calcium seems to be the primary ion affected by cyclic nucleotides[488,490] since the phenomena may be diminished or prevented by pretreatment with organic calcium channel inhibitors, e.g., verapamil, or by inorganic ions, e.g., magnesium or cobalt.[488,148,515] Acetylcholine does not seem to act via this midzone system, since its effects are not changed by drugs that act on the cAMP system, but other neurohormones, notably norepinephrine and related catecholamines, enhance the release of transmitter,[57,45,209,343,496,497] apparently through a presynaptic alpha-adrenoceptor linked to the cyclic nucleotide system.[57]

The nerve ending also bears receptors that respond to morphine and naloxone,[503] 5-hydroxytryptamine,[306,251] dopamine,[434,210,208] adenosine[80,532,485] and other putative transmitters, but little is known about these. They probably respond to appropriate drugs, but their physiologic function is obscure. Since the motor nerve ending is a solitary nerve, there are no connecting autonomic or interneurones that might release transmitters to act on these receptors. The possibility that the receptors respond to circulating transmitters (during stress, for example) to enhance the production, storage and release of acetylcholine has not been explored.

The junctional zone of the nerve ending has been studied extensively, both by electron microscopy and by analysis of miniature endplate potentials.[182,63,264,440,547,548] The membrane is actively involved in the release and recycling of vesicles[247,88,364,593] but drug effects on this process have not been studied. The importance of the entry of calcium to the release of transmitter is established beyond doubt.[395,396,440,332,252] Aspects of this parameter and effects of drugs on it are described separately below. Almost all of this work is based on the hypothesis that transmitter is stored in vesicles[181,264,593,368,88] and released from the nerve in quanta at the active zones. Accordingly, drug actions are described with regard to this hypothetical framework. Far less is known about how drugs might affect the more recently appreciated processes of non-quantal release of neurotransmitter and of spontaneous quanta released from sites other than the active zones.[66,547,548,144]

The regulation of the release zone is an area of great concern physiologically, and also with regard to the major drugs that act at the neuromuscular junction. Since receptors in the nerve ending regulate the release of norepinephrine from sympathetic nerves[522,310,311,523] (but see also Kalsner[285]) and perhaps also the release of acetylcholine from nerves in the parasympathetic nervous system and in the brain,[562,382,538,539,296,322] the question naturally arises as to whether acetylcholine also controls its own release from motor nerve endings, and if so, whether antagonists inhibit the receptor and interfere with the process. Both nicotinic and muscarinic receptors in the nerve ending have been postulated, but present data are conflicting. Some authors do not think such an autoreceptor system is probable in the neuromuscular junction,[335] whether or not it occurs in other cholinergic nerves. There is electron microscopic histochemical data both for[457,324,173] and against[280] the existence in the nerve ending of cholinoceptors that might participate in the process. Similarly, it has been claimed[128,210,434,146,150,151] and denied[233] that the muscarinic agonist, oxotremorine, changes the release of acetylcholine. There is some evidence,[367,369] but not uncontested,[211] that the release of acetylcholine is increased by alpha-bungarotoxin, the snake toxin that blocks nicotinic acetylcholine sites on the alpha subunits of postjunctional receptors.

In short, the prejunctional system is more complicated and remains more cryptic than the postjunctional one. It is intuitively obvious that alterations in the nerve must contribute to changes in neuromuscular transmission, and for almost fifty years we have known with certainty that drugs can modify the behavior of the nerve ending and transmission. Yet our knowledge remains still more descriptive, i.e., what happens when a drug is given, than analytic, i.e., how the drug produces its effect. In this state, ignorance can be blissful and it is easy to forget about the possibility of prejunctional action of a particular drug, even though such action may be a major part of a drug's effect on the neuromuscular junction.

Cation Flux

Ions, both cations and anions, clearly are active participants in all stages of neuromuscular transmission, but the subject is much too large to discuss here. Instead, a few areas of current research and clinical interest related to cations will be presented to illustrate how drugs may affect ionic processes by actions on the nerve terminal or motor endplate, or both.

Only three physiologic cations are involved: sodium, potassium and calcium; but they regulate complicated physiologic systems, including the modulation of each other's flux, and their control presents a variety of potential substrates for drug action. Postjunctional actions are best known, partly because the recent advances in this area have produced a major improvement in insight, and partly because the postjunctional system is simpler than the prejunctional one. Ion flow through postjunctional ion channels mainly produces a depolarizing current to create the endplate potential that triggers muscle contraction. All physiologic cations are involved simultaneously and the actions of drugs are primarily to modify this depolarization by acting on the receptors, in the ion channel or the channel protein, in the lipid membrane about the channel, or on one of the processes that usually maintain the homeostatic balance of electrolytes across the endplate membrane. Many of these processes and the drugs that modify them are described or referenced above.

Prejunctional actions of ions are both more complicated and less well understood. Consequently, drug actions are only partly understood. Sodium has two major functions: conduction of an action potential and participation in metabolic events, especially those related to synthesis, storage, and mobilization of transmitter. In the former role, the rate of influx of sodium is critical and drugs that depress it by obstructing the sodium channel (e.g., local anesthetics, cocaine, phenytoin, pancuronium, aminopyridines, or propranolol) or those that embed themselves in the membrane about the channel (e.g., barbiturates, alcohol and volatile anesthetics) reduce the amplitude of the prejunctional action potential and its capacity to activate release systems in the more distal terminal. Many of these effects, especially those on the channel, are use-dependent; that is, the rate of stimulation may influence the degree of impairment they produce.[109] Other drugs, notably veratroidine and its derivatives, act on the channel to prolong and enhance sodium flux and so intensify the effects of normal conduction. As a consequence, they are among the most effective antagonists of neuromuscular blockade. Strangely, germerine, a veratroidine derivative, is equally effective against blockades produced by *d*-tubocurarine or by succinylcholine.[513,156] The mechanism of the latter is not known, since an increased release of acetylcholine should theoretically not improve neuromuscular transmission blocked by another agonist. It may be that inhibition of prejunctional sodium channels is an important contributor to the action of succinylcholine and germine overcomes this inhibition.

Potassium, the other major physiologic cation, is best known for its roles in maintaining the normal potential of resting nerve and muscle membranes. Less well understood are the reactions between potassium and calcium, in a cascade of events to control each other's flow into and out of the nerve ending. This process has not been well studied directly at the neuromuscular junction but can be extrapolated from the similar interactions that occur in more easily studied neural membranes.

Potassium is the ion that restores the equilibrium when a membrane potential is disturbed by an action potential. It is known that slowing potassium flux, for instance by administering 4-aminopyridine, gallamine, or tetraethylammonium ion, will prolong the recovery cycle of the nerve.[20,245,495] Since the entry of calcium into the nerve and the release of transmitter from it is proportional to the depolarization of the membrane,[328] drugs that slow potassium influx *ipso facto* prolong and increase transmitter release,[291,549,259] Such increased transmitter release may be great enough to antagonize *d*-tubocurarine and/or may cause increased synaptic activity in the central nervous system and autonomic nervous system.

Drug modification of calcium flux is a primary example of a major action on a cation about which we know too little. An enormous amount of effort has been expended to learn the processes by which calcium enters the nerve ending and how that entrance causes the release of acetylcholine. A great deal more is known about the physiology[332,303,439,543,166] than the pharmacology. Inorganic divalent cations apparently mimic calcium in its entry and release roles, but the mimicry is incomplete; actions range from calcium-like releasing actions to calcium blocking actions.[315,397,484] Barium and strontium, calcium-like releasing agents, apparently partly substitute for calcium by entering the nerve and cause an increase in the spontaneous and evoked release of transmitter. Cadmium, cobalt, manganese and lanthanum are agents that can block the flux of calcium into the nerve ending and block the release of transmitter. These effects are not pure; under the proper conditions some inorganic substances, notably cobalt, can transiently cause an increase in transmitter release. Magnesium is most interesting because, like calcium, it enters into the nerve ending, but it has an opposite action at the acetylcholine release sites: it antagonizes calcium, preventing release. Magnesium has long been used as a primary tool to quantitatively antagonize calcium at the release area in studying the physiology and pharmacology of the neuromuscular junction. Magnesium is usually described as a specific agent for this purpose, but like other xenobiotics it actually has a multitude of biologic actions, including some that depress endplate and muscle phenomena. These inorganic ions do not necessarily act only on the nerve endings, calcium entry, and release sites. Some influence calcium by less direct mechanisms. Lead and cobalt, for example, can act on neural enzymes such as adenylate cyclase and through it change calcium flux. Lanthanides may influence calcium by inhibiting a sodium/calcium antiporter that normally moves calcium out of the cell; but, depending on the instantaneous state of the membrane potential, they may reverse and move calcium into the nerve.[392]

Calcium flux and the consequent release of transmitter can be hampered by organic compounds, but these actions are by no means understood. Certain drugs, such as verapamil, its methoxy derivative D-600, nifedepine, and similar agents are known primarily for their capacity to block the entry of calcium into cells through ion channels. On this basis they would be expected to decrease or stop the release of transmitter from the nerve ending, but they do not. To the contrary, they have surprisingly little effect on the release of transmitter from stimulated nerves.[49] The reason is not known. Blockade of calcium entry via voltage-dependent channels seems to occur and to be subject to antagonism (as evidenced by the blockade produced by inorganic ions), but the organic materials of this group are inadequate to impede it. However, these organic calcium blockers will prevent the increased calcium flux promoted by cyclic AMP and they will attenuate the prejunctional component of the anticurare action of edrophonium and neostigmine. It has been postulated that invertebrates, and possibly also vertebrates, have a two-phase calcium channel; the initial voltage-dependent segment may be supplemented by a cyclic nucleotide dependent booster.[418] The nucleotide-dependent component, but not the voltage-dependent part, may be subject to blockade by verapamil. Alternatively, the organic materials may affect a totally different channel, a second channel that opens later than the first.[393] Drugs that act selectively on the second, slow system might not affect transmitter release due to the initial channel opening, but may abolish prolongation of release related to flux through the late opening channel.

It should also be noted that the effects of verapamil and related drugs are not limited to prejunctional action or to calcium flux. They also act on the postjunctional system to produce unrelated phenomena that are easily confused with blockade of calcium entry into the nerve ending. These include entry into and inhibition by drug of the postjunctional ion channel,[67,370] modification of postjunctional kinetics, and, if the concentration of drug is high, inhibition of sodium flow through sodium channels. These effects on the muscle membrane may change contraction characteristics, and can be observed in muscles stimulated directly, independent of neuromuscular transmission.

Dantrolene acts on calcium quite differently from those drugs described above. Its primary effect is to reduce the flow of calcium across the muscle's sarcoplasmic reticulum;[138,174] hence it weakens muscles[402,318,325] and reduces spastic contractions. It may also reduce spontaneous and stimulated release of acetylcholine from the nerve ending[489,432,433,157] and can, in this manner, interact with nondepolarizing blocking drugs to produce a greater than expected depression of neuromuscular transmission during surgery.

The entry of calcium into the nerve ending is related so tightly to the release of transmitter that any drug that reduces the former is bound to reduce the latter. Accordingly, many otherwise unrelated drugs can impede normal neuromuscular transmission. Prominent among these are some antibiotics, particularly the aminoglycosides, tetracyclines and polypeptides.[189] The mechanisms by which the compounds work are not known well, but prejunctional calcium flux is apparently involved. The clinical importance of the action of these drugs, alone or in combination with anesthetics and nondepolarizing neuromuscular blocking drugs, is recognized.

The action of phenytoin on calcium is of particular interest because the neuromuscular junction has been used as a model in which to study antiepileptic action.[175,442,443] Phenytoin clearly changes sodium flux into and out of the nerve[583,430,134,135,85] apparently by antagonizing the activation of sodium channels in preterminal nerve branches, but phenytoin also inhibits both potassium and veratroidine-induced calcium uptake into isolated nerve terminals.[187] The latter effect is reflected in nerve-muscle preparations in which phenytoin reduces the peak amplitude of the evoked and spontaneous endplate potential and decreases the average quantal content of the evoked potential.[204,587] These actions of phenytoin are coupled to the production of neural action potentials because, at a time when evoked postsynaptic depolarizations are blocked by phenytoin, spontaneous potentials can still be recorded at the endplate. The rate of spontaneous depolarizations is, paradoxically, increased at the same time quantal content and mepp and epp amplitudes are markedly decreased.

Attempts have been made to reconcile a discrepancy between spontaneous and evoked release of acetylcholine by studying the effects of phenytoin on calcium flux across membrane surfaces in isolated terminal synaptosomes. Phenytoin antagonizes potassium-depolarized ^{45}Ca uptake across synaptosomal membranes, but does not influence resting flux. Mitochondrial accumulation of ^{45}Ca, which could be antagonized by ruthenium red or mitochondrial inhibitors, is not reduced by phenytoin at the same dose level, but sodium-dependent ^{45}Ca efflux from synaptosomes is reduced. Pincus and Hsiao[428,429] concluded that phenytoin blocks calcium uptake through the slow voltage-dependent calcium channel associated with depolarization secretion mechanisms, but had little effect on the uptake into intracellular organelle calcium buffering systems. These observations suggest the net effect of phenytoin is to reduce calcium uptake during evoked stimulus and to have the greatest effect on repeated stimulation or on slow membrane phenomena (such as the events thought to occur in epilepsy). As for the mechanism, phenytoin in lower than therapeutic concentrations inhibits the phosphorylation of membrane-bound receptors, and phosphorylation may play an important role in the release of transmitter;[225] however, phenytoin also interacts with presynaptic ionic calcium calmodulin-dependent phosphorylation processes linked to transmitter release,[133] and phenytoin has been shown to be an active inhibitor of the calcium-stimulated phosphorylation of protein kinases associated with synaptic vesicles.[133] Since spontaneous release is less sensitive to external and internal calcium ion concentrations, phenytoin would be expected to have less influence on mepps than on ionic calcium-coupled, depolarization-coupled release.

Although most attention has been focused on its neural actions, phenytoin also acts on other parts of the neuromuscular system. Gage[204] suggested that phenytoin could reduce postsynaptic sensitivity by both a presynaptic and a channel blocking effect on the postsynaptic acetylcholine receptors, since the time course of the endplate potential is reduced from control. Braswell et al[64] found in isolated acetylcholine receptor membrane preparations, phenytoin did not antagonize agonist-stimulated cation efflux through agonist-activated acetylcholine receptor channels, but in the presence of phenytoin the [³H] acetylcholine binding to receptor ligand binding sites was decreased by half. Phenytoin enhances agonist-induced postsynaptic desensitization.[82]

Precisely timed and properly sequenced transmembrane flux of cations is essential to the accomplishment of neuromuscular transmission. Understanding how the proper flux of ions is accomplished, how ionic flows are related to biochemical processes, and how drugs affect the processes are among the major problems addressed by current research. Many of the important relationships between ion flow and synaptic function are described in preceding sections of this article and in other chapters of this book, and from them it should be apparent that if a drug modifies an ionic phenomenon, it will modify neuromuscular transmission. It should also be apparent that modification of ionic phenomena by drugs is commonplace. Of the drugs usually thought to affect the neuromuscular junction, the depolarizing and nondepolarizing agonists and antagonists are recognized as having special effectiveness, but this special character is conferred by the specific manner in which they influence ions; the drugs act via receptors making their action highly specific and greatly amplified. Other drugs may affect ion flow, even if they do not operate via receptors, and these will modify the function of the neuromuscular apparatus. The possible sites of action are many, e.g., ion channels, antiporters, lipid or protein in the membrane, ATPase and other restorative properties, noncholinergic receptors, or ion-controlled metabolic processes; equally numerous are the chemical structures that can act on one or more of these systems. In practice, this means that most drugs used clinically or experimentally will have some effect on neuromuscular transmission. The effect may be too small to be significant or too subtle to be noticed until the junction is stressed by disease or by the simultaneous presence of other drugs such as may occur during surgery. The effect on the neuromuscular apparatus may be a laboratory curiosity, an investigator's tool or a clinically important occurrence, but some degree of drug modification of ionic processes, and consequently of neuromuscular transmission, occurs with virtually every available membrane active drug.

Cholinesterases

The body contains a number of enzymes that are capable of catalyzing the hydrolysis of acetylcholine, but two of these are of particular importance in the pharmacology of the neuromuscular junction. The first is acetylcholinesterase (EC 3.1.1.7), sometimes referred to as tissue esterase or true esterase. Acetylcholinesterase is a membrane-bound enzyme found in many tissues, including the synapses in the peripheral and central cholinergic nervous systems. Of the several variants located synaptically, one (the 16S fragment) is thought to be responsible for the destruction of acetylcholine released at the synapse.[351] This enzyme is an essential part of synaptic transmission. When it is depressed by drugs, acetylcholine accumulates and synaptic activity is exaggerated. In small doses, inhibitors or cholinesterase are used medically to increase the concentration and lifetime of acetylcholine in synaptic clefts. For instance, cholinesterase inhibitors are used in the treatment of myasthenia gravis, or to reverse the antagonism of transmission produced by *d*-tubocurarine or similar drugs that compete with acetylcholine for receptors. When inhibition of the enzyme is great, synaptic function can be so completely disrupted that the nervous system cannot operate and the organism dies; it is for this reason that inhibitors of acetylcholinesterase are the major products used throughout the world as insecticides and as potential war "nerve" gases.

The other cholinesterase is butyrylcholinesterase (EC 3.1.1.8), sometimes referred to as plasmacholinesterase or pseudocholinesterase. It is a soluble protein made in the liver and circulated in the plasma. Butyrylcholinesterase is clinically important because it destroys succinylcholine and is responsible for the rapid elimination of that compound. The physiologic function of butyrylcholinesterase is not known, although it apparently is not essential for normal life since there are no detectable signs or symptoms in people genetically lacking butyrylcholinesterase, or in whom the enzyme has been inhibited by drugs. The synthesis of the enzyme is under genetic control with four known allelic genes and ten combinations of these. Most individuals have a pair of normal genes, but at least one person in twenty-five has one normal and one atypical gene[524,409] with resultant reduced amounts of the enzyme that destroys succinylcholine. Most of these people have only mildly (and usually unnoticeably) prolonged responses to succinylcholine. However, about one in 2500 people have two abnormal genes and hydrolyze succinylcholine slowly enough to exhibit a prolonged response to that drug. An extremely rare form of atypical butyrylcholinesterase occurs in one in 100,000 people; these individuals have little or no measurable esteratic activity and consequently have a markedly prolonged paralysis following succinylcholine.[573, 558-560,405]

Functionally, acetylcholinesterase has two active areas: an anionic site and an esteratic (or catalytic) site. Both of these active areas are used in the hydrolysis of acetylcholine, and blocking one or both will prevent enzymic activity. The anionic site contains negatively charged amino acids and serves to attract and temporarily hold positively charged groups such as the quaternary nitrogen of acetylcholine. Held in this way, acetylcholine lines up on the protein and its ester falls into place upon the catalytic site where a chemical reaction transfers the acetate to a serine of the enzyme. The freed choline drifts away, leaving an acetylated enzyme. The acetylated enzyme protein is labile, being readily attacked by hyroxyl ions in the local water to cleave the acetate. The enzyme is thus regenerated and ready for a new reaction. Formation of acetylated enzyme and regeneration of the resting molecule requires only a few microseconds, making acetylcholinesterase one of the most rapidly acting enzymes known.

Most of the compounds used to inhibit acetylcholinesterase form covalently bound ester groups with the serine of the esteratic site and thereby prevent the reaction with acetylcholine. Differences in inhibitors relate primarily to the lability of the covalent bond. An acetylated enzyme is highly susceptible to attack and regeneration by a hydroxyl group. A carbamylated enzyme, such as that formed by neostigmine, pyridostigmine, physostigmine or the carbamate-containing insecticides, is more resistant and the enzyme may remain inactivated for a half-hour[578,298] before the carbamate bond is successfully cleaved and the enzyme regenerated. Phosphorylated enzyme, such as that formed by phosphate insecticides or by the phosphate-containing war gases, is still more resistant, and in many cases the bond is never broken; new enzyme must be synthesized before cholinesterase activity can be restored.

Masking the anionic site also prevents acetylcholine from reacting with the enzyme. Masking is only part of the process by which neostigmine, pyridostigmine or physostigmine react with the enzyme, but it is the single mechanism of inhibition by edrophonium. The last compound has a quaternary nitrogen that is attracted by electrostatic forces, but since the molecule has no ester group it cannot react with the esteratic site. As a result, edrophonium is held in place by a weak electrostatic bond and the inhibitor enzyme complex is only briefly held together. This brevity of action is very apparent in the laboratory and because of it edrophonium has gained a reputation as an anticholinesterase of short duration. Now it appears that this reputation should not be extended to the clinical use of the compound. Binding to the enzyme determines the chemical half-life of the edrophonium-acetylcholinesterase complex, and indeed it is short, but elimination from the body determines the biologic half-life of edrophonium and in this regard the compound is eliminated by the kidneys at about the same rate as neostigmine[118,390] and pyridostigmine.[117,119] As predicted from this analysis it has been demonstrated clinically that in human beings edrophonium produces an antagonism of nondepolarizing relaxants that lasts as long as that of its carbamate analogues.[185,375]

While minor increases in acetylcholine at cholinergic synapses are valuable in certain therapeutic situations, neither ubiquitous synaptic activity nor excessive synaptic activity is ever beneficial. An overdose of anticholinesterase will increase cholinergic activity at the neuromuscular junction, throughout the autonomic nervous system, and in the central nervous system. The results are devastating, with death due to paralysis of respiratory muscles, impairment of airways by bronchoconstriction and secretion, and diminished central respiratory drive. The extreme toxicity, and the speed with which it can occur, has made these compounds favorites not only as insecticides, but also among the world's military establishments which stockpile organophosphates as "nerve gases."

In the event of over-inhibition of cholinesterase, it is desirable to return the enzyme to normal function as quickly as possible. Hydroxyl from body water is the ion that ordinarily breaks the carbamate or phosphate bonds to the enzyme; but an organic molecule, hydroxyamine, is more efficient in breaking the bonds. For this reason, hydroxyamine, incorporated into oxime molecules, has been used to reactivate acetylcholinesterase in human endplates poisoned by an inhibitor.[579,491,580,574] Pralidoxime, or 2 PAM, is available for this purpose in the United States. Pralidoxime works more efficiently than hydroxyl to free the esterified enzyme, and the quaternary nitrogen of the pyridime ring of the pralidoxime molecule draws the compound to the enzyme and positions it properly for the hydroxyamine attack on the phosphate bond.[95,471,528] Although pralidoxime is an effective material and should be used when needed, several caveats should be borne in mind. Pharmacotherapy is no substitute for mechanical ventilation, and respiration must be supported until normal function returns. Pralidoxime does not obviate the need for an antimuscarinic agent such as atropine. Also, pralidoxime is a quaternary ammonium compound that is poorly absorbed from the

GI tract,[323] is not very effective in penetrating into the brain,[52] and is actively secreted by the kidney. (Clearance is about 600 ml/min.) [535,483,473,480] Pralidoxime must be given parenterally and may have to be given repeatedly. Since the phosphate-enzyme bond is more protected by the steric effects of some substituent groups than others, the oxime is less effective treatment for poisoning by some agents than for others. Finally, some organophosphate-enzyme complexes undergo a second reaction called "aging" which renders the inhibited enzyme invulnerable to cleavage by an oxime. The aging process is complex, involving removal of one of the carbon groups from the phosphate and subsequent rearrangement of the whole complex. It occurs more rapidly with the military compounds than with commonly used insecticides and is particularly rapid in the case of soman, the choice of the Soviet military.[35,132]

The actions of drugs that inhibit cholinesterase are almost always assumed to be due to the acetylcholine that accumulates, but there is evidence that this is not so. It has been known for several decades[456] that neostigmine can act directly to depolarize muscle, apparently because its three methyl groups form a quaternary ammonium which resembles that of acetylcholine. Much more recently, neostigmine and edrophonium have been shown to act on isolated nicotinic receptors as agonists, causing the channel to open, and acting inside the opened channel to block it.[26] Some organophosphorus cholinsterase inhibitors prevent 80−90% of agonist binding to the receptor activation sites,[167] and in high concentrations soman causes an irreversible depolarization of the endplate.[76] In agonist-activated channels, organophosphorus molecules compete for binding sites within the open channel[167] and the compound isofluorphate (DFP) seems to block open channels.[305] The drugs also have been known for a half century to have prejunctional actions. They will cause the nerve ending to fire spontaneously, producing fasciculations, and they will cause a slowly stimulated nerve to fire repetitively, producing an increase in the force of contraction of the innervated muscle. It is generally agreed that these are neural phenomena, but there is controversy over whether they are direct actions of the drugs or are secondary to the accumulation of acetylcholine around the nerve ending. This latter view is widely accepted,[301,381] but investigators who have studied acetylcholine do not think that its accumulation could produce the observed neural effects[452,453,261,266] or that it could release enough potassium from the surroundings to cause neural depolarization[261, 266] (but see also Hohlfeld[254]). It seems likely that the anticholinesterase compounds work on something besides a cholinesterase system in the nerve,[519,454] but the exact substrate remains obscure. There also are hints that different substrates are involved in the neural actions of neostigmine, pyridostigmine and edrophonium.[145]

An increased flow of depolarizing ions is necessary to produce the initial depolarization which leads to fasciculations, or to produce the prolonged after-negativity which is needed to produce repetitive activity in stimulated nerves.[455] Some clues as to how this might be produced are available in the observations that the neural effects are attenuated or prevented by drugs that reduce the activity of cyclic AMP in the nerve[515] or that reduce calcium entry into the nerve[488,490] but are not affected by pretreatment with the sodium-blocking material, tetrodotoxin.[509] Physostigmine has been found to be a potent inhibitor of neural phosphodiesterase,[123,124] and this could account for the increased flux of calcium, but physostigmine is unusual in this regard, since none of the other major compounds inhibit phosphodiesterase; neostigmine, edrophonium, isofluorphate and echothiophate are essentially inert in this regard.[123] Since all of these produce similar neural effects, it is not likely that the inhibition of phosphodiesterase accounts for the depolarizing phenomena that characterize this group of drugs. Parenthetically, inhibition of phosphodiesterase by physostigmine may be relevant to another of physostigmine's actions, the capacity to increase release of acetylcholine.[40,41] Further, this may account for the sharper than expected central nervous system actions of physostigmine. In this regard it is noteworthy that among the compounds we tested, tetraaminoacidine is the only other active inhibitor of phosphodiesterase. Tetraaminoacidine is not widely used but it also inhibits cholinesterase,[243] increases muscle force, antagonizes d-tubocurarine,[213,451] and has strong central nervous system actions.[272]

The prejunctional actions of anticholinesterases may be of more than theoretical significance.[137] Laskowski et al,[312–314] Wecker,[568,569] and Dettbarn[184] showed that rats treated with paraoxon, an organophosphate cholinesterase inhibitor insecticide, rapidly develop areas of degeneration in the subjunctional muscle and in the nerve ending. These changes are particularly severe in diaphragm.[568] Although the experiments were done in animals, these workers found similar changes postmortem in a human being accidently poisoned by a single dose of organophosphate.[569] Similar neuromyopathy is produced in rats treated with neostigmine in doses just above those used clinically to treat myasthenia gravis.[267] The lesions seem to be reversible, but possibly only by regeneration of the affected cells. The mechanism is not known, but may be due to the excessive activity that occurs in junctions treated in this way, the accumulation of acetylcholine in and around the junction, or the increased influx of calcium that might be produced by these materials.[42,568,294,465]

In another neural phenomenon that does not appear to be related to acetylcholinesterase, many of the organophosphate compounds produce an irreversible sensorimotor neuropathy that seems to be due to a delayed distal axonal degeneration in the peripheral and central nervous system.[15,1,130] A number of episodes, some involving hundreds of people, have been reported following accidental ingestion of certain organophosphates.[77,493,388,586] The mechanism is not known but the capacity of a compound to produce the lesion is correlated with inhibition of an esterase that is present in axons, the poorly named enzyme known as "neurotoxic esterase" (EC 3.1.1.1). The inhibition of this enzyme is similar to that of acetylcholinesterase at the neuromuscular junction involving the production of a covalent bond between the organophosphate and the enzyme.[97] The inhibition of "neurotoxic esterase" is prevented by pretreatment with other groups of compounds, e.g., carbamates, that do not form such a prolonged inhibition of the esterase, but otherwise is distinct from the synaptic actions of anticholinesterases. Likewise, "neurotoxic esterase" is an intraneuronal enzyme, not a synaptic one, and it does not appear to have a role in the hydrolysis of either synaptic acetylcholine or succinylcholine.[276–279]

Specific Drugs

Nondepolarizing Blocking Drugs

Traditionally, this is a term that is applied to drugs that compete with acetylcholine for the recognition site on the nicotinic cholinergic receptor where, by preventing the usual depolarization of the endplate by acetylcholine, they cause paralysis of neuromuscular transmission. It is now known that these compounds can have additional actions at the neuromuscular junction and that they can affect other organs of the body.

d-Tubocurarine, an active compound in the plant extracts used by Amazonian arrow hunters and the active ingredient of the crude curare first studied by Bernard,[36] is the prototype drug of this group. It was purified by King in 1935 and introduced into anesthetic prac-

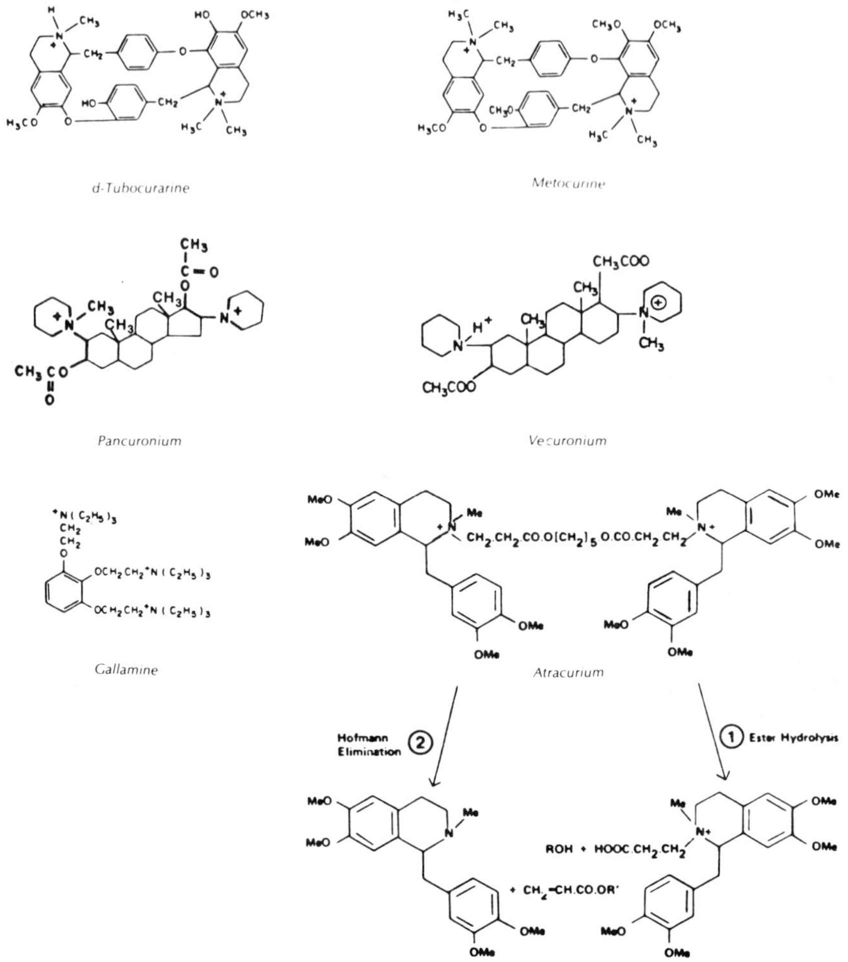

Figure 4.3. Representative nondepolarizing neuromuscular blocking drugs.

tice in 1940.[358,223] Its success led to an enormous investigative effort and a constant flow of potentially useful compounds. Originally, *d*-tubocurarine was described as containing two quaternary nitrogen groups; all of the subsequently synthesized compounds also had at least two quaternary nitrogen groups separated by approximately ten atoms, the same number as in *d*-tubocurarine. The more recent discovery, that actually only one nitrogen of *d*-tubocurarine is quaternized,[176,98] has only just now been paralleled by the introduction into clinical use of a monoquaternary synthetic drug, vecuronium.

d-Tubocurarine has been investigated more than all other nondepolarizing blocking agents. According to usual theory, it acts primarily as a competitive antagonist of acetylcholine at the recognition site of the endplate cholinergic receptor. Its affinity for the receptor is moderate (Kd = 0.34 uM) and on the average it is bound less than 1 msec before it dissociates.[104] Nevertheless, this binding is long enough and strong enough to occlude acetylcholine released in a burst from the nerve and to prevent the agonist from binding to cause the ion channel to open and depolarize the muscle. Muscles are accordingly quiescent and paralyzed in a patient who has received *d*-tubocurarine. In addition, there is recent knowledge that *d*-tubocurarine, in somewhat higher concentrations, also may enter the opened ion channel and add a noncompetitive component to the blockade.[101, 106,107,149,421,477] The exact contribution of the channel blocking action to the clinical paralysis is not known. Postulated action is based on extrapolation of the experimentally determined ratio of concentrations that act on the recognition site to those that act in the channel. Although at minimal concentration, blockade of transmission may be due predominantly to the competition with acetylcholine, the concentrations needed to produce a full clinical blockade may be great enough to cause a significant amount of drug to enter ion channels. Since the latter action blocks transmission but is not a competitive action, transmission would not be easily or fully restored by anticholinesterase.

It also has been postulated that the postjunctional channel blocking action of *d*-tubocurarine is use-dependent,[149,421] an idea that is compatible with the many observations that *d*-tubocurarine becomes more potent as the frequency of nerve stimulation is increased.[570, 71,460,412,431,48,214,16,338,509–511] While there is some evidence of use-dependent channel activity by the drug,[149] a direct demonstration has not yet been published. *d*-Tubocurarine is known to act on motor nerve endings[329,32,506,262,263,215,62,509–511] and it has been postulated that the apparently increased potency in high-frequency stimulated situations is due to a drug-induced decrease in release of transmitter.[263,59] Specifically, it is postulated that *d*-tubocurarine, possibly acting on a prejunctional receptor,[62] interferes with the flux of sodium into the nerve ending and by doing so, prevents the nerve ending from synthesizing and mobilizing transmitter rapidly enough to replenish what is lost during stimulation.[509–511]

Such a notion is also compatible with the many observations of greater potency of *d*-tubocurarine when the nerve is active, the muscle recordings that suggest that the nerve loses its effectiveness when it is stimulated rapidly in the presence of *d*-tubocurarine, the direct observations that *d*-tubocurarine reduces the release of acetylcholine from rapidly stimulated nerves, but not from slowly stimulated ones,[32,510,511] and the lack of significant effect on the spontaneous release of acetylcholine (mepps) from resting nerves.

It seems likely that all of these mechanisms of action are operative in the clinical use of *d*-tubocurarine, but in different proportions in different circumstances. That is, the traditional receptor blocking actions account for the action of *d*-tubocurarine on resting or slowly stimulated preparations exposed to minimally effective concentrations of drug, but more mechanisms become contributory as the concentration of the drug and/or the frequency of stimulation is increased. Postjunctional channel blockade may contribute to the effects of high doses and to the response to short bursts of stimuli to the motor nerve, such as the clinically used "train-of-four," while prejunctional effects to reduce transmitter release may become significant during longer periods of high-frequency stimulation such as those that are used to produce a tetanus. The distinction has practical implications because the impulses in the phrenic nerve that normally drive respiration may be of the appropriate frequency and duration to evoke prejunctional effects.

It has long been said that individual muscles differ in their susceptibility to the actions of *d*-tubocurarine, with the eye muscles being paralyzed by the lowest concentrations of the drug, the diaphragm with the highest, and other muscles failing at various intermediate concentrations, but the reason for such differential susceptibility is not known. In addition, a number of authors have reported that *d*-tubocurarine is more effective in blocking transmission at fast-twitch muscles (e.g., gastrocnemius) than at slow-twitch ones (e.g., soleus).[275,14,336,476,131] Again, the mechanism is not known. The junctions of fast-twitch and slow-twitch muscles are distinctly different in appearance,[170,529] content of acetylcholinesterase,[24,230] glucose utilization,[426] physiology,[246,96,371,139,529] and fatty acid composition of the lipid membrane,[217,191] but none of these has been specifically linked to the difference in susceptibility to nondepolarizing compounds.

d-Tubocurarine is bound to receptors for less than 1 msec, yet the paralysis produced by the administration of the drug intravenously during surgery lasts for up to 2 hours. This large discrepancy occurs because two different processes are at work. At the molecular level the *d*-tubocurarine leaves the recognition site rapidly, but is almost immediately replaced by another molecule from the environment. Thus, as long as the drug remains at the neuromuscular junction

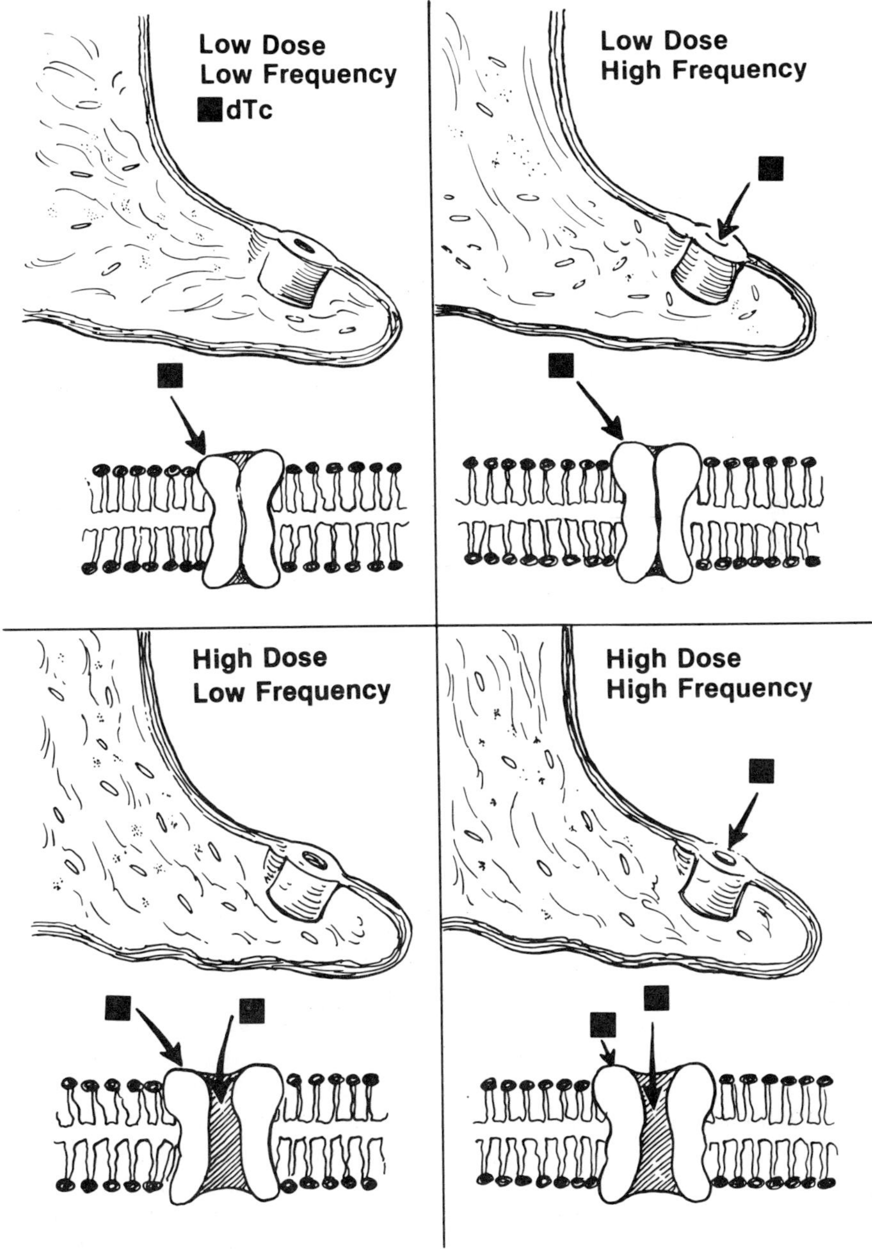

Figure 4.4. Sites of action of *d*-tubocurarine as a function of dose and stimulation frequency.

some molecule of d-tubocurarine almost continuously is present on the receptor. The length of time d-tubocurarine is present at the neuromuscular junction is determined not by molecular phenomena but by the pharmacokinetic properties of the drug. d-Tubocurarine, given intravenously, is 30 to 77% bound to plasma proteins,[160,194,389] but is rapidly distributed to central body compartments, including neuromuscular junctions (alpha distribution $t_{1/2}$ = 8 min).[521] Thence it is distributed to less vascular compartments (Vd_{ss} = 0.30 l/kg). In normal adult human beings, about 45% is eliminated unchanged by the kidneys within 24 hours (elimination $T_{1/2}$ = 89 min);[193] significant amounts of the drug are stored and slowly eliminated.[354,353] Biliary excretion, measured in man, accounts for 12% after 48 hours.[362] Since d-tubocurarine is a quaternary ammonium compound, drug excreted with bile is poorly reabsorbed from the gut. The exact ratio of the renal and hepatic elimination routes varies. In normal young adults most of the drug is filtered out of the blood and into the urine, but the ratio of biliary and renal excretion is changed by anything that reduces glomerular filtration, e.g., drugs, disease or age. The most extreme case, total renal failure, shifts all elimination to the hepatic system and produces an estimated beta $t_{1/2}$ of about 330 min.[376] The relationship between concentration in blood and degree of neuromuscular blockade is fairly well understood.[11,501,239,556,444,353,116] The important practical concern of the immediate effects of a rapidly administered intravenous injection are more complicated and are just beginning to be studied.[520, 521]

While a very valuable drug, d-tubocurarine is not fully specific for cholinergic receptors at the motor endplate and actions at other sites can produce undesirable actions. For example, d-tubocurarine can release histamine[391] and block autonomic ganglia.[43,241] In doses used clinically, the combination of direct histamine release and ganglionic blockade produces a significant reduction in peripheral resistance and a decrease in blood pressure.[467,468] d-Tubocurarine also has been reported to cause a change in central nervous system activity.[90,60] The mechanism of ganglionic blockade was long thought to be due to a classical competitive blockade of acetylcholine at nicotinic cholinergic receptors; however, recent experiments by Ascher et al[21] suggest that ganglionic receptors are not the same as those of the endplate and that at ganglionic receptors d-tubocurarine acts entirely in the ion channel and not at the recognition site.[449,450] There is a debate about the decrease in central respiratory drive that may be produced by d-tubocurarine. As a quaternary ammonium compound, d-tubocurarine would not be expected to penetrate the blood brain barrier, but there is some evidence to the contrary.[90] Alternatively, it has been suggested that *d*-tubocurarine blocks nicotinic receptors on muscle spindles,[492,60] reducing stretch receptor discharges into the central nervous system and may produce effects on behavior that can be misinterpreted as central nervous system actions.[441] Clearly not mediated via cholinergic receptors is the capacity of *d*-tubocurarine to release histamine. This effect occurs with doses used clinically and may occasionally cause signs and symptoms due to histamine, including, in rare individuals, significant respiratory difficulties.

Pancuronium, the other nondepolarizing neuromuscular blocking drug important in present clinical practice, closely resembles *d*-tubocurarine. Although pancuronium is a synthetic product, it is based upon the natural compound, malouetine, found in arrow poisons used by primitive Africans. Pancuronium also acts both on the nicotinic receptor recognition site and in the ion channel. Its alpha and beta $t_{1/2}$s and Vd_{ss} are similar to those of tubocurarine in normal human beings, 20, 140 min, and 0.26 1/kg, respectively,[116] as is the time course of the neuromuscular blockade during a constant infusion. However, attention to the detailed differences between the two drugs may be important to the individual to whom the drugs are administered. With regard to mechanism of action, pancuronium has not been studied as well as *d*-tubocurarine, but is reported to act as a more specific antagonist at the receptor recognition site. It does not enter the open ion channel as readily as *d*-tubocurarine and apparently leaves it more readily[288,421] so as to produce less use-dependent blockade of the channel. Pancuronium is also reported to have less effect in reducing the release of transmitter from nerves stimulated with brief trains or at tetanic frequencies[59,575] and to be less effective than *d*-tubocurarine in opposing the neural actions (e.g., fasciculations) induced by succinylcholine or neostigmine.[567] In clinical doses pancuronium does not produce ganglionic blockade or affect peripheral resistance. Conversely, pancuronium impedes the vagal innervation of the heart and may cause tachycardia and an increase in blood pressure and cardiac output.[346,99,467,468,172,122,470] This vagolytic action usually is ascribed to an inhibitory action on muscarinic cholinergic receptors in the atrium.[469,60,326,152] However, there is evidence that the vagus nerve modulates, via nicotinic receptors on the sympathetic nerve endings, the release of norepinephrine from cardiac sympathetic nerves[61,346,141,60] and blockade of these receptors by pancuronium would lead to an increased release of norepinephrine.[346,467,469] Pancuronium increases plasma catecholamine levels but does not cause release of histamine.[122] Pancuronium does inhibit serum cholinesterase[194] and may interact with substances, notably succinylcholine, that depend upon this enzyme for elimination.

Pancuronium is hydrolyzed in the liver into deacetylated products. The 3-deacetylated-hydroxypancuronium metabolite is 50% as active as the parent compound, while the 17 deacetylated and the 3-17 deactylated metabolites are essentially inactive.[373,345] Despite the fact that the drug can be metabolized by the liver,[10,502,521] the kidney is responsible for eliminating most of a dose.[359,502] The beta $t_{1/2}$, and consequently the duration of neuromuscular blockade, is greatly prolonged in patients with renal failure.[502,359,126,37]

There are a number of other nondepolarizing drugs in clinical use in the United States. They are all similar to d-tubocurarine in their general mechanisms and effects, but they differ from it, and from each other, in important details. For example, metocurine, the derivative of d-tubocurarine, with methyl groups on both nitrogens, as well as two more that form methoxy groups, has almost twice the neuromuscular blocking potency action of d-tubocurarine in humans,[468,353] but only one-half the capacity of d-tubocurarine to release histamine.[468] The blocking effect of metocurine on other cholinergic receptor sites in the autonomic nervous system is considerably less, by a factor of three, than that of d-tubocurarine. Since it causes less vagolytic actions, ganglionic blockade, and histamine release, metocurine has fewer hemodynamic effects[19] than d-tubocurarine and may be preferred in cardiovascular surgery.[531] Metocurine is rapidly removed from the plasma with a plasma clearance of 1.1 ml/kg/min (compared to 1.9 ml/kg/min for d-tubocurarine), but when equipotent doses of metocurine and d-tubocurarine are given, no difference in time to 50% recovery of evoked muscle twitch can be observed. Elimination rate constants are 345 min for metocurine and 190 min for d-tubocurarine. The volume of distribution is little different, 0.51 1/kg with metocurine and 0.47 1/kg for d-tubocurarine.[353] Metocurine is primarily eliminated by renal excretion, with less than 2% eliminated in the bile[362] hours after recovery from paralysis.

Gallamine, another synthetic nondepolarizing drug that blocks neuromuscular transmission, is distinctly different from its pharmacologic relatives. It was designed according to the then prevalent idea that two or more quaternary nitrogens separated by a distance equivalent to that occupied by about ten atoms are necessary for activity. Gallamine does produce the expected type of neuromuscular blockade, but unlike the other compounds, it has ethyl groups, not methyl groups, on the nitrogens. Gallamine has a Vd_{ss} of about 207 ml/kg and is eliminated entirely by the kidney[11] with a beta $t_{1/2}$ of about 135 min.[447]

Although superficially the neuromuscular blockade produced by gallamine is like that produced by *d*-tubocurarine, it is not the same in detail. The differences are subtle, but great enough that most anesthesiologists decline to use gallamine, except in special circumstances. Two features are outstanding. One is a strong vagolytic effect that occurs in almost every recipient;[73,321,413,60] the other is a persistent decrement in neuromuscular function after successive doses that cannot be readily overcome by the usual regimen of anticholinesterase.[376] Occasional patients given gallamine may develop increased peripheral vascular resistance which, when combined with the tachycardia, may cause a troublesome increase in blood pressure.

The mechanisms of these anomalous effects of gallamine are not known, but recent experiments are providing insight into some of them. Gallamine occludes the acetylcholine recognition site, as expected, but it also has significant channel blocking activity.[288,103,105,106] Recognition site occlusion and channel blockade occur in the same range of concentrations and therefore, both effects are always present. The drug has prejunctional effects,[417,499] but depending on the circumstances of its use, these may be distinctly different from those of *d*-tubocurarine. They key seems to be in the ethonium groups that dominate the molecule. In essence, gallamine is three triethylammonium groups attached to a ring, and is more analogous to tetraethylammonium than to any other simple compound. Gallamine, like tetraethylammonium, has been shown to have actions on neural potassium channels to delay the efflux of potassium from stimulated nerves.[494,495] This confers at least some of the special properties. Gallamine, for instance, by blocking potassium, delays the recovery of stimulated nerve endings.[499] This delay of recovery, in turn, causes a prolonged action potential in the nerve ending and a corresponding prolongation of transmitter release, which would tend to antagonize the postjunctional receptor recognition site actions of the compound. In other words, gallamine has built-in mechanisms for self-antagonism. A similar increase in ganglionic transmission may lead to increased sympathetic activity and an increase in peripheral resistance. The vagolytic action is generally ascribed to a blockade by gallamine of muscarinic receptors in the atria,[60,530,152,467] but a direct blocking influence on the vagus, through inhibiting the potassium flux that determines its recovery cycle, has not been ruled out.

One of the anomalies of this series of drugs is that the different agents are not all merely additive in their effects, as would be expected if they all acted in the same way. Combinations of pancuronium and metocurine or of pancuronium and d-tubocurarine (but not of metocurine and d-tubocurarine) produce more intense blockade of neuromuscular transmission in human beings and in animals than would be expected from their individual potencies.[317] The mechanism of this superadditivity, or potentiation, is not known, but obvious mechanisms have been ruled out. There is no change in the elimination kinetics of the combinations[317] or of tissue or plasma protein binding.[348] It has been reported that d-tubocurarine binds at a slightly different point of the alpha subunit of receptor protein than the other compounds.[487] This observation would fit the presumption that the superadditivity results because the members of the pair are acting at different sites, even though the net results—blockade of transmission—is the same. Also, nondepolarizing compounds can act at many parts of the pre- and postjunctional apparatus and differential activity at any, or many, parts could be the explanation of the phenomenon. It is too soon to settle on one of the many possibilities.

Two new nondepolarizing compounds are expected soon to appear in the United States: vecuronium[56] and atracurium.[416] Both have been investigated in animal experiments[51,268] and during clinical trials in human beings.[177,414,30,293,270,269,459,171,116,193] While essentially nothing is known of their molecular mechanism of action, it is presumed to be similar to the older compounds. Both compounds seem to be more specific for the neuromuscular junction than their predecessors in that only weak cardiovascular effects or histamine-releasing capacity has been demonstrated.[268,320,241,28,459,345,172] Both compounds are chemically unstable and need to be mixed into solution or kept refrigerated until just before use. Both are eliminated more rapidly than other clinically used nondepolarizing compounds and have shorter lasting effects than the standard agents. Because of the rapid elimination, both may be given in large doses to hasten the onset of blockade and to induce paralysis more rapidly than older agents; even so, they do not act as rapidly as the depolarizing compound, succinylcholine.[236]

Although alike in major effects on whole organisms, the two compounds are completely different chemically and biochemically. Vecuronium is the monoquaternary analog of pancuronium. It binds to plasma protein,[160,194] but has a Vd_{ss} of about 0.27 1/kg. It is eliminated mostly by liver hydrolysis (beta $t_{1/2}$ = 71 min),[116] but also by renal filtration. Hence, its duration of action is influenced by those factors that influence renal filtration such as age or disease. Atracurium, an isoquinolin like *d*-tubocurarine, is eliminated by molecular self-destruction by means of a Hofmann reaction.[92,268] This reaction, which cleaves the molecule into inert products, is independent of any organ or biochemical process, but is dependent on the pH of the solution and the temperature. Atracurium has a volume of distribution of 157 ml/kg^{-1}, total clearance 5.5 ml/min^{-1}/kg^{-1}, and a beta $t_{1/2}$ of 20 min.[564] Its elimination rate is the same in patients of all ages and states of health,[127,271] but might be modified by factors that cause blood pH to deviate significantly from normal.

Depolarizing Neuromuscular Blocking Drugs

Acetylcholine is the prototypic agonist at the neuromuscular junction, but the compound is hydrolyzed so rapidly and has so many actions in the body that it has no clinical usefulness as a neuromuscular drug. However, several analogues, specifically succinylcholine and decamethonium, are used as neuromuscular blocking drugs. Both drugs were synthesized when it was first thought that *d*-tubocurarine contained two quaternary ammonium groups separated by a distance roughly equal to that occupied by ten carbon or oxygen atoms. It was surprising to investigators that the blockades produced by these two compounds were quite different from that of *d*-tubocurarine in that blockade was preceded by a period of intense stimulation and excitatory phenomena.[411,592,79,411] In retrospect, of course, this is what should be expected of acetylcholine and its analogues.

Succinylcholine is the more important of the two agents, and is, in fact, the most commonly employed neuromuscular blocking drug in the United States. Structurally it is a bis-acetylcholine, with two acetylcholine molecules joined through their acetic acid moieties. The esters are labile and succinylcholine is rapidly hydrolyzed by the cholinesterase in normal plasma (mean half-life of 2.6 min).[365] The first choline is removed rapidly, the second more slowly; but the removal of the first choline effectively ends the pharmacologic action because succinylmonocholine is only one-twentieth as potent as its parent. Succinylcholine is quite resistant to the acetylcholinesterase found in synapses. It is also not destroyed in those patients whose plasma esterase is incompetent because of genetic absence of the normal allele or in those whose plasma esterase has been inhibited by concomitantly used drugs.

Succinylcholine usually is given intravenously to facilitate endo-

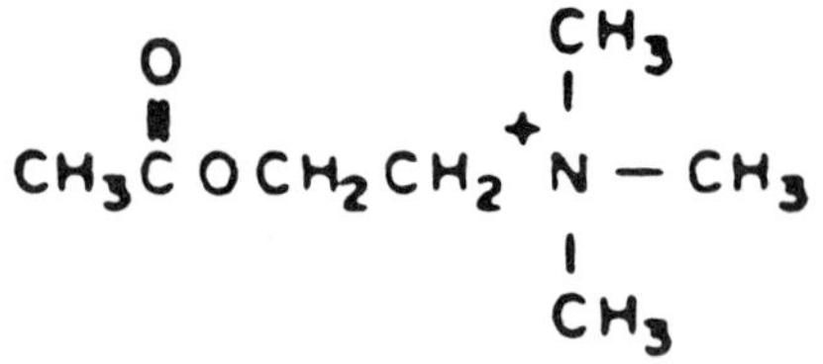

$$CH_3\overset{\overset{O}{\|}}{C}OCH_2CH_2\overset{+}{N}(CH_3)_3$$

Acetylcholine

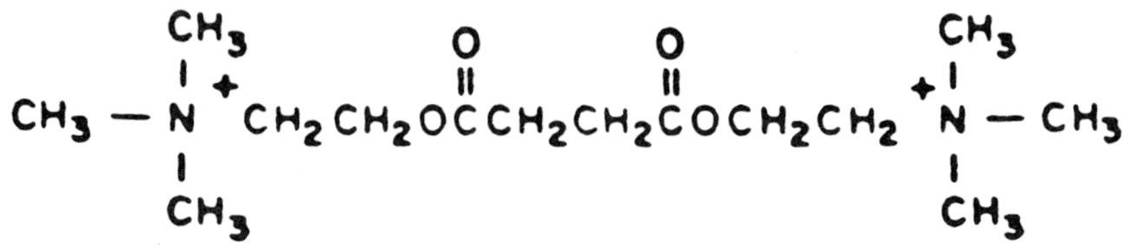

$$(CH_3)_3\overset{+}{N}CH_2CH_2O\overset{\overset{O}{\|}}{C}CH_2CH_2\overset{\overset{O}{\|}}{C}OCH_2CH_2\overset{+}{N}(CH_3)_3$$

Succinylcholine

$$(CH_3)_3\overset{+}{N}-(CH_2)_{10}-\overset{+}{N}(CH_3)_3$$

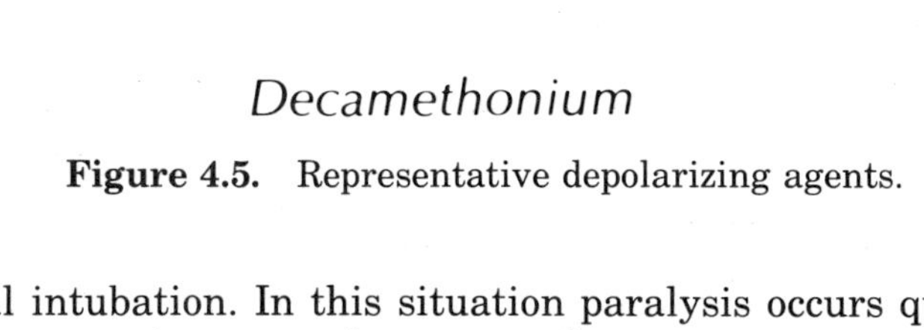

Decamethonium

Figure 4.5. Representative depolarizing agents.

tracheal intubation. In this situation paralysis occurs quickly—in less than one minute—and recovery of spontaneous respiration also is rapid, normally in less than fifteen minutes. This rapidity of offset is due to the rapid hydrolysis of succinylcholine by plasma cholinesterase. However, it is not as well appreciated that the speed of onset of action is also due to the quick hydrolysis by cholinesterase (see Fig. 4.6). Most drugs are administered in doses designed to produce systemic effects that are tolerable. Since most drugs are eliminated slowly by liver or kidney, an intravenous dose of these drugs must be

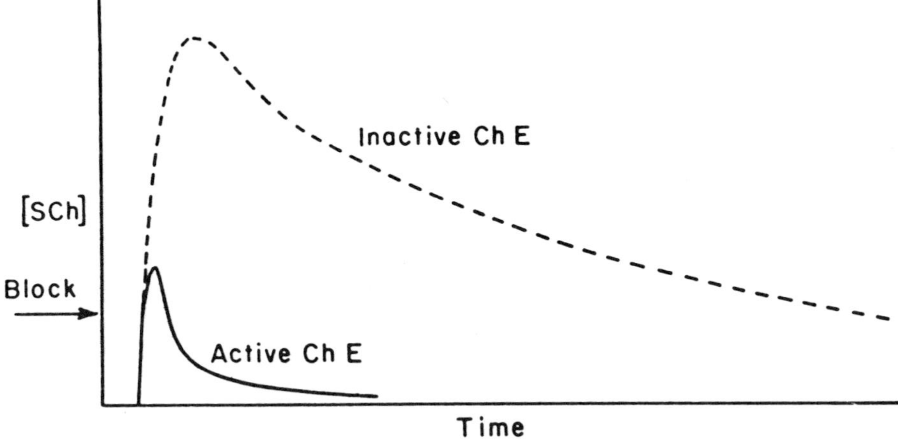

Figure 4.6.   Sketch of different concentrations of succinylcholine that can be produced at the neuromuscular junction when plasma cholinesterase is active and when it is inactive. In the latter case, drug is not destroyed in transit in the plasma and a greater amount is present in the junction for much longer than normally. Adapted from Waud.[565]

small in order not to exceed the maximum total dose tolerated by the recipient. Succinylcholine is different because the drug is rapidly delivered to the neuromuscular junction (one of the organs in the core compartment), blocks the junction quickly, and is destroyed by cholinesterase before it is delivered to most other organs. Because of this, a large dose may be given—one that will have large effects on organs that receive direct and immediate blood supply, such as the neuromuscular junction—but which will have small effect on tissues that are slowly supplied by blood and do not receive much drug in the time before hydrolysis occurs. Succinylcholine also immediately depolarizes nerve terminals, and the consequent release of acetylcholine may augment the initial action of the drug.[512] If necessary, succinylcholine may also be given intramuscularly, but the onset of action is slow (2 to 3 min). For intramuscular injection the pH of the solution is appropriate, and succinylcholine is safer by this route than some of the acidic nondepolarizing compounds.

Succinylcholine frequently is administered as a constant intravenous infusion in order to maintain the muscle relaxation needed by the surgeon,[136,541] yet to permit rapid recovery of respiration after the infusion is stopped. This system is advantageous in that the anesthetist only has to use one drug, but it is disadvantageous if a Phase II block occurs and spontaneous respiration does not appear as

rapidly as expected. The problem can be obviated by using succinylcholine to intubate, and when subsequent paralysis is needed, using a
nondepolarizing agent followed by an antagonist.

Succinylcholine, like the nondepolarizing compounds, has no anesthetic properties and cannot substitute for adequate anesthesia. The
inadequately anesthetized patient may not be able to communicate
with the physicians, but may be painfully aware of the environment
and surgical procedure.[163,347]

In addition to the effect on the muscle endplate, succinylcholine
acts at many other sites in the body to produce an array of undesired
effects. It depolarizes the motor nerve terminal and creates neural
repetitive discharges, which in turn cause fasciculations. The innoc-
uous appearance of rippling of muscle is misleading, appearing in-
nocuous only because the individual motor units are asynchronous in
their discharge. At the cellular level, a muscle cell is subjected to a
barrage of three to seven high-frequency nerve discharges and is
driven to a full, maximum tetanic contraction that may be great
enough to rip or damage muscle cells.[100,197,155] Postoperative
muscle pain is commonly observed, particularly in muscular individuals. This succinylcholine-induced muscle activity may also be great
enough to increase intra-abdominal pressure[18,307,378,394,155] and
is risky in an individual with a full stomach who may vomit. The drug
also may increase intracranial pressure and is a poor choice for
neurosurgical procedures, particularly where increased intracranial
pressure preexists or may jeopardize the patient.[238,360]

It also has been shown that succinylcholine affects intrafusal as
well as the extrafusal muscle fibers. In this case, neural discharges
course through the sensory nerves and spinal cord to repetitively
activate motoneurones and cause fasciculations.[94,413,70,492,287,159]
The fasciculatory activity can be attentuated or prevented by prior
administration of a small dose of nondepolarizing compound that
blocks the action of succinylcholine on the nerve endings[121,33,155,
188,349] (but see also Masey[350]). Unfortunately, the nondepolarizing
compound also antagonizes succinylcholine at the endplate and atten-
uates its depolarizing action there.[199,72,350] Since blockade is dependent on depolarization, the price of attenuation of fasciculations
is a less than optimal paralysis of skeletal muscle.

The rapid conversion of depolarization of the endplate to a flaccid
paralysis of skeletal muscle is due to the special geometry of skeletal
muscle and the rapid development of an accommodation blockade in
the muscle. Other targets of succinylcholine do not have this special
geometry. Particularly important is denervated muscle which makes

and inserts extrajunctional receptors all over its surface.[165,179] These extrajunctional receptors respond to succinylcholine by allowing potassium to leave the cell. Since there is no geometry to produce accommodation block, the discharge of potassium may persist; if a large enough surface of muscle is involved, the discharge may be sufficient to produce hyperkalemia and serious cardiac ventricular dysrhythmias.[533,550,227,498,186,331] Muscle contractures may also develop. Since the extrajunctional receptors are sensitive to agonists but much more resistant to antagonists than endplate receptors, attempted prophylaxis or therapy with a nondepolarizing compound reduces but does not prevent the drug-induced hyperkalemia.[550]

Succinylcholine increases intraocular pressure[2,54,257,155] and is contraindicated for surgery on eye injuries or where an elevation of intraocular pressure may be injurious. The mechanism is not fully known, but probably involves a change in fluid dynamics as well as contraction of the extraocular muscles to compress the eye against the orbit. The latter is especially interesting since the extraocular muscles differ from other skeletal muscle and are especially affected by agonists. Mixed among the ordinary striated muscle cells are bands of unique muscle cells, tonic fibers, that have several neuromuscular junctions per cell and a total sarcolemmal surface that is chemically sensitive. They do not undergo accommodation blockade and flaccid paralysis, but instead are driven to prolonged slow but strong contractures that shorten the muscle and compress the eye.[162,155]

Succinylcholine is less specific for neuromuscular junctions than the nondepolarizing compounds; it depolarizes peripheral nerves that are not protected by myelin and acts at nicotinic receptors of postganglionic sympathetic nerve endings.[401] As a result, norepinephrine is discharged, and cardiac dysrhythmias and alterations in blood pressure or heart rate are common.

Despite the disadvantages of succinylcholine in terms of unwanted effects and the possibility of engendering a Phase II blockade, succinylcholine remains the favorite drug among practitioners, primarily because of its speed of action. Because of the unique elimination mechanism for succinylcholine, it is possible to give the drug rapidly and in large doses to produce an immediate, but short-lived muscle paralysis. However, this advantage may be lost when the patient is one of the few who do not have normal esterase, is receiving other drugs that incidentally inhibit serum cholinesterase, or receives the drug long enough to develop a Phase II blockade.[319,155] Genetic absence of normal serum cholinesterase can be predicted from genetic family studies or detected by relatively simple laboratory procedures. Genetic or laboratory studies are in order when there is reason to suggest an individual is at risk, but since the genetic inability to hydrolyze succinylcholine is so rare, it is not economically practical to test everyone who will receive anesthesia. Since prolonged apnea and the corresponding need for assisted ventilation are the consequence of failure of hydrolysis, cautious observation and, if needed, continued ventilatory assistance and anesthesia usually are adequate to deal with such problems as might occur.[559,560,573,405,409]

It is not usually recognized that serum cholinesterase is subject to inhibition by a great many drugs and chemicals with a diversity of chemical structures. In addition, the pharmacodynamics of succinylcholine can also be altered, with paralysis extended by as much as 30 minutes to several hours when anticholinesterase agents, i.e., pyridostigmine[34] or neostigmine[34,415,536] are given prior to the depolarizing relaxant. Drugs that are not expected to have neuromuscular actions but have been reported to interact with consequent prolongation of succinylcholine paralysis include codeine, morphine, serotonin, epinephrine, LSD, procaine, phenelzine, trimethaphan, hexafluorenium, chlorpromazine, imipramine, and reserpine.[507] The primary effect of an interaction is slowed elimination of succinylcholine, with more powerful and longerlasting effects of the drug. However, only a major degree of enzyme inhibition would be clinically significant, since the duration of respiratory paralysis seems little influenced by plasma levels of serum cholinesterase unless there is 80% or more inhibition.[196]

Decamethonium resembles succinylcholine in that it is an agonist with ten atoms between the quaternary ammonium groups, but since it does not have ester links, decamethonium is not hydrolyzed. Therefore, decamethonium has the disadvantages of succinylcholine, but without the offsetting advantage of a short duration of action, and is rarely used in modern anesthetic practice. Decamethonium acts as an agonist at nicotinic receptors but is capable of blocking ion channels at both neuromuscular junctions[5,379] and ganglionic synapses.[21] It also penetrates the muscle and may be found in the sarcoplasm.[544,113] The neuromuscular blockade produced by decamethonium is long-lasting and usually cannot be reversed by anticholinesterases, either in the early or late stages. However, like other agonists, the action of the drug is complex and poorly understood, and there may be a period in the midpoint of the drug action where anticholinesterases are effective in producing a return of neuromuscular transmission.

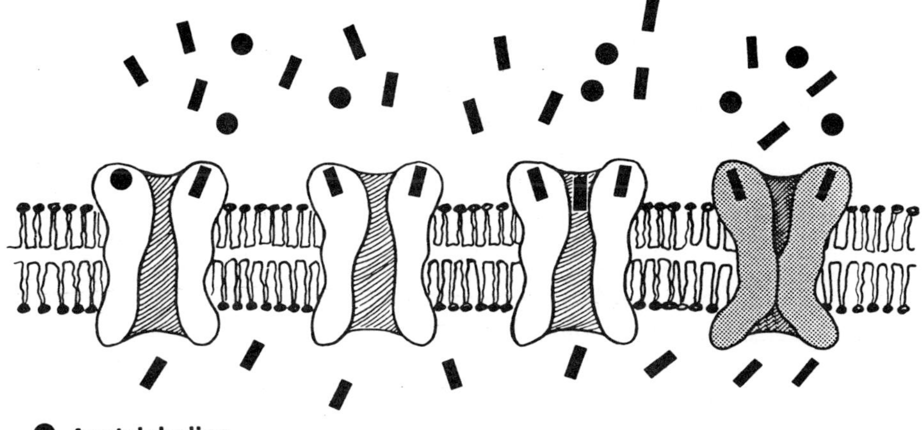

Figure 4.7. Sketch of sites of action of the depolarizing relaxant decamethonium.

Other slender agonist molecules, nicotine, carbachol, and suberyldicholine, an analog of succinylcholine, open receptor channels; but in high concentrations suberyldicholine,[5,3] carbachol, and nicotine[3] enter open channels to block current flow in voltage-clamped muscle membrane. Eldefrawi[168] found decamethonium fifteen times more potent as nicotine in competing for intrachannel binding sites with known channel blocking drugs. Succinylcholine was weakly competitive, causing a greater inhibition of receptor channel permeability by converting receptors to the desensitized state in a voltage-independent manner.[168]

Many attempts have been made to synthesize compounds that would have the speed of action of succinylcholine and the specificity of action of nondepolarizing agents.[466,120] Several nondepolarizing compounds that are hydrolyzed like succinylcholine have emerged from the laboratory, but none have survived to marketability. Although the new nondepolarizing compounds, vecuronium and atracurium, are more rapidly eliminated, and hence are faster and shorter acting than the older agents, they are not as rapidly destroyed as succinylcholine. While the new compounds may replace succinylcholine in some clinical circumstances, they are not likely to replace it entirely.

Anticholinesterases

The commonly used synthetic carbamate anticholinesterases, neostigmine and pyridostigmine, are structurally related to the natural product, physostigmine. Edrophonium is essentially a hydrolysis product of neostigmine (Fig. 4.8). They are similar in their effects, but are different in some ways that affect their use. Physostigmine, a naturally occurring carbamate, is not a quaternary amine. It is true that physostigmine ionizes at biologic pH to acquire a proton and quaternary status, but in its nonionized form it is readily capable of penetrating biologic membranes. This means that it is readily ab-

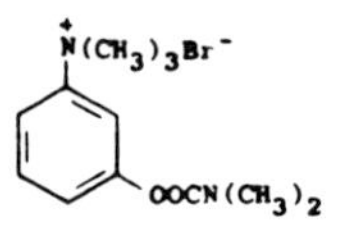

Neostigmine

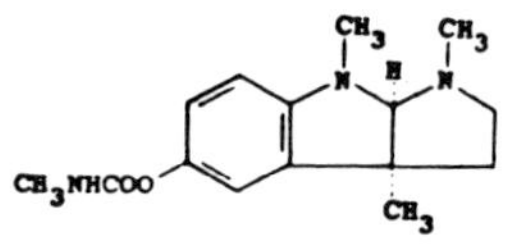

Physostigmine

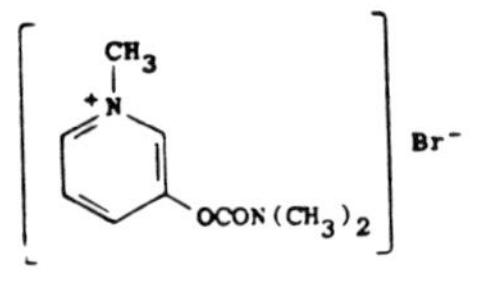

Pyridostigmine

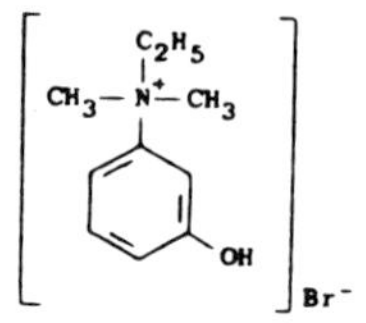

Edrophonium

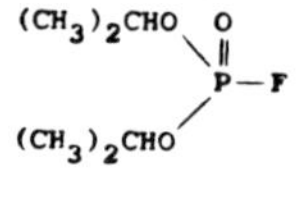

DFP

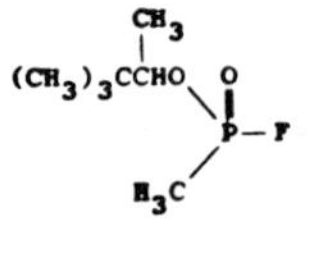

Soman

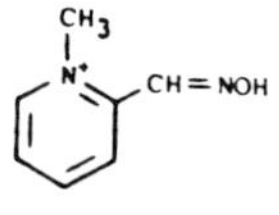

2 PAM

Figure 4.8.   Representative acetylcholinesterase inhibitors and a reactivator.

sorbed from the gastrointestinal tract and, most importantly, it crosses the blood brain barrier. Thus, its use is associated with strong excitation of the central nervous system. This property is useful when there is a need to increase cholinergic activity in the brain, as in cases of poisoning by atropine, antidepressants or other anticholinergic substances, but the central nervous system action may be deleterious when the need for inhibition of cholinesterase exists mainly in the periphery, as in myasthenia gravis and the antagonism of muscle paralysis by neuromuscular blocking drugs.

The commonly used cholinesterase inhibitors are said to act to prolong acetylcholine by slowing its destruction in the synaptic cleft, and giving it a competitive advantage over *d*-tubocurarine and related drugs in competing for the cholinergic receptor. In a similar manner, these drugs have found use in the treatment of myasthenia gravis where inhibition of enzyme would augment the action of acetylcholine and increase its effectiveness at the damaged endplate (see Chapter 6). However, there is substantial evidence that these compounds also act on the nerve ending to increase its activity and augment the release of transmitter.

The three quarternary compounds are similar clinically and resemble each other except for detail. As mentioned previously, pyridostigmine and neostigmine inhibit acetylcholinesterase by carbamylating the active site of the enzyme; the carbamylated product is the same no matter which parent compound is involved. Edrophonium forms an electrostatic attraction with the anionic site of the enzyme. Edrophonium reacts more quickly than its analogues and is suitable for administration in diagnostic tests of neuromuscular function in myasthenia gravis. The termination of action is due to redistribution of the initial bolus of the drug throughout the body such that the synaptic concentration quickly drops below threshold for action. If edrophonium is given more slowly, and in a greater amount, the duration of action depends on elimination from the body instead of redistribution and in this respect it is similar to pyridostigmine and perhaps longer lasting than neostigmine: beta $t_{1/2}$ (minutes) = 110 for edrophonium; 80 for neostigmine; and 112 for pyridostigmine.[117] Both carbamates, neostigmine and pyridostigmine, are metabolized by the liver,[117] but in normal individuals this metabolism is slow and renal elimination of the unchanged molecule is the primary process for removing the drugs.[521]

Although all the compounds can inhibit synaptic acetylcholinesterase and therefore would be presumed to have equivalent effects, there is reported to be a difference among them in their predilection for other autonomic synapses and in their undesired actions when used to enhance neuromuscular transmission. The actions of physostigmine on the central nervous system and the absence of these actions in its quaternary derivatives has already been remarked upon. Among the other three, neostigmine is reported to be most likely, and edrophonium the least likely, to produce troublesome effects via the muscarinic acetylcholine receptor systems of the heart, gut and bronchial tree.[25,117] Perhaps the difference among them is due to the more direct depolarizing action of neostigmine because of its trimethylated quaternary nitrogen. Nonetheless, all of the muscarinic actions can be prevented or terminated by adequate doses of an antimuscarinic such as atropine. Since atropine easily penetrates the central nervous system, a synthetic quaternary ammonium analog of atropine such as glycopyrrolate may be more useful, except when dealing with physostigmine, to specifically offset peripheral signs and symptoms of cholinesterase blockade.[237,406,111,23]

Among the organophosphates, only echothiophate is used clinically and only then for certain ophthalmologic disorders such as glaucoma and certain esotropias that can be improved by prolonged activation of cholinergic systems. Usually the effects of the topical therapy are restricted to the eyes, but occasionally enough of the drug can be absorbed to cause systemic problems, usually involving inhibition of plasma cholinesterase, and so becoming apparent in patients given succinylcholine. Rarely, enough echothiophate is absorbed to produce systemic poisoning.

In contrast to the limited clinical use of organophosphates is the vast agricultural and military use. Large quantities of these compounds are used as insecticides on farms and in buildings and homes. Usually the specific compound and means of use are chosen to limit any hazard to human beings, but accidental exposures occur and sometimes result in death. The world's military establishments have stocked the most lethal of the organophosphates as "nerve gases" since early in World War II.[366] The quantities stored around the world are huge and the lethal potential is enormous, particularly since the chosen materials, especially soman (the Soviet nerve gas of choice), are resistant to therapy by enzyme regenerating agents such as oximes. Even though the muscarinic effects of these "nerve gases" might theoretically be countered by adequate doses of atropine, paralysis of the neuromuscular junction and actions in the central nervous system would be fatal.

References

1. Abou-Donia MB: Organophosphorus ester-induced delayed neurotoxicity. *Ann Rev Pharmacol Toxicol* 21:511–548, 1981.
2. Adams AK, Barnett KC: Anaesthesia and intraocular pressure. *Anaesthesia* 21:202–210, 1966.
3. Adams DJ. Colquhoun D: Current relaxations with high agonist concentration. Do acetylcholine and suberyldicholine block ion channels in frog muscles? *J Physiol* 341:22P–23P, 1983.
4. Adams DJ, Dwyer TM, Hille B: The permeability of endplate channels to monovalent and divalent metal cations. *J Gen Physiol* 75:493–510, 1980.
5. Adams PR, Sakmann B: Decamethonium both opens and blocks endplate channels. *Proc Natl Acad Sci USA* 75:2994–2998, 1978.
6. Adams PR: Acetylcholine receptor kinetics. *J Membr Biol* 58:161–174, 1981.
7. Adams PR: Ion movements in endplate channels. *Brain Res Bull* 4: 147–149, 1979.
8. Adams PR: Voltage jump analysis of procaine action at frog endplate. *J Physiol* 268:291–318, 1977.
9. Adler M, Oliveira AC, Albuquerque EX, Mansour NA. Eldefrawi AT: Reaction of tetraethylammonium with the open and closed conformations of the acetylcholine receptor ionic channel complex. *J Gen Physiol* 74:129–152, 1979.
10. Agoston GA,Vermeer GA, Kersten UW, Meijer DKF: The fate of pancuronium bromide in man. *Acta Anaesth Scand* 17:267–275, 1973.
11. Agoston S, Vermeer GA, Kersten UW, Scaf AHJ: A preliminary investigation of the renal and hepatic excretion of gallamine triethiodide in man. *Br J Anaesth* 50:345, 1978.
12. Aizenman E, Millington WR, Zarbin MA, Bierkamper GG: ^{125}I-α-bungarotoxin binding sites undergo axonal transport in rat sciatic nerve. *Fed Proc* 42:1147, 1983.
13. Albuquerque EX, Tsai MC, Aronstam RS, Eldefrawi AT, Eldefrawi ME: Sites of action of phencyclidine II. Interaction with the ionic channel of the nicotinic receptor. *Mol Pharmacol* 18:167–178, 1980.
14. Alderson AM, MacLagan J: The action of decamethonium and tubocurarine on the respiratory and limb muscles of the cat. *J Physiol* 173: 38–56, 1964.
15. Aldridge WN, Barnes JM, Johnson MK: Studies on delayed neurotoxicity produced by some organophosphorus compounds. *Ann NY Acad Sci* 160:314–322, 1969.
16. Ali HH, Savarese JJ: Stimulus frequency and dose-response curve to *d*-tubocurarine in man. *Anesthesiology* 52:36–39, 1980.
17. Anwyal R, Narahashi T: Desensitization of the acetylcholine receptor of denervated rat soleus muscle and the effect of calcium. *Br J Pharmacol* 69:91–98, 1980.
18. Andersen N: Changes in intragastric pressure following the administration of suxamethonium. *Br J Anaesth* 34:363–367, 1962.

19. Antonio RP, Philbin DM, Savarese JJ: Comparative hemodynamic effects of *d*-tubocurarine and metacurarine in the dog. *Anesthesiology* 51:S281, 1979.
20. Armstrong C: Inactivation of the potassium conductance and related phenomena caused by quaternary ammonium ion injected in squid axons. *J Gen Physiol* 54:519–535, 1976.
21. Ascher P, Large WA, Rang HP: Studies on the mechanism of action of acetylcholine antagonist on rat parasympathetic ganglion cells. *J Physiol* 295:139–170, 1979.
22. Atwood HL, Charlton MP, Thompson CS: Neuromuscular transmission in crustaceans is enhanced by sodium ionophore, monensin, and by prolonged stimulation. *J Physiol* 335:179–196, 1983.
23. Azar I, Pham AN, Karambelkar DJ, Lear E: The heart rate following edrophonium-atropine and edrophonium-glycopyrrolate mixtures. *Anesthesiology* 59:139–141, 1983.
24. Bacou F, Vigneron P, Massoulie J: Acetylcholinesterase forms in fast and slow rabbit muscle. *Nature* 296:661–664, 1982.
25. Baird WLM, Bowman WC, Kerr WJ: Some actions of ORG 45 and of edrophonium in the anaesthetized cat and in man. *Br J Anaesth* 54: 375–385, 1982.
26. Bakry NM, Eldefrawi AT, Eldefrawi ME, Riker WF: Interactions of quaternary ammonium drugs with acetylcholinesterase and acetylcholine receptors of Torpedo electric organ. *Molec Pharmacol* 22: 63–71, 1982.
27. Bali IM, Dundee JW, Assaf RAS: Immediate changes in plasma potassium, sodium and chloride concentrations induced by suxamethonium. *Br J Anaesth* 47:393–397, 1981.
28. Barnes PK, Brindel Smith G, White WD, Tennant R: Comparison of the effect of ORG NC45 and pancuronium bromide on heart rate and arterial pressure in anaesthetized man. *Br J Anaesth* 54:435–439, 1982.
29. Barton SB, Cohen IS, van der Kloot W: The calcium dependence of spontaneous and evoked quantal release at the frog neuromuscular junction. *J Physiol* 337:735–751, 1983.
30. Basta SJ, Ali HH, Savarese JJ, Sunder N, Gionfriddo M, Cloutier G, Lineberry C, Cato AE: Clinical pharmacology of atracurium besylate (BW 33A): A new non-depolarizing muscle relaxant. *Anesth Analg* 61:723–729, 1982.
31. Beach RL, Vaca K, Pilar G: Ionic and metabolic requirements for high affinity choline uptake and acetylcholine synthesis in nerve terminals at a neuromuscular junction. *J Neurochem* 34:1387–1398, 1980.
32. Beani L, Bianchi C, Ledda F: The effect of tubocurarine on acetylcholine release from motor nerve terminals. *J Physiol* 174:172–183, 1964.
33. Bennetts FE, Khalil KI: Reduction of post-suxamethonium pain by pretreatment with four non-depolarizing agents. *Br J Anaesth* 53: 531–536, 1981.
34. Bentz EW, Stoelting RK: Prolonged response to succinylcholine following pancuronium reversal with pyridostigmine. *Anesthesiology* 44: 258–260, 1976.
35. Berends F, Posthumas CH, Van der Sheys I, Deirhauf FA: The chemical basis of the "aging process" of DFP-inhibited pseudocholinesterase. *Biochem Biophys Acta* 34:576–578, 1958.

36. Bernard C: Analyse physiologique des propriétés des systemes musculaire et nerveux au moyen du curare. *C R Acad Sci* (Paris) 43:825–829, 1856.
37. Bevan DR: Reversal of pancuronium with edrophonium. *Anesthesia* 34:614–619, 1979.
38. Bevan S, Steinbach JH: Denervation increases the degradation rate of endplates in vivo and in vitro. *J Physiol* 336:159–177, 1983.
39. Bever CT, Chang WH, Penn AS, Jaffe IA, Bock E: Penicillamine-induced myasthenia gravis: Effects of penicillamine on acetylcholine receptor. *Neurology* 32:1077–1082, 1982.
40. Bierkamper GG, Goldberg AM: Release of acetylcholine from the isolated perfused diaphragm. In Hanin I, Goldberg Am (eds): *Progress in Cholinergic Biology: Model Cholinergic Synapses.* New York, Raven Press, 1982, pp 113–137.
41. Bierkamper GG, Millington WR: Physostigmine and *d*-tubocurarine have presynaptic actions at the neuromuscular junction. *Soc Neurosci Abstr* 8:495, 1982.
42. Binder N, Landon EJ, Wecker L, Dettbarn W-D: Effect of parathion and its metabolites on calcium uptake activity of rat skeletal muscle sarcoplasmic reticulum in vitro. *Biochem Pharmacol* 25:835–839, 1975.
43. Birmingham AT, Hussain SZ: A comparison of the skeletal neuromuscular and autonomic ganglion-blocking potencies of five non-depolarizing relaxants. *Br J Pharmacol* 70:501–506, 1980.
44. Blaber LC, Bowman WC: The effects of some drugs on the repetitive discharges produced in nerve and muscle by anticholinesterases. *Int J Neuropharmacol* 6:473–484, 1967.
45. Blaber LC, Gallagher JP: The facilitatory effects of catechol and phenol at the neuromuscular junction of the cat. *Neuropharmacol* 10:153–159, 1971.
46. Blaber LC: The prejunctional action of some non-depolarizing blocking drugs. *Br J Pharmacol* 47:109–116, 1973.
47. Blackman JG, Gauldie RW, Milne RJ: Interaction of competitive antagonist: The anti-curare action of hexamethonium and other antagonists at the skeletal neuromuscular junction. *Br J Pharmacol* 54:91–100, 1975.
48. Blackman JG: Stimulus frequency and neuromuscular block. *Br J Pharmacol Chemother* 20:5–16, 1963.
49. Blake GJ, Dretchen KL: Quantal release in cut muscle: Effects of limited calcium availability. *Life Sci* 27:2535–2540, 1980.
50. Blaustein MP, Ickowicz RK: Phencyclidine in nanomolar concentrations binds to synaptosomes and blocks certain potassium channels. *Proc Natl Acad Sci USA* 80:3855–3859, 1983.
51. Booij LHDJ, Edwards RP, Sohn YJ, Miller RD: Cardiovascular and neuromuscular effects of Org NC45, pancuronium, metacurarine, and *d*-tubocurarine in dogs. *Anesth Analg* 59:26–34, 1980.
52. Boskovic B, Tadic V, Kusic R: Reactivating and protective effects of Pro-2-PAM in mice poisoned with paraoxon. *Tox Appl Pharmacol* 55:32–36, 1980.
53. Bostock H, Sears TA, Sherratt RM: The effects of 4-aminopyridine and tetraethylammonium ions on normal and demyelinated mammalian nerve fibres. *J Physiol* 313:301–315, 1981.

54. Bowen DJ, McGrand JC, Hamilton AG: Intraocular pressure after suxamethonium and endotracheal intubation. *Anaesthesia* 33: 518–522, 1978.
55. Bowman WC, Harvey AL, Marshall IG: The actions of aminopyridines on avian muscle. *Naunyn-Schmiedeberg's Arch Pharmacol* 297: 99–103, 1977.
56. Bowman WC, Norman J (ed): Symposium on ORG NC 45. *Br J Anaesth* 52: 1S–72S, 1980.
57. Bowman WC, Nott MW: Actions of sympathomimetic amines and their antagonists on skeletal muscle. *Pharmacol Rev* 21:27–72, 1969.
58. Bowman WC, Savage AO: Pharmacological actions of aminopyridines. *Rev Pure Appl Pharmacol Sci* 2:317–369, 1981.
59. Bowman WC, Webb SN: Tetanic-fade during partial transmission failure produced by non-depolarizing neuromuscular blocking drugs in the cat. *Clin Exp Pharmacol Physiol* 3:545–555, 1976.
60. Bowman WC: Non-relaxant properties of neuromuscular blocking drugs. *Br J Anaesth* 54:147–160, 1982.
61. Bowman WC: *Pharmacology of the Neuromuscular Junction*. Bristol, John Wright Sons, 1980, pp 71–121.
62. Bowman WC: Prejunctional and postjunctional cholinoceptors at the neuromuscular junction. *Anesth Analg* 59:935–943, 1980.
63. Boyd IA, Martin AR: Spontaneous subthreshold activity at mammalian neuromuscular junctions. *J Physiol* 132:61–73, 1956.
64. Braswell LM, Miller KW, Sauter JF: Differential effects of nonspecific pertubers on the acetylcholine receptor from *Torpedo* and its ionophore. *Br J Pharmacol* 73:187P–188P, 1981.
65. Braswell LM, Miller KW: A binding site of pentobarbitone on cholinergic membrane from *Torpedo californica*. *Br J Pharmacol* 75S:171P, 1982.
66. Bray JJ, Forrest JW, Hubbard JI: Evidence for the role of non-quantal acetylcholine in the maintenance of the membrane potential of rat skeletal muscle. *J Physiol* 326:285–296, 1982.
67. Bregestovski PD, Miledi R, Parker I: Blocking of frog endplate channels by the organic calcium antagonist D600. *Proc R Soc London Ser B* 211:15–24, 1980.
68. Brenner HR, Sakmann B: Neurotrophic control of channel properties at neuromuscular synapses of rat muscle. *J Physiol* 337: 159–171, 1983.
69. Brigant JL, Mallard A: Presynaptic currents in mouse motor endings. *J Physiol* 333:619–636, 1982.
70. Brinling JC, Smith CM: A characteristic of the stimulation of mammalian muscle spindles by succinylcholine. *J Pharmacol Exp Ther* 129: 56–60, 1960.
71. Briscoe G: Selective action of small doses of curarine for certain rates and strengths of stimulation. *J Physiol* 84:43P–44P, 1935.
72. Brodsky JB, Brock-Utne JG, Samuels SI: Pancuronium pretreatment and postsuccinylcholine myalgias. *Anesthesiology* 51:259–261, 1979.
73. Brown BR, Crout JR: The sympathomimetic effects of gallamine on the heart. *J Pharmacol Exp Ther* 172:266–273, 1970.

74. Brown MC, Hopkins WG, Keynes RJ: Comparison of effects of denervated and botulinum toxin paralysis on muscle properties in mice. *J Physiol* 327:29–37, 1982.

75. Brown RD, Taylor P: The influence of antibiotics on agonist occupation and functional states of the nicotinic acetylcholine receptor. *Molec Pharmacol* 23:8–16, 1983.

76. Bullock JO, Farquharson DA, Hoskin FCG: Soman and receptor-ligand interaction in electrophorus electroplaques. *Biochem Pharmacol* 26:337–343, 1977.

77. Burley BT: Polyneuritis from tricresylphosphate. *JAMA* 98:298–304, 1932.

78. Burley ES, Jacobs RS: Effects of 4-aminopyridine on nerve terminal action potentials. *J Pharmacol Exp Ther* 219:268–272, 1981.

79. Burns B, Paton WDM: Depolarization of the motor end-plate by decamethonium and acetylcholine. *J Physiol* 115:41–73, 1951.

80. Burnstock G: Purinergic modulation of cholinergic transmission. *Gen Pharmacol* 11:15–18, 1980.

81. Cahalan M: Molecular properties of sodium channels in excitable membranes. *Cell Surface Rev* 6:1–47, 1980.

82. Carney L, Gundfest S: Excitability membrane stabilization by diphenylhydantoin and calcium. *Neuropharmacol* 13:1097–1108, 1974.

83. Carp JS, Aronstam RS, Witkop B, Albuquerque EX: Electrophysiological and biochemical studies on enhancement of desensitization by phenothiazine neuroleptics. *Proc Nat Acad Sci USA* 80:310–314, 1983.

84. Carter FG, Sokoll MD, Gergis SD: Effect of spinal cord transection on neuromuscular function in the rat. *Anesthesiology* 55:542–546, 1981.

85. Catterall WA: Inhibition of voltage-sensitive sodium channels in neuroblastoma cells by antiarrhythmic drugs. *Molec Pharmacol* 20:356–362, 1981.

86. Ceccarelli B, Grohavaz F, Hurlbut WP, Iezzi N: Freeze-fracture studies of frog neuromuscular junction during intense release of neurotransmitter. I. Effects of black widow spider venom and Ca-free solutions on the structure of the active zone. *J Cell Biol* 81:163–177, 1979.

87. Ceccarelli B, Hurlbut WP: Calcium-dependent recycling of synaptic vesicles at the frog neuromuscular junction. *J Cell Biol* 87:297–303, 1980.

88. Ceccarelli B, Hurlbut WP: Vesicle hypothesis of the release of quanta of acetylcholine. *Physiol Rev* 60:396–441, 1980.

89. Chang CC, Chuang ST, Huang MC: Effects of chronic treatment with various neuromuscular blocking agents on the number and distribution of acetylcholine receptors in the rat diaphragm. *J Physiol* 250:161–173, 1975.

90. Chang HT: Similarity in action between curare and strychnine on cortical neurons. *J Neurophysiol* 16:221–233, 1953.

91. Chang RSL, Potter LT, Smith DS: Postsynaptic membranes in the electric tissue of Narcine: IV. Isolation and characterization of the nicotinic receptor protein. *Tiss Cell* 9:623–644, 1977.

92. Chapple DJ, Clark JS: Pharmacological action of breakdown products of atracurium and related substances. *Br J Anaesth* 55:11S–16S, 1983.

93. Chestnut TJ: Two-component desensitization at the neuromuscular junction of the frog. *J Physiol* 336:229–241, 1983.
94. Churchill-Davison HC: Suxamethonium (succinylcholine) chloride and muscle pains. *Br Med J* 1:74–75, 1954.
95. Clement JG: Toxicology and pharmacology of bispyridinium aldoximes. Insight into the mechanism of action vs soman poisoning in vivo. *Fundam Appl Toxicol* 1:193–202, 1981.
96. Close RI: Dynamic properties of mammalian skeletal muscles. *Physiol Rev* 52:129–197, 1972.
97. Clothier B, Johnson MK: Rapid aging of neurotoxic esterase after inhibition by di-isopropyl phosphorofluoridate. *Biochem J* 177:549–558, 1979.
98. Codding PW, James MNG: The crystal and molecular structure of a potent neuromuscular blocking agent: d-tubocurarine dicholoride pentahydrate. *Acta Crystallogr* 29B:935–954, 1973.
99. Coleman AJ, Downing JW, Leary WP, Styles M: The immediate cardiovascular effects of pancuronium, alcuronium, and tubocurarine in man. *Anaesthesia* 27:415–422, 1972.
100. Collier C: Suxamethonium pains and fasciculations. *Proc R Soc Med* 68:105–108, 1975.
101. Colquhoun D, Dreyer F, Sheridan RE: The actions of tubocurarine at the frog neuromuscular junction. *J Physiol* 293:247–284, 1979.

102. Colquhoun D, Sheridan RE: Kinetic effects of tubocurarine on skeletal muscle at high agonist concentrations. *Br J Pharmacol* 68:143P–144P, 1980.
103. Colquhoun D, Sheridan RE: Modes of action of gallamine at the neuromuscular junction. *Br J Pharmacol* 66:78P–79P, 1979.
104. Colquhoun D, Sheridan RE: The effect of tubocurarine competition on the kinetics of agonist action on the nicotinic receptor. *Br J Pharmacol* 75:77–86, 1982.
105. Colquhoun D, Sheridan RE: The modes of action of gallamine. *Proc R Soc London Ser B* 211:181–203, 1981.
106. Colquhoun D: Competitive block and ion channel as mechanisms of antagonist action on the skeletal muscle endplate. *Adv Psychopharmacol* 21:67–80, 1980.
107. Colquhoun D: The kinetics of conductance changes at nicotinic receptors of the muscle endplate and of ganglia. In *Drug Receptors and Their Effectors*. London, Macmillan, 1981, pp 107–126.
108. Cooperman IH: Succinylcholine-induced hyperkalemia in neuromuscular disease. *JAMA* 213:1867–1871, 1970.
109. Courtney KR, Kendig JT, Cohen EN: Frequency dependent conduction block: The role of nerve impulse patterns in local anesthetic potency. *Anesthesiology* 48:111–117, 1978.
110. Couteaux R: Structure of the subsynaptic sarcoplasm in the interfolds of the frog neuromuscular junction. *J Neurocytol* 10:947–962, 1981.
111. Cozanitis DA, Dundee JW, Merrett JD, Jones CJ, Mirakhur RK: Evaluation of glycopyrrolate and atropine as adjuncts to reversal of nondepolarizing neuromuscular blocking agents in a "true-to-life" situation. *Br J Anaesth* 52:85–89, 1980.

112. Creese R, Humphrey PPA, Mitchell LD: Recovery from decamethonium in rat muscle and denervated guinea-pig diaphragm. *J Physiol* 334:365–377, 1983.
113. Creese R, MacLagan J: Autoradiography of decamethonium in rat muscle. *Nature* (London) 215:988–989, 1967.
114. Creese R, MacLagan J: Entry of decamethonium in rat muscle studied by autoradiography. *J Physiol* 210:363–386, 1970.
115. Creese R, MacLagan J: Labelled decamethonium in cat muscle. *Br J Pharmacol* 58:141–148, 1976.
116. Cronnelly R, Fisher DM, Miller RD, Gencarelli P, Nguyen-Gruenke L, Castagnoli N: Pharmacokinetics and pharmacodynamics of vercuronium (ORG NC45) and pancuronium in anesthetized humans. *Anesthesiology* 58:405–408, 1983.
117. Cronnelly R, Morris RB: Antagonism of neuromuscular blockade. *Br J Anaesth* 54:183–194, 1982.
118. Cronnelly R, Stanski DR, Miller RD, Sheiner LB, Sohn YJ: Renal function and the pharmacokinetics of neostigmine in anesthetized man. *Anesthesiology* 51:222–226, 1979.
119. Cronnelly R, Stanski DR, Miller RD, Sheiner LB: Pyridostigmine kinetics with and without renal function. *Clin Pharmacol Ther* 28:78–81, 1980.
120. Crul JF: Relaxant drugs: From native drugs to the selective agents of today. *Acta Anaesth Scand* 26:409–415, 1982.
121. Cullen DJ: The effect of pretreatment with nondepolarizing muscle relaxants on the neuromuscular blocking action of succinylcholine. *Anesthesiology* 35:572–578, 1971.
122. Cummings MF, Russell WJ, Frewin DB: Effects of pancuronium and alcuronium on the changes in arterial pressure and plasma catecholamine concentrations during tracheal intubation. *Br J Anaesth* 55:619–623, 1983.
123. Curley WH, Dretchen KL, Standaert FG: Inhibition by physostigmine of neural phosphodiesterase. *Fed Proc* 39:410, 1980.
124. Curley WH, Standaert FG, Dretchen KL: Physostigmine inhibition of 3′-5′-cAMP phosphodiesterase from cat sciatic nerve. *J Pharmacol Exp Ther* (in press).
125. D'Hollander AA, Agoston S, DeVille A, Cuvelier F: Clinical and pharmacological actions of a bolus injection of suxamethonium: Two phenomena of distinct duration. *Br J Anaesth* 55:131–134, 1983.
126. D'Hollander AA, Camu F, Sanders M: Comparative evaluation of neuromuscular blockade after pancuronium administration in patients with and without renal failure. *Acta Anaesth Scand* 22:21–26, 1978.
127. D'Hollander AA, Luyckx C, Barvais L, DeVille A: Clinical evaluation of atracurium besylate requirement for a stable muscle relaxation during surgery. Lack of age-related effects. *Anesthesiology* 59:237–240, 1983.
128. Das M, Ganguly DK, Vedasiromoni JR: Enhancement by oxotremorine of acetylcholine release from the rat phrenic nerve. *Br J Pharmacol* 62:195–198, 1978.
129. David CJF, Montgomery A: The effect of prolonged inactivity upon the contraction characteristics of fast and slow mammalian twitch muscle. *J Physiol* 270:581–594, 1977.

130. Davis CS, Richardson RJ: Organophosphorus compounds. In Spencer PS, Schaunberg HH (eds): *Experimental and Clinical Neurotoxicology.* Baltimore, Williams and Wilkins, 1980, pp 527–544.

131. Day NS, Blake GJ, Standaert FG, Dretchen K: Characteristics of the train-of-four response in fast and slow muscles: Effect of *d*-tubocurarine, pancuronium, and vercuronium. *Anesthesiology* 58:414–417, 1983.

132. De Jong LPA, Wolring GZ: Reaction of acetylcholinesterase inhibited by 1, 2, 2′-trimethylpropyl methylphosphonofluoridate (Soman) with HI-6 and related oximes. *Biochem Pharmacol* 29:2379–2387, 1980.

133. DeLorenzo RJ: Phenytoin: Calcium- and calmodulin-dependent protein phosphorylation and neurotransmitter release. *Adv Neurol* 27: 399–414, 1980.

134. DeWeer P: Antiepileptic drugs. Phenytoin blockage of resting sodium channels. *Adv Neurology* 27:353–361, 1980.

135. DeWeer P, Greduldig D: Electrogenic sodium pump in squid axons. *Science* 79:1326–1328, 1973.

136. Delisle S, Lebrun M, Bevan DR: Plasma cholinesterase activity and tachyphylaxis during prolonged succinylcholine infusion. *Anesth Analg* (Cleveland) 61:941–944, 1982.

137. Derache R: The toxicity of organophosphorus compounds in man. In *Organophosphorus Pesticides: Criteria (Dose/Effect) Relationship for Organophosphorus Pesticides.* Commission of the European Communities. Oxford, Pergamon Press, 1979, pp 87–98.

138. Desmedt JE, Hainaut K: Dantrolene and A23187 ionophore: Specific action on calcium channels revealed by acquorin method. *Biochem Pharmacol* 28:957–964, 1979.

139. Dionne VE, Parsons RL: Characteristics of the acetylcholine-operated channel in twitch and slow fiber neuromuscular junction of the garter snake. *J Physiol* 310:145–158, 1981.

140. Dionne VE: Acetylcholine receptor kinetics at slow fiber neuromuscular junctions. *Fed Proc* 40:2614–2617, 1981.

141. Docherty JR, McGrath JC: A comparison of the relaxant and autonomic effects of pancuronium and its monoquaternary derivative Organon NC45 in the pithed rat. *Br J Pharmacol* 68:140P–141P, 1980.

142. Docherty JR, McGrath JC: Sympathomimetic effects of pancuronium bromide in the cardiovascular system of the pithed rat. A comparison with the effects of drugs blocking the neuronal uptake of noradrenaline. *Br J Pharmacol* 64:589–599, 1978.

143. Dodson BA, Miller KW: Structurally specific modulation of acetylcholine receptor binding by various barbiturates. *Soc Neurosci Abstr* 8: 340, 1982.

144. Dolezal V, Tucke S: The synthesis and release of acetylcholine in normal and denervated rat diaphragms during incubation in vitro. *J Physiol* 334:461–474, 1983.

145. Donati F, Ferguson A, Bevan DR: Twitch depression and train-of-four ratio after antagonism of pancuronium with edrophonium, neostigmine, or pyridostigmine. *Anesth Analg* 62:314–316, 1983.

146. Dowall MJ, Golds PR, Strange PG: Properties of Torpedo electric organ muscarinic receptors. *J Physiol* (Paris) 78:378–384, 1982.

147. Dretchen KL, Sokoll MD, Gergis SD, Long JP: The actions of pancuronium on the motor nerve terminal. *Fed Proc* 31:535, 1972 (abstract).

148. Dretchen KL, Standaert FG, Skirboll JR, Morgenroth VH: Evidence for a prejunctional role of cyclic nucleotides in neuromuscular transmission. *Nature* 264:79–81, 1976.

149. Dreyer F: Acetylcholine receptor. *Br J Anaesth* 54:115–130, 1982.

150. Dunant Y, Jones GJ, Schaller-Clostre F: Acetylcholine release in the electric organ of Torpedo. *J Physiol* 78:357–365, 1982.

151. Dunant Y, Walker AI: Cholinergic inhibition of acetylcholine release in the electric organ of Torpedo. *Eur J Pharmacol* 78:201–212, 1982.

152. Dunlap J, Brown JM: Heterogeneity of binding sites on cardiac muscarinic receptors induced by the neuromuscular blocking agents gallamine and pancuronium. *Molec Pharmacol* 24:15–22, 1983.

153. Dunn SMJ, Blanchard SG, Raftery MA: Effects of local anesthetics and histrionicotoxin on the binding of carbamoylcholine to membrane-bound acetylcholine receptors. *Biochemistry* 21:5617–5624, 1981.

154. Dunn SMT, Raftery MA: Activation and desensitization of Torpedo acetylcholine receptor: Evidence for separate binding sites. *Proc Nat Acad Sci USA* 79:6757–6761, 1982.

155. Durant NN, Katz RL: Suxamethonium. *Br J Anaesth* 54:195–208, 1982.

156. Durant NN, Lee C, Katz RL: Germine monoacetate, 4-aminopyridine and succinylcholine. *Anesthesiology* 53:S280, 1980.

157. Durant, NN, Lee C, Katz RL: The action of dantrolene on transmitter mobilization at the rat neuromuscular junction. *Eur J Pharmacol* 68:403–408, 1980.

158. Durant NN, Nyuyen N, Lee C, Katz RL: A comparison of 3, 4-diaminopyridine and 4-aminopyridine in the anaesthetized cat. *Eur J Pharmacol* 48:215–219, 1982.

159. Dutia MB: Activation of cat muscle spindles primary, secondary and intermediate sensory endings by suxamethonium. *J Physiol* 304:315–330, 1980.

160. Duvaldestin P, Henzel D: Binding of tubocurarine, fazadinium, pancuronium and ORG NC 45 to serum proteins in normal man and in patients with cirrhosis. *Br J Anaesth* 54:513–516, 1982.

161. Dwyer TA, Adams DJ, Hille B: The permeability of the endplate channel to organic cations in frog muscle. *J Gen Physiol* 75:469–492, 1980.

162. Eakins KE, Katz RL: The action of succinylcholine on the tension of extraocular muscle. *Br J Pharmacol* 26:205–211, 1966.

163. Editorial: On being aware during anaesthesia. *Br J Anaesth* 51:611–712, 1979.

164. Edwards C: Pore size analysis of an electrically excitable membrane. *Brain Res Bull* 4:153–154, 1979.

165. Edwards C: The effects of innervation on the properties of acetylcholine receptors in muscle. *Neuroscience* 4:565–582, 1979.

166. Edwards C: The selectivity of ion channels in nerve and muscle. *Neuroscience* 7:1335–1366, 1982.

167. Eldefrawi AT, Mansour NA, Eldefrawi ME: Insecticides affecting acetylcholine receptor interactions. *Pharmacol Ther* 16:45–65, 1982.

168. Eldefrawi AT, Miller ER, Eldefrawi ME: Binding of depolarizing drugs to the ionic channel sites of the nicotinic acetylcholine receptor. *Biochem Pharmacol* 31:1819–1822, 1982.

169. Eldridge L, Liebhold M, Steinbach JH: Alterations in cat skeletal neuromuscular junctions following prolonged inactivity. *J Physiol* 313:529–545, 1981.

170. Ellisman MH, Rash JE, Staehelin LA, Porter KR: Studies of excitable membranes II. A comparison of specializations at neuromuscular junctions and nonjunctional sarcolemmas of mammalian fast and slow twitch fibers. *J Cell Biol* 68:752–774, 1976.

171. Engbaek J, Ording H, Viby-Morgensen J: Neuromuscular blocking effects of vercuronium and pancuronium during halothane anaesthesia. *Br J Anaesth* 55:497–500, 1983.

172. Engbaek J, Ording H, Sorensen B, Viby-Morgensen J: Cardiac effects of vecuronium and pancuronium during halothane anaesthesia. *Br J Anaesth* 55:501–505, 1983.

173. Engel AG, Linstrom JM, Lambert EJ, Lennon VA: Ultrastructural localization of the acetylcholine receptor in myasthenia gravis and in its experimental autoimmune model. *Neurology* (Cleveland) 27:307–315, 1977.

174. Erlij D, Shen WK, Reinach P, Schoen H: Effects of dantrolene and D_2O on K-stimulated respiration of skeletal muscle. *Am J Physiol* 243:C87–C95, 1982.

175. Esplin D: Effect of diphenylhydantoin on synaptic transmission in the cat spinal cord and stellate ganglion. *J Pharmacol Exp Ther* 120:301–323, 1957.

176. Everett AJ, Lowe LA, Wilkinson S: Revision of the structure of (+)-tubocurarine chloride and (+)-chondrocurine. *Chem Commun* 16:1020–1021, 1970.

177. Fahey MR, Morris RB, Miller RD, Sohn YJ, Cronnelly R, Gencarelli P: Clinical pharmacology of ORG NC 45 (Norcuron): A new non-depolarizing muscle relaxant. *Anesthesiology* 55:6–11, 1981.

178. Fambrough DM: Biosynthesis and turnover of nicotinic acetylcholine receptors. In Birdsall NJM (ed): *Drug Receptors and Their Effectors.* New York, MacMillan, 1981, pp 155–163.

179. Fambrough DM: Control of acetylcholine receptors in skeletal muscle. *Physiol Rev* 59:165–226, 1979.

180. Farley JM, Yeh JZ, Watanabe S, Narahashi T: Endplate channel block by guanidine derivatives. *J Gen Physiol* 77:273–293, 1981.

181. Fatt P, Katz B: Some observations on biological noise. *Nature* (London) 66:597–598, 1950.

182. Fatt P, Katz B: Spontaneous subthreshold activity at motor nerve endings. *J Physiol* 117:109–128, 1952.

183. Feltz A, Trautmann A: Desensitization at the frog neuromuscular junction a biphasic process. *J Physiol* 322:257–272, 1982.

184. Fenichel GM, Kibler WB, Olson WH, Dettbarn W-D: Chronic inhibition of cholinesterase as a cause of myopathy. *Neurology* 22:1026–1033, 1972.

185. Ferguson A, Egerszegi P, Bevan DR, Chir B: Neostigmine, pyridostigmine, and edrophonium as antagonists of pancuronium. *Anesthesiology* 53:390–394, 1980.

186. Fergusson RJ, Wright DJ, Willey RF, Crompton GK, Grant IWB: Suxamethonium is dangerous in polyneuropathy. *Br Med J* 282:298–299, 1981.

187. Ferrendelli JA, Daniels-McQueen S: Comparative actions of phenytoin and other anticonvulsant drugs on potassium- and veratroidine-stimulated calcium uptake in synaptosomes. *J Pharmacol Exp Ther* 220: 29–34, 1982.

188. Ferres CJ, Mirakhur RK, Craig HJL, Browne ES, Clarke RSJ: Pretreatment with vercuronium, as a prophylactic against post-suxamethonium muscle pain. *Br J Anaesth* 55:735–741, 1983.

189. Fiekers JF: Effects of the aminoglycoside antibiotics, streptomycin and neomycin, on neuromuscular transmission. I. Presynaptic consideration. *J Pharmacol Exp Ther* 225:487–495, 1983.

190. Fischbach GD, Robbins N: Effects of chronic disuse of rat soleus neuromuscular junctions on postsynaptic membrane. *J Neurophysiol* 34: 562–569, 1971.

191. Fischbeck KH, Bonilla E, Schotland DL: Freeze-fracture analysis of plasma membrane cholesterol in fast- and slow-twitch muscles. *J Ultrastruc Res* 81:117–123, 1982.

192. Fischer DM, Miller RD: Neuromuscular effects of vecuronium (ORG NC45) in infants and children during nitrous oxide, halothane anesthesia. *Anesthesiology* 58:123–519, 1983.

193. Fisher DM, O'Keeffe C, Stanski DR, Cronnelly R, Miller RD, Gregory GA: Pharmacokinetics and pharmacodynamics of *d*-tubocurarine in infants, children and adults. *Anesthesiology* 57:203–208, 1982.

194. Foldes F, Deery A: Protein binding of atracurium and other short-acting neuromuscular blocking agents and their interaction with human cholinesterases. *Br J Anaesth* 55:31S–34S, 1983.

195. Foldes F, Morita K, Nagashima H, Duncalf D: Type of stimulus and reversal of neuromuscular block in vivo. *Anesthesiology* 53:S264, 1980.

196. Foldes FF, Swerdlow M, Lipschitz E, van Hees GR, Shanor SP: Comparison of respiratory effects of suxamethonium and suxethonium in man. *Anesthesiology* 17:559–568, 1956.

197. Foster CA: Muscle pains that follow administration of suxamethonium. *Br Med J* 2:182, 1960.

198. Frank E, Fischbach GD: Early events in neuromuscular junction formation in vitro. *J Cell Biol* 83:143–158, 1979.

199. Freud FC, Rubin AP: The need for additional succinylcholine after *d*-tubocurarine. *Anesthesiology* 36:182–187, 1972.

200. Furukawa T, Sasaoka T, Hosoya Y: Effects of tetrodotoxin on the neuromuscular junction. *Jpn J Pharmacol* 9:143–152, 1959.

201. Gage PW, Hamill OP, Wachtel RE: Sites of action of procaine at the motor endplate. *J Physiol* 335:123–137, 1983.

202. Gage PW, Hamill OP: Effects of anesthetics on ion channels in synapses. *Int Rev Physiol* 25:1–45, 1981.

203. Gage PW, Hamill OP: Lifetime and conductance of acetylcholine-activated channels in normal and denervated toad sartosium muscle. *J Physiol* 298:525–538, 1980.

204. Gage PW, Lonergan M, Torda TA: Presynaptic and postsynaptic depressant effects of phenytoin sodium at the neuromuscular junction. *Br J Pharmacol* 69:119–121, 1980.

205. Galindo A: The role of prejunctional effects in myoneural transmission. *Anesthesiology* 36:598–608, 1972.

206. Galindo A: Depolarizing neuromuscular block. *J Pharmacol Exp Ther* 178:339–349, 1971.
207. Galindo A: Prejunctional effect of curare: Its relative importance. *J Neurophysiol* 34:289–301, 1971.
208. Gallager JF, Karczmar AG: A direct facilitatory effect for dopamine at the neuromuscular junction. *Neuropharmacol* 12:783–791, 1973.
209. Gallagher JP, Blaber LC: Catechol, a facilitatory drug that demonstrates only a prejunctional site of action. *J Pharmacol Exp Ther* 184: 129–135, 1972.
210. Ganguly DK, Das M: Effects of oxotremorine demonstrate presynaptic muscarinic and dopaminergic receptors on motor nerve terminals. *Nature* 278:645–646, 1979.
211. Gelsema AJ: Apparent lack of effect of alpha-bungarotoxin on the spike-induced release of acetylcholine at the mammalian motor endplate. *Neurosci Letts* 20:189–193, 1980.
212. Gergis SD, Dretchen KL, Sokoll MD, Long JP: Effects of pancuronium bromide on acetylcholine release. *J Pharmacol Exp Ther* 139:74–76, 1972.
213. Gershon S, Shaw FH: Tetrahydroaminacrin as a decurarising agent. *J Pharmac Pharmacol* 10:638, 1958.
214. Gissen AJ, Katz RL: Twitch, tetanus, posttetanic potentiation as indices of neuromuscular block in man. *Anesthesiology* 30:481–487, 1969.
215. Glavinovic MI: Presynaptic action of curare. *J Physiol* 290:499–506, 1979.
216. Glover WE: The aminopyridines. *Gen Pharmacol* 13:259–285, 1982.
217. Gonzales-Ros JM, Llanillo M, Praschos A, Martinez-Carrion M: Lipid environment of acetylcholine receptor from Torpedo californica. *Biochemistry* 21:3467–3474, 1982.
218. Gordon AS, Milfay D, Diamond I: Phosphorylation of the membrane-bound acetylcholine receptor inhibition by diphenylhydantoin. *Ann Neurol* 5:201–203, 1979.
219. Gotti C, Conti-Tronconi BM, Raftery MA: Mammalian muscle acetylcholine receptor purification and characterization. *Biochem* 21: 3148–3154, 1982.
220. Graham EH: Monitoring neuromuscular block may be unreliable in patients with upper motor-neuron lesion. *Anesthesiology* 52:74–75, 1980.
221. Granit R, Skoglund S, Thesleff S: Activation of muscle spindles by acetylcholine and decamethonium: The effects of curare. *Acta Physiol Scand* 28:134–151, 1953.
222. Gray EG: Neurotransmitter release mechanisms and microtubules. *Proc R Soc London Ser B* 218:253–258, 1983.
223. Gray TC: Exciting and dangerous days. *Br J Anaesth* 55:227–228, 1983.
224. Green DM, Smith AP: The reversal by pyridostigmine of soman induced neuromuscular blockade in primate respiratory muscle. *Br J Pharmacol* 79S:252P, 1983.
225. Greengard P: Cyclic nucleotides, phosphorylated proteins, and the nervous system. *Fed Proc* 38:2208–2217, 1979.

226. Grohovaz F, Limbrick AR, Miledi R: Acetylcholine receptors at the rat neuromuscular junction as revealed by deep etching. *Proc R Soc London Ser B* 215:147–154, 1982.
227. Gronert GA, Kanbert EH, Theye RA: The response of denervated skeletal muscle to succinylcholine. *Anesthesiology* 39:13–22, 1973.
228. Gronert GA, Theye RA: Pathophysiology of hyperkalemia induced by succinylcholine. *Anesthesiology* 43:43–99, 1975.
229. Gronert GA: Disuse atrophy with resistance to pancuronium. *Anesthesiology* 55:547–549, 1981.
230. Groswald DE, Dettbarn W-D: Nerve crush induced changes in molecular forms of acetylcholinesterase in soleus and extensor digitorum muscles. *Exp Neurol* 79:519–531, 1983.
231. Gullisck WJ, Lindstrom JM: Structural similarities between acetylcholine receptors from fish electric organs and mammalian muscle. *Biochem* 21:4563–4569, 1982.
232. Gundersen CB: The effects of botulinum toxin on the synthesis, storage, and release of acetylcholine. *Prog Neurobiol* 14:99–119, 1980.
233. Gunderson CB, Jenden DJ: Oxotremorine does not enhance acetylcholine release from rat diaphragm preparations. *Br J Pharmacol* 70:8–10, 1980.
234. Guth L, Kemerer VF, Samaras TA, Warnick JE, Albuquerque EX: The roles of disuse and loss of neurotrophic function in denervation atrophy of skeletal muscle. *Exp Neurol* 73:20–36, 1981.
235. Guy HR, Maeno T, Morello R, Dekin MS: Acetylcholine-activated permeability of normal and denervated muscles to organic cations. *Biophys J* 16:211A, 1976.
236. Gyasi H, Williams A, Melloni C: ORG NC45 for short intra-abdominal operations: A comparison with succinylcholine. *Can Anaesth Soc* 30:132–135, 1983.
237. Gyermek L: Clinical pharmacology of the reversal of neuromuscular block. *Int J Clin Pharmacol* 15:356–362, 1977.
238. Haldin M, Wahlin A: Effect of succinylcholine on the intraspinal fluid pressure. *Acta Anaesth Scand* 3:155–161, 1959.
239. Ham J, Miller RD, Sheiner LB, Matteo RS: Dosage-schedule independence of *d*-tubocurarine pharmacokinetic and pharmacodynamics, and recovery of neuromuscular function. *Anesthesiology* 50:528–532, 1979.
240. Hamitt OP, Marty A, Neher E, Sakmann B, Sigworth FJ: Improved patch-clamp techniques for high resolution current recording from cells and cell-free membrane patches. *Pfluegers Arch* 391:85–100, 1981.
241. Healy TEJ, Palmer JP: In vitro comparison between the neuromuscular and ganglionic blocking potency ratios of atracurium and tubocurarine. *Br J Anaesth* 54:1307–1311, 1982.
242. Heidmann T, Oswald RE, Changeux J-P: Multiple sites of action for noncompetitive blockers on acetylcholine receptor rich membrane fragments from Torpedo marmorata. *Biochem* 22:3112–3217, 1983.
243. Heilbronn E: Inhibition of cholinesterases by tetrahydroxyaminoacrine. *Acta Chem Scand* 15:1386, 1961.
244. Heinonen E: Effects of dopamine and dibutyryl cyclic adenosine monophosphate on delayed release of transmitter at the rat neuromuscular junction. *Pfluegers Arch* 393:144–147, 1982.

245. Hermann A, Groman ALF: Effects of 4-aminopyridine on potassium currents in a molluscan neuron. *J Gen Physiol* 78:63–86, 1981.

246. Hess A, Pilar G: Slow fibres in the extraocular muscles of the cat. *J Physiol* 169:780–799, 1963.

247. Heuser JE, Reese TS, Dennis MJ, Jan JL, Evans L: Synaptic vesicle exocytosis captured by quick freezing and correlated with quantal release. *J Cell Biol* 81:275–300, 1979.

248. Heuser JE, Reese TS: Structural changes after transmitter release at the frog neuromuscular junction. *J Cell Biol* 88:564–580, 1981.

249. Heuser JE, Salpeter SR: Organization of acetylcholine receptors in quick frozen deep etched and rotary-replicated Torpedo postsynaptic membrane. *J Cell Biol* 82:150–173, 1979.

250. Hilgenberg JC: Comparison of the pharmacology of vercuronium and atracurium with that of other currently available muscle relaxants. *Anesth Analg* (Cleveland) 62:524–531, 1983.

251. Hirai K, Koketsu K: Presynaptic regulation of the release of acetylcholine by 5-hydroxytryptamine. *Br J Pharmacol* 70:499–500, 1980.

252. Hirokawa H, Heuser JE: Structural evidence that botulinum toxin blocks neuromuscular transmission by impairing the calcium influx that normally accompanies nerve depolarization. *J Cell Biol* 88:160–171, 1981.

253. Hirokawa N, Heuser JE: Internal and external differentiations of the postsynaptic membrane at the neuromuscular junction. *J Neurocytol* 11:487–510, 1982.

254. Hohlfeld R, Sterz R, Peper K: Prejunctional effects of anticholinesterase drugs at the endplate. *Pfluegers Arch* 391:213–218, 1981.

255. Hohlfeld R, Sterz R, Kalies I, Peper K, Wekerle H: Neuromuscular transmission in experimental autoimmune myasthenia gravis. Quantitative ionophoresis and current fluctuation analysis of normal and myasthenic rat endplates. *Pfluegers Arch* 390:156–160, 1981.

256. Holley EO: Relaxant resistance in disuse atrophy. *Anesthesiology* 57:142–144, 1982.

257. Holloway KB: Control of the eye during general anaesthesia for intraocular surgery. *Br J Anaesth* 52:671–679, 1980.

258. Holtzman E, Wise D, Wall J, Karlin A: Electron microscopy of complexes of isolated acetylcholine receptors, biotinyl-toxin and avidin. *Proc Nat Acad Sci* 79:310–314, 1982.

259. Horn AS, Lambert JJ, Marshall IG: A comparison of the facilitatory actions of 4-aminopyridine methiodide and 4-aminopyridine on neuromuscular transmission. *Br J Pharmacol* 65:53–62, 1979.

260. Horn R, Brodwick MS, Dickey WD: Asymmetry of the acetylcholine channel revealed by quaternary anesthetics. *Science* 210:205–207, 1980.

261. Hubbard JI, Schmidt RF, Yokota T: The effect of acetylcholine upon mammalian motor nerve terminals. *J Physiol* (London) 181:810–829, 1966.

262. Hubbard JI, Wilson DF, Miyamoto M: Reduction of transmitter release by *d*-tubocurarine. *Nature* (London) 223:531–533, 1969.

263. Hubbard JI, Wilson DF: Neuromuscular transmission in mammalian preparation in the absence of blocking drugs and the effect of *d*-tubocurarine. *J Physiol* 228:307–325, 1973.

264. Hubbard JI: Physiology and pharmacology of synaptic transmission: Mechanism of transmitter release from nerve terminals. *Ann NY Acad Sci* 183:131–146, 1971.
265. Hubbard JI: Repetitive stimulation of the mammalian neuromuscular junction, and the mobilization of transmitter. *J Physiol* 169:641–662, 1963.
266. Hubbard JI: The origin and significance of antidromic activity in motor nerves. In Curtis DR, McIntyre, JC (eds): *Studies in Physiology*. New York, Springer Verlag, 1965, pp 85–92.
267. Hudson CS, Rash JE, Tiedt TN, Albuquerque EX: Neostigmine-induced alterations at the mammalian neuromuscular junction. II. Ultrastructure. *J Pharmacol Exp Ther* 205:340–356, 1978.
268. Hughes R, Chappel DJ: The pharmacology of atracurium: A new competitive neuromuscular blocking agent. *Br J Anaesth* 53:31–44, 1981.
269. Hughes R, Payne JP: Clinical assessment of atracurium using the single twitch and tetanic responses of the adductor pollicis muscle. *Br J Anaesth* 55:47S–52S, 1983.
270. Hunter JM, Jones RS, Utting JE: Use of atracurium during general surgery monitored by the train-of-four stimuli. *Br J Anaesth* 54:1243–1250, 1982.
271. Hunter JM, Jones RS, Utting JE: Use of atracurium in patients with no renal function. *Br J Anaesth* 54:1251–1258, 1982.
272. Itil T, Fink M: Anticholinergic drug induced delirium: Experimental modifications, quantitative EEG and behavioral correlation. *J Nerv Ment Dis* 143:492, 1966.
273. Jackson MB, Lecar H, Askanas V, Engel WK: Single cholinergic receptor channel currents in cultured human muscle. *J Neurosci* 2:1465–1473, 1982.
274. Jenden DB, Kamijo K, Taylor DB: The action of decamethonium on the isolated rabbit lumbrical muscle. *J Pharmacol Exp Ther* 111:229–240, 1954.
275. Jewell PA, Zaimis EJ: A differentiation between red and white muscle in the cat based on responses to neuromuscular blocking agents. *J Physiol* 124:417–428, 1954.
276. Johnson MK: Organophosphorus esters causing delayed neurotoxic effects: Mechanism of action and structure activity relationship. *Arch Toxicol* 34:259–288, 1975.
277. Johnson MK: The delayed neuropathy caused by some organophosphorus esters. Mechanism and challenge. In *CRC Critical Reviews in Toxicology*. Cleveland, CRC Press, 1975, pp 289–316.
278. Johnson MK: The mechanism of delayed neuropathy caused by some organophosphorus esters: Using the understanding to improve safety. *J Environ Sci Health (B)* 15:823–841, 1980.
279. Johnson MK: The primary biochemical lesion leading to the delayed neurotoxic effects of some organophosphorus compounds. *J Neurochem* 23:785–789, 1974.
280. Jones SW, Salpeter MM: Absence of ^{125}I-α-bungarotoxin binding to motor nerve terminals of frog, lizard, and mouse muscle. *J Neurosci* 3:326–331, 1983.
281. Jope RS: Acetylcholine turnover and compartmentation in rat brain synaptosomes. *J Neurochem* 36:1712–1721, 1981.

282. Jope RS: High affinity choline transport and acetylCoA production in brain and their roles in regulation of acetylcholine synthesis. *Brain Res Rev* 1:313–344, 1979.
283. Judge SE: Effect of general anaesthetics on synaptic ion channels. *Br J Anaesth* 55:191–200, 1983.
284. Juel C: Presynaptic function in Helix pomatia is changed by phosphodiesterase inhibitors, cyclic nucleotide derivatives, and neurotransmitter induced cAMP. *Comp Biochem Physiol C* 68:21–27, 1980.
285. Kalsner S: Evidence against the unitary hypothesis of agonist and antagonist action at presynaptic adrenoceptors. *Br J Pharmacol* 77:375–380, 1982.
286. Karlin A, Holtzman E, Yodh N, Lobel P, Wall J, Hainfeld J: The arrangement of the subunits of the acetylcholine receptor of Torpedo californica. *J Biol Chem* 258:6678–6681, 1983.
287. Kato M, Bunichi F: On the mechanism of fascicular twitching following administration of succinylcholine chloride. *J Pharmacol Exp Ther* 149:124–130, 1965.
288. Katz B, Miledi R: A re-examination of curare action at the motor endplate. *Proc R Soc London Ser B* 203:119–133, 1978.
289. Katz B, Miledi R: Does the motor nerve impulse evoke non-quantal transmitter release. *Proc R Soc London Ser B* 212:131–137, 1981.
290. Katz B, Miledi R: Tetrodotoxin and neuromuscular transmission. *Proc R Soc Biol* 167:8–22, 1967.
291. Katz B, Miledi R: Estimates of 'quantal potentiation' of transmitter release. *Proc R Soc London Ser B* 205:369–378, 1979.
292. Katz B, Miledi R: Transmitter leakage from motor nerve endings. *Proc R Soc London Ser B* 196:59–72, 1977.
293. Katz RL, Stirt J, Murray AL, Lee C: Neuromuscular effects of atracurium in man. *Anesth Analg* (Cleveland) 61:730–734, 1982.
294. Kawabuchi M: Neostigmine myopathy is a calcium ion-mediated myopathy initially affecting the motor endplate. *J Neuropath Exp Neurol* 41:298–314, 1982.
295. Kelly RB, Deutsch JW, Carlson SS, Wagner JA: Biochemistry of neurotransmitter release. *Ann Rev Neurosci* 2:399–446, 1979.
296. Kilbinger H, Wessler I: Inhibition by acetylcholine of the stimulation-evoked release of [^{3}H] acetylcholine from the guinea-pig myenteric plexus. *Neuroscience* 5:1331–1340, 1980.
297. Kistler J, Stroud RM, Klymkowsky MW, LaLancette RA, Fairclough RH: Structure and function of an acetylcholine receptor. *Biophys J* 37:371–383, 1982.
298. Kitz RJJ: Human tissue cholinesterase: Rates of recovery after inhibition by neostigmine: Michaelis-Menton constant. *Biochem Pharmacol* 13:1275–1282, 1964.
299. Koblin DD, Lester HA: Voltage-dependent and voltage-independent blockade of acetylcholine receptors by local anesthetics in Electrophorus electroplaques. *Molec Pharmacol* 15:559–580, 1979.
300. Kocsis JD, Ruiz JA, Waxman SG: Maturation of mammalian myelineated fibers: Changes in action-potential characteristics following 4-aminopyridine application. *J Neurophysiol* 50:449–463, 1983.
301. Koelle GB: A new general concept of the neurohumoral functions of acetylcholine and acetylcholinesterase. *J Pharm Pharmacol* 14:65–90, 1962.

302. Koketsu K, Miyagawa M, Akasu T: Catecholamine modulates nicotinic acetylcholine receptor sensitivity. *Brain Res* 236:487–491, 1982.
303. Kostyuk PG: Calcium ionic channels in electrically excitable membrane. *Neuroscience* 5:945–959, 1980.
304. Krueger BK, Blaustein MP: Sodium channels in presynaptic nerve terminals. *J Gen Physiol* 76:287–313, 1980.
305. Kuba K, Albuquerque EX, Daly J, Barnard EA: A study of the irreversible cholinesterase inhibitor, diisopropylfluorophosphate on time course of end-plate currents in frog sartorious muscle. *J Pharmacol Exp Ther* 189:499–512, 1974.
306. Kuba K: Effects of catecholamines on neuromuscular function in the diaphragm. *J Physiol* 211:551–570, 1970.
307. La Cour D: Rise in intragastric pressure caused by suxamethonium fasciculation. *Acta Anaesthsiol Scand* 13:255–261, 1969.
308. Lambert JJ, Durant NN, Henderson EG: Drug-induced modifications of ionic conductance at the neuromuscular junction. *Ann Rev Pharmacol Toxicol* 23:505–539, 1983.
309. Lambert JJ, Volle RL, Henderson EG: An attempt to distinguish between the actions of neuromuscular blocking drugs on the acetylcholine receptor and its associated ionic channel. *Proc Nat Acad Sci USA* 77:5003–5007, 1980.
310. Langer SZ: Presynaptic receptors and modulation of neurotransmission: Pharmacological implications and therapeutic relevance. *Trends in Neuroscience.* 110–111, 1980.
311. Langer SZ: Presynaptic receptors and their role in the regulation of transmitter release. *Br J Pharmacol* 60:481–497, 1977.
312. Laskowski MB, Olson WH, Dettbarn WD: Ultrastructural changes at the motor end-plate produced by an irreversible cholinesterase inhibitor. *Exp Neurol* 47:290–306, 1977.
313. Laskowski MB, Dettbarn W-D: Presynaptic effects of neuromuscular cholinesterase inhibition. *J Pharmacol Exp Ther* 194:351–361, 1975.
314. Laskowski MB, Dettbarn W-D: The pharmacology of experimental myopathies. *Ann Rev Pharmacol Toxicol* 17:387–409, 1977.
315. Laskowski MB, Thies R: Interactions between calcium and barium on the spontaneous release of transmitter from mammalian motor nerve terminals. *Intern J Neurosci* 4:11–16, 1972.
316. Lavoie PA, Collier B, Tenenhouse A: Comparison of alpha-bungarotoxin binding to skeletal muscles after inactivity or disuse. *Nature* (London) 260:349–350, 1976.
317. Lebowitz PW, Ramsey FM, Savarese JJ, Ali HH: Potentiation of neuromuscular blockade in man produced by combinations of pancuronium and *d*-tubocurarine. *Anesth Analg* 59:604–609, 1980.
318. Lee C, Durant NN, Au E, Katz RL: Reversal of dantrolene sodium-induced depression of skeletal muscle in the cat. *Anesthesiology* 54:61–65, 1981.
319. Lee C: Dose relationships of phase II, tachyphylaxis and train-of-four fade in suxamethonium-induced dual neuromuscular block in man. *Br J Anaesth* 47:841–844, 1975.
320. Lee Son S, Waud BE, Waud DR, Phil D: A comparison of the neuromuscular blocking and vagolytic effects of ORG NC45 and pancuronium. *Anesthesiology* 55:12–18, 1981.

321. Lee Son S, Waud DR: Effects of non-depolarizing neuromuscular blocking agents on the cardiac vagus nerve in the guinea pig. *Br J Anaesth* 52:981–987, 1980.
322. Lehmann J, Lee CR, Langer SZ: Dopamine receptors modulating [³H] acetylcholine release in slices of the cat caudate: Effects of (-)-N-(2-cholorethyl) norapomorphine. *Eur J Pharmacol* 90:393–400, 1983.
323. Lemanowicz EF, Sugita ET, Niebergall PJ, Schnaare RL: Kinetics of absorption and elimination of pralidoxime chloride in dogs. *J Pharmac Sci* 68:141–145, 1979.
324. Lentz TL, Mazurkiewicz JE, Rosenthal L: Cytochemical localization of acetylcholine receptors at the neuromuscular junction by means of horseradish peroxidase labels and alpha-bungarotoxin. *Brain Res* 132:423–442, 1977.
325. Leslie GC, Part NJ: The action of dantrolene sodium on rat fast and slow muscles in vivo. *Br J Pharmacol* 72:665–672, 1981.
326. Leung E, Mitchelson F: Modification by hexamethonium of the muscarinic receptor blocking activity of pancuronium and homatropine in isolated tissues of the guinea-pig. *Eur J Pharmacol* 80:11–17, 1982.
327. Levitt TA, Salpeter MM: Denervated endplates have a dual population of junctional acetylcholine receptors. *Nature* (London) 291:239–241, 1981.
328. Liley AW, North KAK: An electrical investigation of effects of repetitive stimulation on mammalian neuromuscular junction. *J Neurophysiol* 16:509 – 527, 1953.
329. Lilleheil G, Naess K: A presynaptic effect of *d*-tubocurarine in the neuromuscular junction. *Acta Physiol Scand* 52:120–136 1961.
330. Lindstrom J, Anholt R, Einarson B, Engel A, Osame M, Montal M: Purification of acetylcholine receptor reconstituted into lipid vesicles and study of agonist-induced cation channel regulation. *J Biol Chem* 255:8340–8350, 1980.
331. Linter SPK, Thomas PR, Withington PS, Hall MG: Suxamethonium associated hypertonicity and cardiac arrest in unsuspected pseudohypertrophic muscular dystrophy. *Br J Anaesth* 54:1331–1332, 1982.
332. Llinas R, Steinberg IZ, Walton K: Presynaptic calcium currents in squid giant synapse. *J Biophysical Soc* 33:289–322, 1981.
333. Loh HH, Law PY: The role of membrane lipids in receptor mechanics. *Ann Rev Pharmacol Toxicol* 20:201–234, 1980.
334. Loring RH, Salpeter MM: Denervation increases turnover rate of junctional acetylcholine receptors. *Proc Nat Acad Sci USA* 77:2293–2297, 1980.
335. MacIntosh JC: Cholinergic transmission: variations on a theme. In Hanin I, Goldberg, AM (eds): *Progress in Cholinergic Biology. Model Cholinergic Synapses.* New York, Raven Press 1982, pp 1–22.
336. Magazanik LG, Fedorov VV, Snetkov VA: The time course of postsynaptic currents in fast and slow junctions and its alteration by cholinesterase inhibition. *Prog Br Res* 49:225–240, 1979.
337. Magazanik LG, Vyskočil F: The effect of temperature on desensitization kinetics at the post-synaptic membrane of the frog muscle fibre. *J Physiol* 249:285–300, 1975.

338. Magleby KL, Pallotta BS, Terrar DA: The effect of (+)-tubocurarine on neuromuscular transmission during repetitive stimulation in the rat, mouse, and frog. *J Physiol* 312:97–113, 1981.
339. Magleby KL, Pallotta BS: A study of desensitization of acetylcholine receptors using nerve-released transmitter in the frog. *J Physiol* 316: 225–250, 1981.
340. Malathi S, Batmanabane M: Alterations in the morphology of the neuromuscular junction following experimental immobilization in cats. *Experientia* 39:547–549, 1983.
341. Maleque MA, Souccar C, Cohen JB, Albuquerque EX: Meproadifen reaction with the ionic channel of the acetylcholine receptor potentiation of agonist-induced desensitization at the frog neuromuscular junction. *Molec Pharmacol* 22:636–647, 1982.
342. Mallard A, Brigant JL: Electrical activity at motor nerve terminals of the mouse. *J Physiol* (Paris) 78:407–411, 1982.
343. Malta E, McPherson GA, Raper C: Comparison of pre-junctional alpha-adrenoceptors at the neuromuscular junction with vascular post-junctional alpha receptors in cat skeletal muscle. *Br J Pharmacol* 65: 249–256, 1979.
344. March D, Watts A, Barrantes FJ: Phospholipid chain immobilization and steroid rotational immobilization in acetylcholine receptor-rich membranes from Torpedo marmorata. *Biochemica Biophysica Acta* 645: 97–101, 1981.
345. Marshall IG, Gibb AJ, Durant NN: Neuromuscular and vagal blocking actions of pancuronium bromide, its metabolites, and vecuronium bromide (ORG NC 45) and its potential metabolites in the anaesthetized cat. *Br J Anaesth* 55:703–714, 1983.
346. Marshall RJ, Ojewole JAO: Comparison of the autonomic effects of some currently used neuromuscular blocking agents. *Br J Pharmacol* 66:77P–78P, 1979.
347. Martin LVH: Consciousness during anesthesia. *Br J Anaesth* 52:241, 1980.
348. Martyn JAJ, Leibel WS, Matteo RS: Competitive nonspecific binding does not explain the potentiating effects of muscle relaxant combinations. *Anesth Analg* (Cleveland) 62:160–163, 1983.
349. Marx GF, Bassell GM: In defense of the use of *d*-tubocurarine prior to succinylcholine in obstetrics. *Anesthesiology* 59:157, 1983.
350. Masey SA, Glazebrook CW, Goat VA: Suxamethonium: A new look at pre-treatment. *Br J Anaesth* 55:729–733, 1983.
351. Massoulie J, Bon S: The molecular forms of cholinesterase and acetylcholinesterase in vertebrates. *Ann Rev Neurosci* 5:57–106, 1982.
352. Matteo RS, Nishitateno K, Pua EK, Spector S: Pharmacokinetics of *d*-tubocurarine in man: Effect of an osmotic diuretic on urinary excretion. *Anesthesiology* 52:335–338, 1980.
353. Matteo RS, Brotherton WP, Nishitateno K, Khambatta HJ, Dias J: Pharmacodynamics and pharmacokinetics of metocurine in humans. Comparison to *d*-tubocurarine. *Anesthesiology* 57:183–190, 1982.
354. Matteo RS, Nishitateno K, Pua EK: Pharmacokinetics of *d*-tubocurarine in man: Effect of an osmotic diuretic on urinary excretion. *Anesthesiology* 52:335–338, 1980.

355. Matthews-Bellinger AJ, Salpeter MM: Fine structural distribution of acetylcholine receptors at developing mouse neuromuscular junctions. *J Neurosci* 3:644–657, 1983.
356. McIntyre AR, King RE, Dunn AL: Electrical activity of denervated mammalian skeletal muscle as influenced by *d*-tubocurarine. *J Physiol* 8:297–307, 1945.
357. McIntyre AR: Curare and the central nervous system. In *Curare*. Chicago, University of Chicago Press, 1947, pp 174–181.
358. McIntyre AR: The clinical use of curare. In *Curare*. Chicago, University of Chicago Press, 1947, pp 182–208.
359. McLeod K, Watson MJ, Rawlings MD: Pharmacokinetics of pancuronium in patients with normal and impaired renal function. *Br J Anaesth* 48:341–345, 1976.
360. McLeskey CH, Cullen BF, Kennedy RD, Galindo A: Control of cerebral perfusion pressure during induction of anesthesia in high risk aneurosurgical patients. *Anesth Analg* (Cleveland) 53:985–992, 1974.
361. McNamee MG, Ochoa ELM: Reconstitution of acetylcholine receptor function in model membranes. *Neuroscience* 7:2305–2319, 1982.
362. Meijer D, Weitering J, Vermeer GA, Schaf AHJ: Comparative pharmacokinetics of *d*-tubocurarine and metacurarine in man. *Anesthesiology* 51:402–407, 1979.
363. Meiri H, Erulkar SD, Lerman T, Rahaminimoff R: The action of the sodium ionophore, Monensin, on transmitter release at the frog neuromuscular junction. *Brain Res* 204:204–208, 1981.
364. Meldolesi J, Ceccarelli B: Exocytosis and membrane recycling. *Phil Trans R Soc B* 296:55–65, 1981.
365. Merrett RA, Thompson CW, Webb FW: In vitro degradation of atracurium in human plasma. *Br J Anaesth* 55:61–66, 1983.
366. Meselson M, Robinson JP: Chemical warfare and chemical disarmament. *Sci Amer* 242:38–47, 1980.
367. Miledi R, Molenaar PC, Polak RL: Alpha-bungarotoxin enhances transmitter "release" at the neuromuscular junction. *Nature* (London) 272:641–643, 1978.
368. Miledi R, Molenaar PC, Polak RL: Effect of lanthanum ion on acetylcholine in frog muscle. *J Physiol* 309:199–214, 1980.
369. Miledi R, Molenaar PC, Polak RL: Electrophysiological and chemical determination of acetylcholine release at the frog neuromuscular junction. *J Physiol* 334:245–254, 1983.
370. Miledi R, Parker I: Blocking of acetylcholine-induced channels by extracellular or intracellular application of D600. *Proc R Soc London Ser B* 211:143–150, 1980.
371. Miledi R, Uchitel OD: Properties of postsynaptic channels induced by acetylcholine in different frog muscle fibres. *Nature* (London) 291:162, 1981.
372. Miledi R: Intracellular calcium and desensitization of acetylcholine receptors. *Proc R Soc London Ser B* 209:447–452, 1980.
373. Miller RD, Agoston S, Booij IHDJ, Kersten UW, Crul JF, Ham J: The comparative potency and pharmacokinetics of pancuronium and its metabolites in anesthetized man. *J Pharmacol Exp Ther* 207:539–543, 1978.

374. Miller RD, Booij LHDJ, Agoston S, Crul JF: 4-Aminopyridine potentiates neostigmine and pyridostigmine in man. *Anesthesiology* 50: 416–420, 1979.
375. Miller RD, Cronnelly R: A new look at an old drug. *Anesthesiology* 59:84–85, 1983.
376. Miller RD, Larsen CP, Way WC: Comparative antagonism of *d*-tubocurarine, gallamine, and pancuronium induced neuromuscular blockade by neostigmine. *Anesthesiology* 37:503–509, 1972.
377. Miller RD, Matteo RS, Benet LZ, Sohn YJ: The pharmacokinetics of *d*-tubocurarine in man with and without renal failure. *J Pharmacol Exp Ther* 202:1–7, 1977.
378. Miller RD, Way WL: Inhibition of succinylcholine-induced increased intragastric pressure by nondepolarizing muscle relaxants and lidocaine. *Anesthesiology* 34:185–188, 1971.
379. Milne RJ, Byrne JH: Effects of hexamethonium and decamethonium on end-plate current parameters. *Molec Pharmacol* 19:276–281, 1981.
380. Misler S, Hurlbut WP: Post-tetanic potentiation of acetylcholine release at the frog neuromuscular junction develops after stimulation in Ca-free solutions. *Proc Nat Acad Sci USA* 80:515–519, 1983.
381. Miyamoto MD: The actions of cholinergic drugs on motor nerve terminals. *Pharmacol Rev* 29:221–247, 1977.
382. Molenaar PC, Polak RL: Inhibition of acetylcholine release by activation of acetylcholine receptors. *Prog Pharmacol* 34:39–44, 1980.
383. Molgo J, Lemeignan M, Lechat P: Effects of 4-aminopyridine at the frog neuromuscular junction. *J Pharmacol Exp Ther* 203:653–663, 1977.
384. Molgo J, Thesleff S: Electronic properties of motor nerve terminals. *Acta Physiol Scand* 114:271–275, 1982.
385. Momoi MY, Lennon VA: Purification and biochemical characterization of nicotinic acetylcholine receptors of human muscle. *J Biol Chem* 257:12757–12764, 1982.
386. Moortby SS, Hilgenberg JC: Resistance to non-depolarizing muscle relaxants in paretic upper extremities of patients with residual hemiplegia. *Anesth Analg* (Cleveland) 59:624–627, 1980.
387. Morel N, Manaranche R, Isreal M, Gulik-Kryzywicki T: Isolation of pre-synaptic plasma membrane fraction from Torpedo cholinergic synaptasomes: Evidence for a specific protein. *J Cell Biol* 93:349–356, 1982.
388. Morgan JP, Penovich P: Jamaican ginger paralysis. Forty-seven year follow up. *Arch Neurol* 35:530–532, 1978.
389. Morino A, Kitamura K, Katayama K, Kakemi M, Koizumi T: Kinetics of *d*-tubocurarine disposition and pharmacologic response in rats. *J Pharmacokinet Biopharm* 11:47–53, 1983.
390. Morris RB, Cronnelly R, Miller RD, Stanski DR, Fahey MR: Pharmacokinetics of edrophonium and neostigmine when antagonizing *d*-tubocurarine neuromuscular blockade in man. *Anesthesiology* 54:399–402, 1981.
391. Moss J, Rosow CE, Savarese JJ, Philbin D, Kinffen KJ: Role of histamine in the hypotensive action of *d*-tubocurarine in humans. *Anesthesiology* 55:19–25, 1981.

392. Mullins LJ: Steady state calcium fluxes: Membrane versus mitochondrial control of ionized calcium in axoplasm. *Fed Proc* 35:2583–2587, 1976.
393. Mullins LJ, Requena J: The late Ca channel in squid axons. *J Gen Physiol* 78:683–700, 1981.
394. Murarchick S, Burkett L, Gold MI: Succinylcholine-induced fasciculations and intragastric pressure during induction of anesthesia. *Anesthesiology* 55:180–183, 1981.
395. Nachshen DA, Blaustein MP: The effects of some organic "calcium antagonist" on calcium influx in presynaptic nerve terminals. *Molec Pharmacol* 16:579–586, 1979.
396. Nachshen DA, Blaustein MP: Some properties of potassium-stimulated calcium influx in presynaptic nerve endings. *J Gen Physiol* 76:709–728, 1980.
397. Nachshen DA, Blaustein MP: Influx of calcium, strontium, and barium in presynaptic nerve endings. *J Gen Physiol* 79:1065–1087, 1982.
398. Neher E, Sakmann B: Single-channel currents recorded from membrane of denervated frog muscle fibers. *Nature* (London) 260:779–802, 1976.
399. Neher E, Steinbach JH: Local anaesthetics transiently block currents through single acetylcholine-receptor channels. *J Physiol* 277:153–176, 1976.
400. Neubig RR, Boyd ND, Cohen JB: Conformations of Torpedo acetylcholine receptor associated with ion transport and desensitization. *Biochem* 27:3400–3407, 1982.
401. Nigrovic V, McCullough LS, Wajskol A, Levin JA, Martin JTL: Succinylcholine-induced increases in plasma catecholamine levels in humans. *Anesth Analg* (Cleveland) 62:627–632, 1983.
402. Nott MW, Bowman WC: Actions of dantrolene sodium on contractions of the tibialis anterior and soleus muscles of cats under chloralose anaesthesia. *Clin Expl Pharmacol Physiol* 1:113–122, 1974.
403. Olek A, Younkin RM, Slugg RM, Koniesczkoski M, Robbins N: A transient increase in junctional acetylcholine receptors after denervation. *Brain Res* 214:429–432, 1981.
404. Olek AJ, Robbins N: Properties of junctional acetylcholine receptors that appear rapidly after denervation. *Neurosci* 9:226–233, 1983.
405. Oshita S, Sari A, Fujii S, Yonei A: Prolonged neuromuscular blockade following succinylcholine in a patient homozygous for the silent gene. *Anesthesiology* 59:71–73, 1983.
406. Ostheimer GW: A comparison of glycopyrrolate and atropine during reversal of nondepolarizing neuromuscular block with neostigmine. *Anesth Analg* (Cleveland) 56:182–186, 1977.
407. Oswald R, Changeux J-P: Ultraviolet light-induced labeling by non-competitive blockers of acetylcholine receptor from Torpedo marmorata. *Proc Nat Acad Sci USA* 78:3925–3929, 1981.
408. Oswald RE, Heidmann T, Changeux J-P: Multiple affinity states for non-competitive blockers revealed by [^{3}H]Phencyclidine binding to acetylcholine receptor rich membrane fragments from Torpedo marmorata. *Biochemistry* 22:3128–3136, 1983.

409. Owen H, Hunter AR: Heterozygotes for atypical cholinesterase. *Br J Anaesth* 55:315–318, 1983.
410. Parsons RL, Cochrane DE, Schnitzler RM: End-plate desensitization specificity of calcium. *Life Sci* 13:459–465, 1973.
411. Paton WDM, Zaimis EJ: Methonium compounds. *Pharmacol Rev* 4: 219–253, 1952.
412. Paton WDM, Zaimis EJ: The action of *d*-tubocurarine and of decamethonium on respiratory and other muscles in the cat. *J Pharmacol Exp Ther* 107:165–171, 1951.
413. Paton WDM: The effects of muscle relaxants other than muscle relaxation. *Anesthesiology* 20:453–463, 1959.
414. Payne JP, Hughes R: Evaluation of atracurium in anaesthetized man. *Br J Anaesth* 53:45–54, 1981.
415. Payne JP, Hughes R, Azawi SA: Neuromuscular blockade by neostigmine in anesthetized man. *Br J Anaesth* 52:69-76, 1980.
416. Payne JP, Utting JE: Symposium on atracurium. *Br J Anaesth* 55: 1S–140S, 1983.
417. Payton BW, Shand DG: Actions of gallamine and tetraethylammonium at the frog neuromuscular junction. *Br J Pharmacol Chemother* 28: 23–34, 1966.
418. Pellmar TC, Carpenter DO: Cyclic AMP induces a voltage-dependent current in neurons of Aplysia californica. *Neurosci Letts* 22:151–157, 1981.
419. Peng HB: Cytoskeletal organization of the presynaptic nerve terminal and the acetylcholine receptor cluster in cell cultures. *J Cell Biol* 97:489–498, 1983.
420. Pennefather P, Quastel DMJ: Fast desensitization of the nicotinic receptor at the mouse neuromuscular junction. *Br J Pharmacol* 77: 395–404, 1982.
421. Peper K, Bradely RJ, Dreyer F: The acetylcholine receptor at the neuromuscular junction. *Physiol Rev* 62:1271–1340, 1982.
422. Peper K, Sterz R: Effects of drugs and antibodies on the postsynaptic membrane of the neuromuscular junction. *Ann NY Acad Sci* 377:519–543, 1981.
423. Pestronk A, Drachman DB, Stanley EF, Price DL, Griffin JW: Cholinergic transmission regulates extrajunctional acetylcholine receptors. *Exp Neurol* 70:690–696, 1980.
424. Pestronk A, Drachman DD, Griffin JW: Effect of muscle disuse on acetylcholine receptor. *Nature* (London) 260:352–353, 1976.
425. Pestronk A: "Hidden" alpha-bungarotoxin binding sites in rat skeletal muscle in vivo. *Soc Neurosci Abstr* 226:8, 1981.
426. Pickett JB: Nerve terminals are as metabolically different as the muscle fibers they innervate. *Science* 210:927–928, 1980.
427. Pilar G, Beach R, Vaca K, Suszkiw J: Control of acetylcholine synthesis in motor nerve terminals. *Adv Behav Biol* 24:481, 1977.
428. Pincus JH, Hsiao K: Phenytoin inhibits both synaptosomal ^{45}Ca uptake and efflux. *Exp Neurol* 74:293–298, 1981.
429. Pincus JH, Yaari Y, Argov Z: Phenytoin: Electrophysiological effects at the neuromuscular junction. *Adv Neurol* 27:363–376, 1982.

430. Pincus JH: Diphenylhydantoin and ion flux in lobster nerves. *Arch Neurol* 26:4–10, 1972.

431. Preston JB, Van Maanen EF: Effects of frequency of stimulation on the paralyzing dose of neuromuscular blocking agents. *J Pharmacol Exp Ther* 107:165–171, 1953.

432. Publicover SJ, Duncan CJ: Dantrolene and the effect of temperature on the spontaneous release of transmitter at the frog neuromuscular junction. *Experientia* 37:859–860, 1981.

433. Publicover SJ: The effect of dantrolene on tetanic potentiation of mepp frequency in EGTA containing salines. *Brain Res* 253:321–324, 1982.

434. Publicover SJ, Duncan CJ: The effects of oxotremorine demonstrate presynaptic muscarinic and dopaminergic receptors on motor nerve terminals. *Nature* 278:645–646, 1979.

435. Pumplin DW, Fambrough DM: Turnover of acetylcholine receptors in skeletal muscle. *Ann Rev Physiol* 44:319–335, 1982.

436. Pumplin DW: Normal variations in presynaptic active zones of frog neuromuscular junction. *J Neurocytol* 12:317–323, 1983.

437. Raftery MA, Changeux J-P: The nicotinic acetylcholine receptor (AChR). *Neurosci Res Prog Bull* 20:277–293, 1982.

438. Raftery MA, Hunkapiller MW, Strader CD, Hood LE: Acetylcholine receptor: Complex of homologous subunits. *Science* 208:1454–1456, 1980.

439. Rahamimoff R, Lev-Tov A, Meiri H: Primary and secondary regulation of quantal transmitter release: Calcium and sodium. *J Exp Biol* 89:5–18, 1980.

440. Rahaminoff R, Lev-Tov A, Meiri H, Rahaminoff H, Nussinovitch I: Regulation of acetylcholine liberation from presynaptic nerve terminals. *Monog Neural Sci* 7:3–18, 1980.

441. Raines A, Helke CJ, Iadorola MJ, Britton EW, Anderson RJ: Blockade of the tonic hindlimb extensor component of maximal electroshock and pentylenetetrazole-induced seizures by drugs action on muscle and muscle spindle system: A perspective on method. *Epilepsia* 17:395–402, 1976.

442. Raines A, Standaert FG: Effects of anticonvulsant drugs on nerve terminals. *Epilepsia* 10:211–227, 1969.

443. Raines A, Standaert FG: Pre- and postjunctional effects of diphenylhydantoin at the cat soleus neuromuscular junction. *J Pharmacol Exp Ther* 153:361–366, 1966.

444. Ramzam MI, Triggs EJ, Shanks CA: Pharmacokinetic studies in man with gallamine triethiodide: I. Single and multiple clinical doses. *Eur J Clin Pharmacol* 17:135–143, 1980.

445. Ramzan MI, Shanks CA, Triggs EJ: Gallamine disposition in surgical patients with chronic renal failure. *Br J Clin Pharmacol* 12:141–147, 1981.

446. Ramzan MI, Shanks CA, Triggs EJ: Pharmacokinetics of tubucurarine administration by combined i.v. bolus and infusion. *Br J Anaesth* 52:893–899, 1980.

447. Ramzan MI, Triggs EJ, Shanks CA: Pharmacokinetic studies in man with gallamine triethiodide. *Eur J Clin Pharmacol* 17:145–152, 1980.

448. Rang HP, Ritter JM: On the mechanism of desensitization at cholinergic receptors. *Molec Pharmacol* 6:357–382, 1970.

449. Rang HP: Drugs and ionic channels: Mechanisms and implications. *Postgrad Med J* 57:89–97, 1981.
450. Rang HP: The action of ganglionic blocking drugs on the synaptic responses of rat submandibular ganglion cells. *Br J Pharmacol* 75:151–168, 1982.
451. Rees JMH: Anticurare activity of tacrine (THA). *J Pharm Pharmacol* 18:289–293, 1966.
452. Riker WF Jr: Actions of acetylcholine on mammalian motor nerve terminals. *J Pharmacol Exp Ther* 397–416, 1966.
453. Riker WF Jr: Prejunctional effects of neuromuscular blocking and facilitatory drugs. In Katz, R (ed): *Muscle Relaxants*. Amsterdam, Excerpta Medica 1975, pp 59–102.
454. Riker WF Jr, Okamoto M: Pharmacology of motor nerve terminals. *Ann Rev Pharmacol* 9:173–208, 1969.
455. Riker WF, Standaert FG: The action of facilitatory drugs and acetylcholine on neuromuscular transmission. *Ann NY Acad Sci* 135:135–164, 1966.
456. Riker WF Jr, Wescoe WC: The relationship between cholinesterase inhibition and function in a neuro-effector system. *J Pharmacol Exp Ther* 95:515–527, 1949.
457. Ringel SP, Bender AN, Festoff BW, Engel WK: Ultrastructural demonstration and analytical application of extrajunctional receptors of denervated human and rat skeletal muscle fibres. *Nature* 255:730–731, 1975.
458. Robbins N, Fischbach GD: Effect of chronic disuse of rat soleus neuromuscular junctions on presynaptic function. *J Neurophysiol* 34:562–578, 1977.
459. Robertson EN, Booij LHDJ, Fragen RJ, Crul JF: Clinical comparison of atracurium and vercuronium (ORG NC45). *Br J Anaesth* 55:125–129, 1983.
460. Rosenblueth A, Morison RS: Curarization, fatigue, and Wedensky inhibition. *Am J Physiol* 119:236–256, 1937.
461. Ross MJ, Klymkowsky MW, Agard DA, Stroud RM: Structural studies of a membrane-bound acetylcholine receptor from Torpedo californica. *J Mol Biol* 116:635–659, 1977.
462. Ruff RL: The kinetics of local anesthetic blockade of end-plate channels. *Biophys J* 37:625–631, 1982.
463. Sakmann B, Adams PR: Biophysical aspects of agonist action at frog endplate. *Adv Pharmacol Ther* 1:81–91, 1978.
464. Salpeter MM, Harris R: Distribution and turnover rate of acetylcholine receptors throughout the junction folds at a vertebrate neuromuscular junction. *J Cell Biol* 96:1781–1785, 1983.
465. Salpeter MM, Leonard JP, Kasprzak H: Agonist-induced postsynaptic myopathy. *Neuroscience Commentaries* 1:73–83, 1982.
466. Savarese JJ, Kitz RJ: Does clinical anesthesia need new neuromuscular blocking agents. *Anesthesiology* 42:236–238, 1975.
467. Savarese JJ: Cardiovascular and autonomic effects of muscle relaxants. In *American Society of Anesthesiologists Annual Refresher Course Lectures*. Am Soc Anesth Ann Meeting, New Orleans, 1980, pp 220 (1–13).

468. Savarese JJ: The autonomic margins of safety of metocurarine and *d*-tubocurarine in the cat. *Anesthesiology* 50:40–46, 1979.
469. Saxena PR, Bonta IL: Mechanism of selective cardiac vagolytic action of pancuronium bromide, specific blockade of cardiac muscarine receptors. *Eur J Pharmacol* 11:332–341, 1970.
470. Saxena PR, Dhasmana KM, Prakash O: A comparison of systemic and regional hemodynamic effects of *d*-tubocurarine, pancuronium, vecuronium. *Anesthesiology* 59:102–108, 1983.
471. Schoene K: Reactivation of soman inhibited acetylcholinesterase in vitro and protection against soman in vivo by bispyridinium-2-aldoximes. *Biochem Pharmacol* 32:1649–1651, 1983.
472. Schofield GG, Witkop B, Warnick JE, Albuquerque EX: Differentiation of the open and closed states of the ionic channels of nicotinic acetylcholine receptors by tricyclic antidepressants. *Proc Nat Acad Sci USA* 78:5340–5244, 1981.
473. Schwartz RD, Sidell FR: Renal tubular secretion of pralidoxime in man. *Proc Soc Exp Biol Med* 146:419–424, 1974.
474. Schwarz JR, Spielmann RP: Flurazepam: Effects on sodium and potassium currents in myelinated nerve fibers. *Eur J Pharmacol* 90:359–366, 1983.
475. Scott RPF, Goat VA: Atracurium: Its speed of onset in comparison with suxamethonium. *Br J Anaesth* 54:909–911, 1982.
476. Secher NH, Rube N, Secher O: Effect of tubocurarine on human soleus and gastrocnemous muscles. *Acta Anaesth Scand* 26:231–234, 1982.
477. Shaker N, Eldefrawi AT, Aguayo LG, Warnick JE, Albuquerque EX, Eldefrawi ME: Interactions of *d*-tubocurarine with the nicotinic acetylcholine receptor/channel molecule. *J Pharmacol Exp Ther* 220:172–177, 1982.
478. Shanks CA, Somogyi AA, Triggs EJ: Dose-response and plasma concentration-response relationships of pancuronium in man. *Anesthesiology* 51:111–118, 1979.
479. Shayevitz JR, Matteo RS: Altered response to metocurarine in patients with upper motoneuron disease. *Anesthesiology* 59:A287, 1983.
480. Shek E, Higuchi T: Improved delivery through biological membranes. 2. Distribution, excretion, metabolism of N-methyl-1, 6-dihydropyridine-2-carbaldoxime hydrochloride, a pro-drug of N-methylpyridinium 2-carbaldoxime chloride. *J Med Chem* 19:108–112, 1976.
481. Sheridan RE, Lester HA: Functional stoichiometry at the nicotinic receptor. *J Gen Physiol* 80:449–515, 1982.
482. Shotton DM, Heuser JE, Reese BF, Reese TS: Postsynaptic membrane folds of the frog neuromuscular junction visualized by scanning electron microscopy. *Neuroscience* 4:427–435, 1979.
483. Sidell FP, Groff WA, Kaminskis A: Pralidoxime methanesulfonate: Plasma levels and pharmacokinetics after oral administration in man. *J Pharmac Sci* 61:1136–1140, 1972.
484. Silinsky EM: On the role of barium in supporting the asynchronous release of acetylcholine quanta by motor nerve impulses. *J Physiol* (London) 274:157–171, 1978.
485. Silinsky EM: Evidence for specific adenosine receptors at cholinergic nerve endings. *Br J Pharmacol* 71:191–194, 1980.

486. Sine SM, Taylor P: Local anesthetics and histrionicotoxin are allosteric inhibitors of the acetylcholine receptor. *J Biol Chem* 257:8106–8114, 1982.

487. Sine SM, Taylor P: Relationship between reversible antagonist occupancy and the functional capacity of the acetylcholine receptor. *J Biol Chem* 256:6692–6699, 1981.

488. Skirboll L: *An Electrophysiological Investigation of the Interaction between Ca Ions and a Cyclic Nucleotide System in the Mammalian Motor Nerve Terminal.* Thesis, Georgetown University, 1977.

489. Skirboll L, Dretchen KL: A stimulatory action of dantrolene sodium on the motor nerve terminal. *Fed Proc* 34:751, 1975.

490. Skirboll LR, Standaert FG, Dretchen KL: Effects of calcium on a cyclic system in soleus motor nerve terminals. *Eur J Pharmacol* 54:295–298, 1979.

491. Smith AP, van der Weil HJ, Wolthuis OL: Analysis of oxime-induced neuromuscular recovery in guinea pigs, rat and man following soman poisoning in vitro. *Eur J Pharmacol* 70:371–379, 1981.

492. Smith CM: Neuromuscular pharmacology: Drugs and muscle spindles. *Ann Rev Pharmacol* 3:223, 1963.

493. Smith H, Spalding JMK: Outbreak of paralysis in Morocco due to orthocresyl phosphate poisoning. *Lancet* 2:1019–1021, 1959.

494. Smith KJ, Schauf CL: Effects of gallamine triethiodide on membrane currents in amphibian and mammalian peripheral nerve. *J Pharmacol Exp Ther* 217:719–726, 1981.

495. Smith KJ, Schauf CL: Gallamine triethiodide (Flexedil): Tetraethylammonium- and pancuronium-like effects in myelinated nerve fibers. *Science* 212:1170–1172, 1981.

496. Snider RM, Gerald MC: Noradrenergic-mediated potentiation of acetylcholine release from the phrenic nerve: Evidence for presynaptic $alpha_1$-adrenoceptor involvement. *Life Sci* 31:853–857, 1982.

497. Snider RM, Gerald MC: Studies on the mechanism of (+)-amphetamine enhancement of neuromuscular transmission, muscle contraction, electrophysiological and biochemical results. *J Pharmacol Exp Ther* 221: 14–21, 1982.

498. Sokoll MD, Carter JG, Gergis SD: Spinal cord transection and nerve muscle transmission. *Anesthesiology* 51:S274, 1979.

499. Sokoll MD, Dretchen KL, Gergis SD, Long JP: The effects of gallamine on nerve terminals and endplates. *Anesthesiology* 38:157–165, 1973.

500. Sokoll MD: Neuromuscular disease causing decreased sensitivity to relaxants. Presented to The International Symposium Clinical Neuromuscular Pharmacology, Boston, 1983.

501. Somogyi AA, Shanks CA, Triggs EJ: Combined i.v. bolus and infusion of pancuronium bromide. *Br J Anaesth* 50:575–582, 1978.

502. Somogyi AA, Shanks CA, Triggs EJ: The effect of renal failure on the disposition and neuromuscular blocking action of pancuronium bromide. *Eur J Clin Pharmacol* 12:23–29, 1977.

503. Soteropoulos GC, Standaert FG: Neuromuscular effects of morphine and naloxone. *J Pharmacol Exp Ther* 184:136–141, 1975.

504. Spencer PS, Schaumburg HH: The relationship between the chemical classification of neurotoxic disease. A morphological approach. In

Spencer PS, Schaumburg HH (eds): *Experimental and Clinical Neurotoxicology*. Baltimore, Williams and Wilkins Co, 1980, pp 92–99.
505. Spivak CE, Albuquerque EX: Dynamic properties of the nicotinic acetylcholine receptors ionic channel complex: Activation and blockade. In Hanin I, Goldbery AM, (eds): *Progress in Cholinergic Biology: Model Cholinergic Synapses*. New York, Raven Press, 1982, pp 323–352.
506. Standaert FG: The action of *d*-tubocurarine on the motor nerve terminal. *J Pharmacol Exp Ther* 143:181–186, 1964.
507. Standaert FG: Interactions among neuromuscular blocking agents and other drugs. Refresher Courses in Anesthesiology. Am Soc Anesth, Inc. 1978, pp 111–114.
508. Standaert FG: Cyclic nucleotides and synaptic function. *Fed Proc* 38: 2178–2183, 1979.
509. Standaert FG: Release of transmitter at the neuromuscular junction. *Br J Anaesth* 54:131–145, 1982.
510. Standaert FG: *Sites of Action of Muscle Relaxants*. Refresher Courses in Anesthesiology. Am Soc Anesth, Inc, 1982, pp 226(1–3).
511. Standaert FG: Mechanism of action of neuromuscular blocking drugs. 30th Annual Anesthesiology Review Course Lecture Notes. *Proc Soc Air Force Anesthesiologists*, San Antonio, Texas. 115(1–4), 1983.
512. Standaert FG, Adams JE: The actions of succinylcholine on the mammalian motor nerve terminal. *J Pharmacol Exp Ther* 140:113–123, 1965.
513. Standaert FG, Detwiler PB: The neuromuscular pharmacology of germine-3-acetate and germine-3, 16-diacetate. *J Pharmacol Exp Ther* 171:223–241, 1970.
514. Standaert FG, Dretchen KL: Cyclic nucleotides and neuromuscular transmission. *Fed Proc* 38:2183–2192, 1979.
515. Standaert FG, Dretchen KL: Cyclic nucleotides in neuromuscular transmission. *Anesth Analg* (Cleveland) 60:91–99, 1981.
516. Standaert FG, Dretchen KL, Skirboll LA, Morgenroth VH: Effects of cyclic nucleotides on mammalian motor nerve terminals. *J Pharmacol Exp Ther* 199:544–552, 1976.
517. Standaert FG, Dretchen KL, Skirboll LR, Morgenroth VH: A role of cyclic nucleotides in neuromuscular transmission. *J Pharmacol Exp Ther* 199:553–564, 1976.
518. Standaert FG, Levitt GB, Roberts J: Antagonism of digitalis arrhythmia by pronethalol—A neural phenomenon. *Nature* (London) 210: 742–745, 1966.
519. Standaert FG, Riker WF: The consequences of cholinergic drugs actions on motor nerve terminals. *Ann NY Acad Sci* 144:517–533, 1967.
520. Stanski DR, Sheiner LB: Pharmacokinetics and dynamics of muscle relaxants. *Anesthesiology* 51:103–105, 1979.
521. Stanski DR, Watkins WD: *Disposition in Anesthesia*. New York, Grune Stratton, 1982, pp 97–136.
522. Starke K, Endo T: Presynaptic alpha-adrenoceptors. *Biochem Pharmacol* 7:307–312, 1976.
523. Starke K: Presynaptic receptors. *Ann Rev Pharmacol Toxicol* 21:7–30, 1980.

524. Steegmuller H: On the geographical distribution of pseudocholinesterase variants. *Human Genet* 26:167–185, 1975.

525. Steinbach JH: Developmental changes in acetylcholine receptor aggregates at rat skeletal neuromuscular junctions. *Dev Biol* 94:267–276, 1981.

526. Steinbach JH: Neuromuscular junctions and alpha-bungarotoxin binding sites in denervated and contralateral cat skeletal muscles. *J Physiol* 313:513–528, 1981.

527. Stephenson FA, Harrison R, Lunt GG: The isolation and characterization of the nicotinic acetylcholine receptors from human skeletal muscle. *Eur J Biochem* 115:91–97, 1981.

528. Sterri SH, Lyngaas S, Fonnum FJ: Cholinesterase and carboxylesterase activities in soman poisoned rats treated with bispyridinium monooximes HI-6 and HS-6. *Biochem Pharmacol* 32:1646–1649, 1983.

529. Sterz R, Pagala M, Peper K: Postjunctional characteristics of the endplates in mammalian fast and slow muscles. *Pfluegers Arch* 398:48–54, 1983.

530. Stockton JM, Birdsall NJM, Burgen ASV, Hulme EC: Modification of the binding properties of muscarinic receptors by gallamine. *Molec Pharmacol* 23:551–557, 1983.

531. Stoelting R: Choice of relaxant in patient with heart disease. Presented to the International Symposium Clinical Neuromuscular Pharmacology. Boston, August 1983.

532. Stone TW: Physiological roles of adenosine and adenosine-5-triphosphate in the nervous system. *Neuroscience* 6:523–555, 1981.

533. Stone WA, Bench TF, Hamelberg W: Succinylcholine danger in the spinal cord injured patient. *Anesthesiology* 32:168–169, 1970.

534. Stoyanov E, Vulchev P, Shturbova M, Marinova M: Clinical electromyomechanographic and electromyographic studies in decurarization with pymadine. *Anaesth Resus Inten Therap* 4:139–142, 1976.

535. Sundwall A: Plasma concentration curves of N-methylpyridinium-2-aldoxime methane sulphonate after intravenous, intramuscular, and oral administration in man. *Biochem Pharmacol* 5:225–230, 1960.

536. Sunew KY, Hicks RG: Effects of neostigmine and pyridostigmine on duration of succinylcholine action and pseudocholinesterase activity. *Anesthesiology* 49:188–191, 1978.

537. Swartz RD, Sidell FR: Renal tubular secretion of pralidoxime in man. *Proc Soc Exp Biol Med* 146:419–424, 1974.

538. Szerb JC: Characterization of presynaptic muscarinic receptors in central cholinergic neurons. *Adv Behav Biol* 24:49–60, 1977.

539. Szerb JC: Effect of low calcium and oxotremorine on the kinetics of the evoked release of [^{3}H] acetylcholine from the guinea-pig myenteric plexus: Comparison with morphine. *Naunyn-Schmeideberg's Arch Pharmacol* 311:119–127, 1980.

540. Tamaki M: The effect of streptomycin on the neuromuscular junction of the frog. *Brain Res* 265:241–247, 1983.

541. Tammisto T, Salmenpera M: Neuromuscular blocking properties of dioxonium. *Acta Anaesth Scand* 24:439–443, 1980.

542. Tauc L: Nonvesicular release of neurotransmitter. *Physiol Rev* 62:857–893, 1982.

543. Tauc L, Israel M, Pichon Y, Simonneau M, Stinnakre J: Calcium in synaptic transmission. *J Physiol* (Paris) 76:383–528, 1980.
544. Taylor DB, Creese R, Nedergaard PA Case R: Labelled depolarizing drugs in normal and denervated muscle. *Nature* (London) 208:901–902, 1965.
545. Taylor P, Brown RD, Johnson DA: The linkage between ligand occupation and response of the nicotinic acetylcholine receptor. *Current Topics in Membranes and Transport* 18:407–446, 1983.
546. Taylor P, Weiland G, Sine S, Chignell CF, Brown RD: Cholinergic receptor state transitions and local anesthetic action. *Prog Anesthesiol* 2:175–183, 1980.
547. Thesleff S, Molgo J, Lundh H: Botulinum toxin and 4-aminoquinoline induce a similar abnormal type of spontaneous quantal transmitter release at the neuromuscular junction. *Brain Res* 264:89–97, 1983.
548. Thesleff S, Molgo J: A new type of transmitter release at the neuromuscular junction. *Neurosci* 9:1–8, 1983.
549. Thesleff S: Aminopyridines and synaptic transmission. *Neuroscience* 5:1413–1419, 1980.
550. Tobey RE, Jacobsen PM, Kahle CT, Clubb RJ, Dean MA: The serum potassium response to muscle relaxants in neural injury. *Anesthesiology* 37:332–337, 1972.
551. Torda TA, Gage PW: Postsynaptic effect of i.v. anaesthetic agents at the neuromuscular junction. *Br J Anaesth* 49:771–776, 1977.
552. Trautmann A: Curare can open and block ionic channels associated with cholinergic receptors. *Nature* (London) 298:272–275, 1982.
553. Tucek S: *Acetylcholine Synthesis in Neurons*. New York, John Wiley and Sons, 1978.
554. Tucek S: The synthesis of acetylcholine in skeletal muscles of the rat. *J Physiol* 322:53–69, 1982.
555. Vaca K, Pilar G: Mechanisms controlling choline transport and acetylcholine synthesis in motor nerve terminals during electrical stimulation. *J Gen Physiol* 75:605–628, 1979.
556. Van der Veen F, Bencini A: Pharmacokinetics and pharmacodynamics of ORG NC45 in man. *Br J Anaesth* 52:375–405, 1980.
557. van Helden HPM, van der Weil HJ, Wolthuis OL: Therapy of organophosphate poisoning: The marmoset as a model for man. *Br J Pharmacol* 78:579–589, 1983.
558. Viby-Mogensen J, Handel HK: Increased sensitivity to succinylcholine in a patient heterozygous for the silent and the fluoride-resistant gene. *Anesth Analg* (Cleveland) 57:422–426, 1978.
559. Viby-Mogensen J, Hanel HK: Prolonged apnoea after suxamethonium. *Acta Anaesth Scand* 22:371–380, 1978.
560. Viby-Mogensen J: Correlation of succinylcholine duration of action with plasma cholinesterase activity in subjects with the genotypically normal enzyme. *Anesthesiology* 53:517–520, 1980.
561. Vizi, ES, Vyskočil F: Changes in total and quantal release of acetylcholine in the mouse diaphragm during activation and inhibition of membrane ATPase. *J Physiol* 286:1–14, 1979.
562. Vizi ES: Presynaptic modulation of neurochemical transmission. *Prog Neurobiol* 12:181–290, 1979.

563. Vyskočil F, Nikolsky E, Edwards C: An analysis of the mechanisms underlying the non-quantal release of acetylcholine at the mouse neuromuscular junction. *Neuroscience* 9:429–435, 1983.
564. Ward S, Neill EAM, Weatherley BC, Corall IM: Pharmacokinetics of atracurium besylate in healthy patients (after a single i.v. bolus dose). *Br J Anaesth* 55:113–117, 1983.
565. Waud B: Pharmacokinetics of relaxants. Proceedings Pharmacology of the Anesthesiologist. Emory University, Atlanta, March 1978, pp 29–30.
566. Waud DR: The nature of "depolarizing block." *Anesthesiology* 29:1014–1024, 1968.
567. Webb SN, Bowmann WC: The role of pre- and post-junctional cholinoceptors in the action of neostigmine at the neuromuscular junction. *Clin Exp Pharmacol Physiol* 1:123–134, 1974.
568. Wecker L, Dettbarn W-D: Paraoxon induced myopathy: Muscle specificity and acetylcholine involvement. *Exp Neurol* 51:282–291, 1976.
569. Wecker L, Laskowski B, Dettbarn W-D: Neuromuscular dysfunction induced by acetylcholinesterase inhibition. *Fed Proc* 37:2818–2822, 1978.
570. Wedensky N: *Uber die Beziehung zwischen Reisung und Erregung im Tetanus.* St. Petersburg no. 12. Oct 9, 1886.
571. Weiler M, Roed IS, Whittaker VP: The kinetics of acetylcholine turnover in a resting nerve terminal and the magnitude of the cytoplasmic compartment. *J Neurochem* 38:1187–1191, 1982.
572. Werner G: Spontaneous miniature activity and gradation of transmission at the neuromuscular junction. *Sparatum Experientia* 17:95, 1961.
573. Whittaker M: Plasma cholinesterase variants and the anaesthetist. *Anaesthesia* 35:174–197, 1980.
574. Whorton MD, Obrinsky DL: Persistence of symptoms after mild to moderate acute organophosphate poisoning among 19 farm field workers. *J Toxicol Envir Health* 11:347–354, 1983.
575. Williams NE, Webb SN, Calvey RN: Differential effects of myoneural blocking drugs on neuromuscular transmission. *Br J Anaesth* 52:1111–1115, 1980.
576. Willow M, Catterall VA: Inhibition of binding of [^{3}H] batrachotoxinin A 20-alpha-benzoate to sodium channels by the anticonvulsant drugs diphenylhydantoin and carbamazepine. *Molec Pharmacol* 22:627–635, 1982.
577. Wilson DF: The effects of dibutyryl cyclic adenosine 3, 5-monophosphate, theophylline, and aminophylline on neuromuscular transmission in the rat. *J Pharmacol Exp Ther* 188:447–452, 1974.
578. Wilson IB, Harrison MA, Ginsburg, S: Carbamyl derivatives of acetylcholine. *J Biol Chem* 236:1498, 1961.
579. Wolthuis O, Van Wersch RAP, van der Weil HJ: The efficacy of some dispyridinium oximes as antidotes to soman in isolated muscles of several species including man. *Eur J Pharmacol* 70:355–369, 1981.
580. Wolthuis OL, Berends F, Meeter E: Problems in the therapy of soman poisoning. *Fundam Appl Toxicol* 1:183–192, 1981.
581. Wong BS: Quinidine interactions with Myxicola giant axons. *Molec Pharmacol* 20:98–106, 1981.

582. Wood M, Stone WJ, Wood AJJ: Plasma binding of pancuronium: Effect of age, sex and disease. *Anesthesiology* 53:S286, 1980.
583. Woodbury DM: Effects of diphenylhydantoin on electrolytes and radiosodium turnover in brain and other tissues of normal, hyponatremic and postictal rats. *J Pharmacol Exp Ther* 115:74–95, 1958.
584. Wray D: Noise analysis and channels at the postsynaptic membrane of skeletal muscle. *Prog Drug Res* 24:9–56, 1981.
585. Xavier E, Valle JR: Synergism of cholinesterase inhibitors with acetylcholine on toad rectus abdominis muscle. *Acta Physiol Lat Amer* 13:282–289, 1963.
586. Xintharas C, Burg JR: Screening and prevention of human neurotoxic outbreaks: Issues and problems. In Spencer PS, Schaumberg HH (eds): *Experimental and Clinical Neurotoxicology.* Baltimore, Williams & Wilkins, 1980, pp 663–674.
587. Yaari Y, Pincus JH, Argov Z: Depression of synaptic transmission by diphenylhydantoin. *Ann Neurol* 1:334–338, 1977.
588. Yoshioka K, Miyaya Y: Uneven distribution of extrajunctional ACh sensitivity in the rat soleus muscle after cordotomy. *Neurosci Lett* 18:S4, 1980.
589. Young AP, Sigman DS: Allosteric facilitation of in vitro desensitization of the acetylcholine receptor by volatile anesthetics. *Prog Anesthesiol* 2:209–228, 1980.
590. Young AP, Sigman DS: Conformational effects of volatile anesthetics on the membrane-bound acetylcholine receptor protein: Facilitation of the agonist-induced affinity conversion. *Biochem* 22:2155–2159, 1983.
591. Young SH, Poo M: Topographical rearrangement of acetylcholine receptors alters channel kinetics. *Nature* 304:161–163, 1983.
592. Zaimis EJ: Motor endplate differences as a determining factor in the mode of action of neuromuscular blocking substances. *J Physiol* 122:238–251, 1953.
593. Zimmerman H: Vesicle recycling and transmitter release. *Neurosci* 4:1773–1804, 1979.

Chapter 5

The Effects of Nerve Injury on the Neuromuscular Junction

Robert G. Miller, M.D.

The impact of injury to a motor nerve upon the neuromuscular junction will be reviewed in this chapter. Substantial changes also occur in the dynamic properties of denervated and partially denervated muscle, and in the muscle membrane, and these will also be discussed. The trophic effects of nerve upon muscle are a subject of intense interest and investigation, and this review will attempt to give some perspective on this fascinating area. The orderly sequence of events in repair and regeneration, as well as sprouting, will be delineated. Morphological changes at the neuromuscular junction and the mechanical and electrical responses in reinnervated muscle will be reviewed, both from experimental models and from human diseases of peripheral nerve.

Distal to an axonal transection, the light microscopic changes of Wallerian degeneration (first described by Waller[196] in 1850) are similar in all species, and have recently been reviewed.[175,186] The contents of the axoplasm undergo disruption, and there is loss of longitudinal orientation with fragmentation of neural tubules and neural filaments throughout the axon. Mitochondria become swollen and discontinuities develop in the axolemma. Areas of swelling and narrowing occur in the axon and fragmentation takes place initially between nodes of Ranvier, usually in the smallest fibers first. There is some controversy about whether changes in the axon progress simultaneously along the entire distal segment or whether they move centrifugally from the site of nerve injury. Degenerating axonal fragments are surrounded by myelin, and ellipsoids are formed which subdivide into smaller spheres. Proliferating Schwann cells and macrophages produce further degradation by approximately the fifth day. Digestion of these fragments occurs over the next several weeks. The same sequence of events will occur whether the nerve is injured by a crush or a complete section.

Before these changes of Wallerian degeneration in a damaged axon become apparent, abnormalities at the neuromuscular junction are detectable.[82] Following nerve transection in primates, there is a progressive fall in amplitude of both muscle and nerve action potentials on successive days. Transmission failure occurs first at the neuromuscular junction. The muscle response to nerve stimulation disappears by the fourth or fifth day after nerve section, whereas the ascending nerve action potential is obtainable for five to eight days.[81] In rabbit, guinea pig, cat, dog, baboon and human, neuromuscular transmission fails before conduction failure in the axon.[84] In lower mammals, the time to neuromuscular transmission failure is shorter, and in humans, it may be longer, although insufficient data have been obtained to establish the point.[70,83,95,115,125,165]

Miledi and Slater correlated the functional and structural changes accompanying denervation of the neuromuscular junction following nerve section in the rat.[143] Neuromuscular transmission was normal until eight to ten hours after nerve section, at which point an increasing number of endplates began to fail, and after 20 hours, no endplates transmitted an impulse. Transmission failure occurred abruptly at most endplates and was usually accompanied by cessation of spontaneous miniature endplate potentials, although occasionally miniature endplate potentials persisted after junctional transmission had failed. In some junctions, the frequency of miniature endplate potentials was very low, suggesting an intermediate stage in the failure of miniature endplate potentials. There was a direct relationship between the time of junctional failure and the length of the degenerating nerve stump. For each additional centimeter of nerve in the distal stump, neuromuscular transmission failure was delayed 45 minutes. Ultrastructural changes in nerve endings closely paralleled changes in function. There were no detectable morphological abnormalities at the endplate in the first eight to twelve hours after nerve section. When neuromuscular transmission was failing, some endplates were clearly undergoing structural breakdown. All endplates were morphologically abnormal when neuromuscular failure was complete.

The development of freeze-fracture electron microscopy has made possible the study of large areas of the endplate and structures within the nerve terminal membrane that had otherwise been inaccessible.[56] The active zones on the nerve terminal are the sites for the quantal release of neurotransmitter by synaptic vesicle exocytosis at the neuromuscular junction[46,100,101] (see chapter 2). The active zones lie directly opposite the junctional folds of the postsynaptic membrane, and are usually perpendicular to the longitudinal axis of the nerve terminal (Fig. 5.1). After nerve section, and before neuromuscular transmission failure, no histological abnormality is evident in the active zones or in the remaining portion of the neuromuscular junction with freeze-fracture electron microscopy.[121] As neuromuscular transmission begins to fail, the active zones become disrupted (Fig. 5.2). At a given nerve terminal, once one active zone becomes disrupted, every active zone at that particular terminal becomes disordered. The particles which normally occur in two double rows become disorganized and interrupted and finally vanish. Nerve terminals become fragmented and Schwann cells partially engulf fragmented nerve terminals and begin to occupy large areas of the endplate. Eventually, Schwann cells completely engulf nerve terminals so that the junctions have a new cellular arrangement (Schwann cell and muscle fiber) and neither endplate potentials nor miniature endplate potentials can be recorded from the muscle fiber. Ridges in the Schwann cell occur directly opposite to junctional folds and perpendicular to the longitudinal axis of the junctions, but no organized rows or large particles (corresponding to the active zones at nerve terminals) are found along the Schwann cell ridges.

The disruption of nerve terminal active zones is probably associated with the failure of endplate potentials, and the disappearance of miniature endplate potentials probably corresponds to the engulfment of nerve terminals by Schwann cells. The loss of neuromuscular transmission in the degenerating neuromuscular junction appears to be entirely due to changes at the nerve terminal, since the morphology of the junctional folds and the endplate sensitivity to acetylcholine remain unchanged when transmission first fails after denervation.[16] Although after engulfment of the nerve terminals the Schwann cells develop ridges exactly over the junctional folds, the lack of two double rows of particles suggests that these ridges are not equivalent to the active zones of nerve terminals. However, the ridges may represent the special sites for spontaneous Schwann cell release of acetylcholine, since several days after the complete failure of synaptic activity miniature endplate potentials resume.[16] Schwann cell membranes apparently lack the potential-dependent calcium channels that are thought to correspond to the active zone particles on nerve terminal membranes.

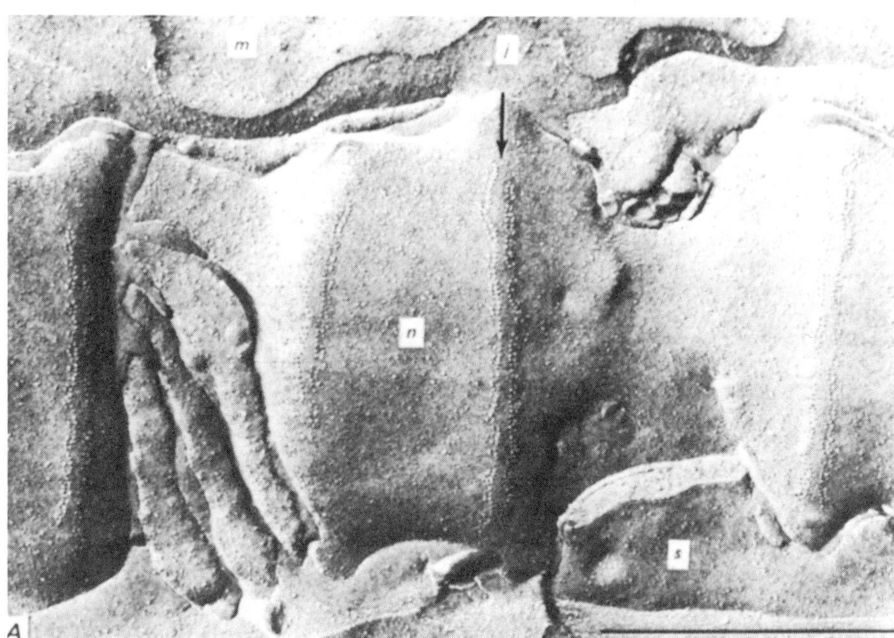

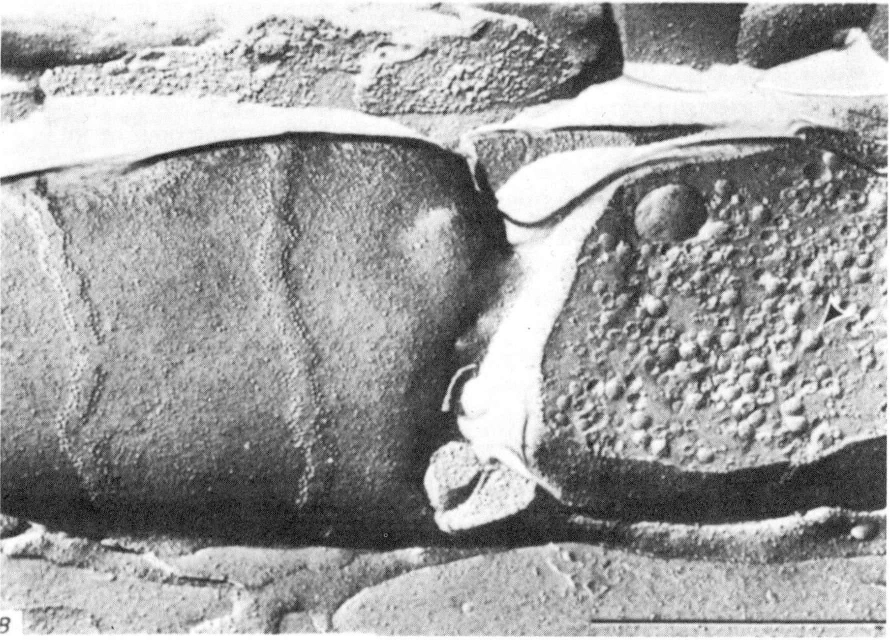

Dynamic Properties of Denervated Muscle

The ultimate purpose of the motor unit (nerve-junction-muscle system) is to produce force. No discussion of the effect of nerve injury upon the neuromuscular junction would be complete without some reference to the alteration of dynamic properties of the muscle following denervation. The story is somewhat complicated by the differences between different species. Three to four weeks after denervation in both fast and slow muscle of the cat, twitch contraction times are prolonged.[117,133,134] In isotonic contractions of denervated cat muscle, the maximum velocity of shortening per sarcomere was determined; for both fast and slow muscles the increase in contraction time in the muscle twitch was accompanied by a decrease in the maximum velocity of shortening. In denervated rabbit muscles, fast-twitch muscle is slowed less than slow-twitch muscle, but the time to peak tension of denervated slow muscle is decreased by 50%.[187] Changes in rat denervated fast muscle are similar to those in denervated cat fast muscle; however, in denervated rat slow muscle only slight changes have been noted.[77,134]

In the rat extensor digitorum longus and soleus muscles, the effects of denervation and botulinum toxin have been compared.[53] Both botulinum treatment and denervation produced progressive slowing of the time to peak tension of the twitch, as well as prolongation of the relaxation time. These changes were more pronounced in the extensor digitorum longus than in the soleus. Both treatments produced slowing of the relaxation curve following tetanic contraction, more marked in the fast muscle than in the slow muscle. The observed slowing of relaxation led the authors to suggest a prolongation of the active state of the muscle. The maximum rate of rise of the tetanus did not change significantly in either muscle after either intervention. Since botulinum toxin and denervation produced virtually iden-

---

Figure 5.1. (A) Endplate in normal frog has a three-cell arrangement: nerve terminal (n), Schwann cell and muscle fiber (m) with junctional folds (j). Opposed to junctional folds, there are active zones (arrow) with two double rows of large intramembrane particles (10 nm in diameter) on the nerve terminal. ×45,000. (B) Endplate in a muscle denervated 36 hr (summer frog). Neuromuscular transmission remained normal in this muscle, every fiber had epps and 80% showed mepps. Active zones still had normal organization of two double rows of large particles. × 45,000. (Compare Fig. 5.2.) Reprinted by permission from the *Journal of Physiology*.[121]

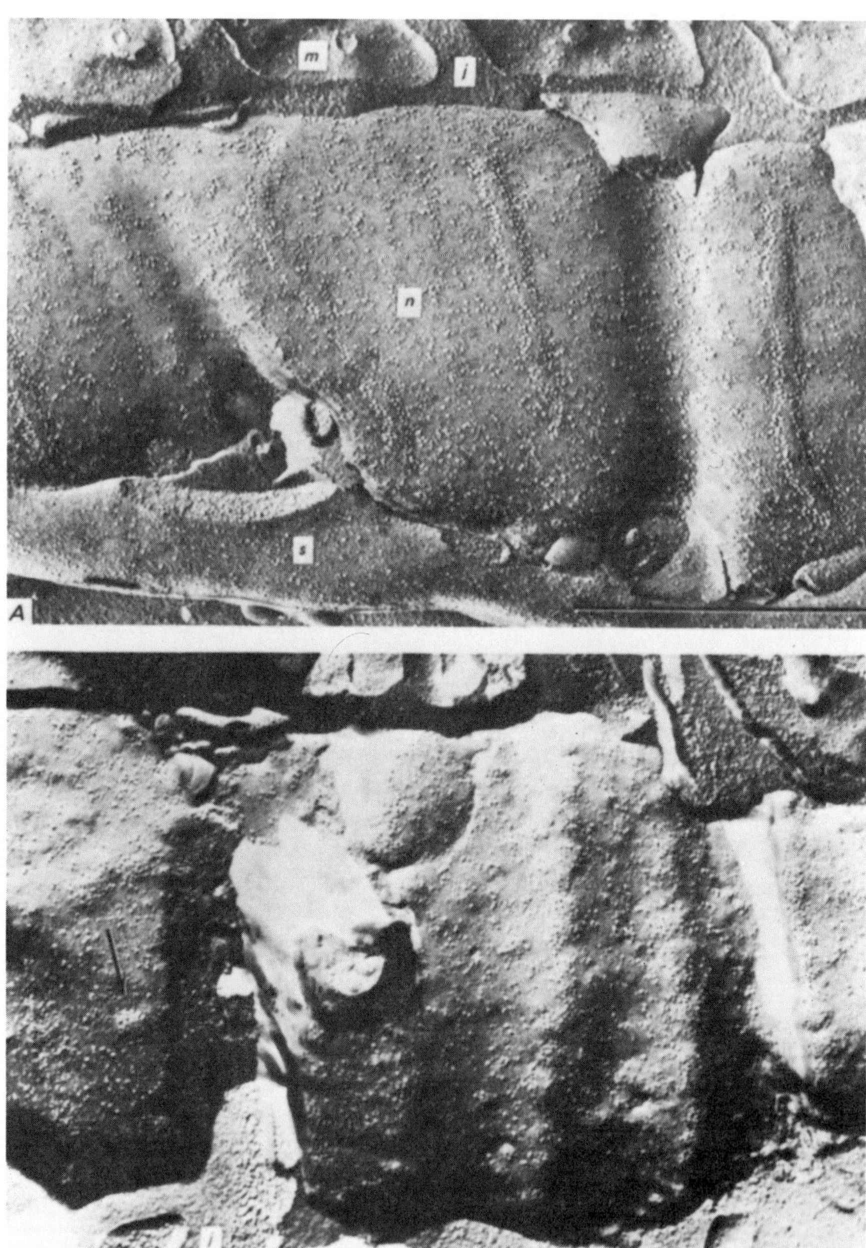

Figure 5.2. Endplates from summer frog muscle denervated 45.5 hr (A) and 41 hr (B). Active zones are disorganized, with loss of normal two double rows of particles or reduction to small fragments (arrow). This was seen before any engulfment of terminals by the Schwann cell could be observed. ×45,000. (Compare Fig. 5.1.) Reprinted by permission from the *Journal of Physiology*.[121]

tical changes in the dynamic properties of these muscles, it was suggested that cholinergic transmission (including muscle usage), or some factor closely related to cholinergic transmission, accounted for the trophic influence of the motor nerve in maintaining dynamic properties of skeletal muscles.[53]

The effect of electrical stimulation upon denervated muscle is important in terms of the dynamic properties. In the rat, the twitch time to peak tension of denervated slow muscle may be markedly decreased by prolonged intermittent direct stimulation at 100 Hz.[138] This result suggests that muscle activity alone is important in determining muscle speed. It should be noted that there was also a very marked fall in the twitch-tetanus ratio. Stimulation at 10 Hz produced a small but significant decrease in twitch time to peak tension. Although many questions remain, it is clear that the activity of muscle is important in the process by which the nerve affects muscle speed, and it seems equally clear that nerve activity can influence force-velocity relationships in muscle. Other aspects of trophism will be considered in more detail below.

In human beings, partial, rather than complete, denervation is by far the most commonly encountered condition. Most denervating diseases affecting human muscle result in some degree of denervation and reinnervation, and unlike the situation in completely denervated animal muscles, many muscle fibers in partially denervated human muscle have intact innervation. In a study of partially denervated human muscle, in which only the responses of innervated muscle fibers were studied, striking similarities were found to the changes encountered in completely denervated muscle from the rat, rabbit and cat.[145] The principal findings in partially denervated human muscle were markedly reduced load-bearing capability and prolonged twitch contraction and relaxation time. Decreased load bearing of partially denervated muscle was observed as a reduction in maximum voluntary contraction strength, the peak amplitude of the twitch, and the peak amplitude of the tension produced by repetitive nerve stimulation at 10, 20, 50 and 100 Hz. The prolongation of contraction time and relaxation time of the muscle twitch has also been observed in individual motor units of partially denervated muscle.[147] Although prolongation of the active state has been postulated to explain the slowing of contraction time and relaxation time in completely denervated muscle in experimental animals,[134] no measurements have been made of active state in partially denervated human muscle. Other factors which may be important in the prolongation of twitch contraction time and half relaxation time include slowed muscle fiber propagation velocity, increased duration of the compound muscle action potential, slowed conduction in immature nerve sprouts, greater atrophy of fast motor units, and alterations in the series elastic element. The pattern of activity of the motor neuron has been postulated as an important factor in twitch contraction speed, but we have observed no difference in mean firing rates in partially denervated human muscle compared to controls.[146]

The maximum rate of rise of tension in partially denervated muscle was not significantly reduced in a voluntary contraction, in a single muscle twitch, or at stimulating frequencies of 10, 20, 50 and 100 Hz. An adjustment was made for the diminished load-bearing capability of weakened muscles in determining the maximum rate of rise of tension. Both the amount and rate of calcium liberation from the sarcoplasmic reticulum, as well as the rate at which calcium is utilized by the contractile proteins, seem important factors in determining the rate of rise of tension. The increase in sarcotubular components noted in histological studies of denervated muscle may be significant in this regard.[69]

A study comparing the dynamic properties of partially denervated muscle with controls and with a group of patients with primary muscle disease suggested different mechanisms for weakness in these two groups.[144] The degree of weakness was not significantly different in the two patient groups, yet the amplitude of the compound muscle action potential recorded with surface electrodes over the belly of an intrinsic hand muscle was markedly different. Mean amplitude of the compound muscle action potential was reduced by only 18% in patients with primary muscle disease, compared with a mean reduction of 61% in patients with partial denervation. Since the compound muscle action potential amplitude recorded over the belly of a small muscle varies directly with the size and number of muscle fibers activated, this finding suggests much greater atrophy for a given degree of weakness in partial denervation compared with primary muscle disease. Even more striking was the analysis of neuromuscular efficiency (the twitch tension in grams divided by the compound muscle action potential in millivolts), which was reduced by a mean of 50% in patients with primary muscle disease, whereas the neuromuscular efficiency of partially denervated muscle was actually increased by 55%. Both a larger twitch tension and a much smaller compound muscle action potential amplitude contributed to the increased neuromuscular efficiency seen in partial denervation. In patients with partial denervation, the finding of neuromuscular efficiency greater than in normal controls suggests partial functional compensation in surviving motor units. This finding is quite consistent with the old clinical aphorism that in denervating diseases, weakness is often much less than would be expected by the degree of wasting. On the other hand, in primary muscle diseases weakness is often much more than one would expect from the relatively slight amount of muscle atrophy.

Denervation is associated with considerable muscle fiber atrophy, and the myofibrillar atrophy is proportional to the reduction in muscle fiber size.[69] During the first few days after denervation, there is an increase in mitochondrial volume and sarcotubular surface, while fiber size and contractile elements decrease rapidly. Within one week of denervation, mitochondria and sarcotubules decrease in amount, but less than the decrease in contractile elements, and the overall effect is that of an increase in the concentration of sarcotubular profiles. Mitochondrial volume returns toward normal during the first month after denervation. The rate of muscle fiber atrophy after denervation is different in different muscles and in different species. In rat limb muscles, there may be a 50% reduction in weight within two weeks of denervation,[180] whereas rat diaphragm may transiently hypertrophy before atrophy occurs.[184] The rapid increase in muscle DNA content after denervation may be attributed to mitosis in interstitial cells, but labelled DNA precursor molecules appear also in satellite cells,[204] and mononucleate myoblasts are seen in interstitial spaces.[129] The general effect of denervation is to decrease the rate of synthesis of muscle proteins and to increase their rate of degradation.[86]

Other Effects of Denervation on Skeletal Muscles

In addition to altered dynamic properties and obvious muscle atrophy, there are at least five other changes in muscle membrane properties that follow denervation. The earliest muscle change that occurs after denervation is a reduction in the resting membrane potential. Soon afterwards, tetrodotoxin fails to block muscle action potentials initiated near old motor endplates and, within a week after denervation, action potentials can be evoked in any part of a muscle fiber despite the presence of tetrodotoxin.[163] Next, there is an increase in the sensitivity of extrajunctional regions of the muscle membrane to acetylcholine. Spontaneous fibrillation activity arises from the endplate region, with a latent interval that depends upon the length of the distal nerve stump.

Finally, an increase in the specific membrane resistance of the muscle develops. Three of these events will be considered in some detail: (1) decrease in resting membrane potential, (2) fibrillation potentials, and (3) increased sensitivity to acetylcholine.

Decreased Resting Membrane Potential

(This has been recently reviewed.[188]) In denervated mouse and rat skeletal muscles, the reduction in resting membrane potential (which occurs after cessation of miniature endplate potentials) amounts to approximately 15 to 20 mv. Using the soleus muscle of the intact rat, highly reproducible results have been obtained with regard to alterations in the resting membrane potential after denervation.[183] The resting potential begins to decrease 18 to 24 hours after nerve transection, and reaches a plateau after about 42 hours, with no further significant change for the next 30 hours in experiments performed with a nerve stump of less than 2 mm. Whereas with the short nerve stump miniature endplate potential activity had virtually ceased at 14 hours and decrease in the muscle resting potential occurred at 18 to 20 hours, with a longer nerve stump of 40 mm the resting potential did not begin to decrease until 22 hours. Because the denervated muscles are inactive regardless of the length of the nerve stump, some factor other than contractile activity must account for the increasing delay, with increasing stump length, from the time of nerve transection to the decrease in the resting membrane potential. In two different studies, the delay was approximately 45 minutes per centimeter of nerve stump,[143,183] a value quite close to the rate of rapid axoplasmic transport. Since it is likely that axonal transport is necessary for the maintenance of nerve terminals, it is not surprising that changes in nerve terminal function, including neuromuscular transmission and the neural influence on muscle resting membrane potential, should follow a time course corresponding to that of rapid axonal transport. More will be said about mechanisms underlying these observed changes in the section on neurotrophism (page 216).

The changes in resting membrane potential occur first in the endplate region and only later appear in the more distal regions of the muscle.[2,22] The observed depolarization is caused by a reduction in the electrogenic activity of the sodium pumping mechanism of the muscle membrane, with decreased resting potassium permeability and increased sodium permeability.[188] The myofiber atrophy appearing after denervation reduces the fiber diameter, contributing to an increase in the input impedance of the fiber. The reduced amount of synaptic current that is needed to depolarize the denervated muscle fiber contributes to the increased sensitivity of the muscle cell to both electrical and chemical stimuli. However, both of these changes (the decrease in resting membrane potential and the increased input impedance of the muscle fiber) are minor in comparison with the appearance of acetylcholine receptors outside the synaptic region[142] (see below).

Fibrillation Waves

In clinical work, the appearance of fibrillations in human muscles characteristically occurs approximately two to three weeks after a nerve injury that results in a functional separation between the nerve terminal and the postsynaptic membrane. Fibrillations may occur as early as two days after experimental denervation of rat muscle.[171] Fibrillations represent the spontaneous and usually asynchronous twitching of individual muscle fibers. Fibrillation waves seen in the clinical electromyography laboratory in patients with nerve injuries are generally taken to indicate the presence of axonal degeneration, and the intensity of fibrillation wave activity correlates in an approximate way with the amount of axonal degeneration. Fibrillation potentials usually arise near old endplates[178] and propagate along the whole length of the muscle fiber.[61] Near points of origin, it is possible to record sub-threshold fibrillation potentials which may be spontaneous events in the transverse tubule system.[162] These potentials may occur at a fixed regular frequency of 5 to 20 Hz or as bursts. It has been shown *in vivo* that only a proportion of denervated fibers are fibrillating at any given time, suggesting a cyclical pattern of activity.[37,189]

Extra-Junctional Acetylcholine Receptors[64,73,154]

The distribution of acetylcholine receptors in mammalian skeletal muscle is to a large extent regulated by motor innervation. In innervated muscles, acetylcholine (ACh) receptors are almost exclusively located at neuromuscular junctions, but following denervation there is a proliferation of "extra-junctional receptors" at sites outside the endplate.[130] The number of acetylcholine receptor molecules per muscle fiber increases 5- to 50-fold after denervation, with the vast majority of new receptors found in extra-junctional sites. The increase in acetylcholine sensitivity that follows denervation can be blocked by compounds that inhibit protein synthesis.[120,175] Blocking RNA synthesis with actinomycin-D prevents the appearance of extrajunctional acetylcholine receptors and the development of denervation hypersensitivity.[39] Evidence both from studies of inhibitors of protein synthesis and from direct labelling experiments indicates that denervation supersensitivity involves the biosynthesis of new acetylcholine receptor molecules.[24,50] The biosynthesis of the multisubunit, integral membrane glycoproteins of the acetylcholine receptors involves translation of messenger RNA molecules, glycosylation of specific amino acyl residues, folding and assembling of polypeptide chains to form the correct subunit structure, and the insertion of functional receptor molecules into the plasma membrane.[73] It has been suggested that some extra-junctional acetylcholine receptors are present in a latent form in the muscle prior to denervation, and that after denervation, invading phagocytic cells unmask the latent receptor sites.[87] However, the contribution of latent receptors to the denervation hypersensitivity must be small, since most receptors appearing after denervation have been demonstrated to be products of *de novo* synthesis. Chang et al[40] reported an increase of about 50% in the number of receptors per endplate region in the week following denervation. Frank et al[79] found that the number of receptors at former endplates declines very slowly following denervation of rat soleus and that after five weeks the number was approximately 50% of innervated muscle.

The stability following denervation of postsynaptic structures, the persistence of clustered junctional acetylcholine receptors, and the low turnover of these receptors provide evidence against the possibility that junctional acetylcholine receptors redistribute after denervation.[73,74] The metabolic turnover of junctional acetylcholine receptors is very slow in both innervated and newly denervated muscles. Postsynaptic structures survive for long periods after denervation. Whereas nerve terminals degenerate within one week, frog muscle junctional folds and postsynaptic densities remain unaltered for up to 130 days after denervation.[16] Postsynaptic structures in mouse muscles and rat diaphragm survive up to four months after denervation. The former postsynaptic areas also retain high acetylcholine receptor density in denervated muscle.[79,98,159]

It has been possible to study the mechanism of degradation of ACh receptors by the use of electron microscopic autoradiography with labelled α-bungarotoxin. Utilizing this technique, internalization of the ACh receptor-toxin complex, followed by proteolytic destruction in secondary lysosomes and generation of iodotyrosine has been demonstrated. This degradation process for ACh receptors appears homologous with processes by which cells ingest and degrade their surface membrane proteins after enzymatic iodination.[110] In denervated mouse muscle, the rate of degradation of receptors at the neuromuscular junction progressively increased, even though the concentration of junctional receptors changed little overall.[132] The increased rate of receptor degradation could be due to a progressive increase in the rate of degradation simultaneously in all junctional receptors or it may reflect the involvement of two separate populations of junctional receptors with different rates of turnover: those existing before denervation and those appearing after denervation. It was found that the original receptors had a half-life of about eight days, which is virtually identical to that of innervated junctional receptors. Within 8 to 10 days after denervation, the half-life fell to about 2.5 days. New junctional receptors appearing after denervation had a half-life of 24 hours. These findings suggest that two separate populations of junctional receptors exist at the neuromuscular junction after denervation.[182] Further, a transient increase in junctional receptors two days after denervation has been recently reported, followed by a decline after 14 days. The release of factors from degenerating nerve terminals was offered as a possible explanation for the early rise in junctional receptors.[153]

Much more is known about the mechanisms and rates of turnover of extra-junctional receptors. Estimates of average receptor lifetimes for extra-junctional receptors range from 6 to 35 hours, with some of the differences reflecting species or cell line differences. The degradation rate of acetylcholine receptors is sensitive to pH, temperature, and protein environment. Because of the relatively short average lifetime, the entire population of extra-junctional receptors must be replaced every few days.[137] It is assumed that the mechanisms for turnover of junctional and extra-junctional receptors are similar, even though the rate of junctional receptor turnover is much slower. The biochemical or structural basis for difference in turnover rates is uncertain. There are slight but definite chemical differences between junctional and extra-junctional receptor molecules.[24] The isoelectric point differs by about 0.1 to 2.0 pH units with extra-junctional receptors having a slightly higher pH value (5.27 to 5.36) compared with the junctional receptor pH value (5.09 to 5.17). This difference in pH may represent a difference of as much as 10 to 30 charges per molecule, considering the large size of the receptors. Both receptors have been shown to bind concanavalin A. They are not different in immuno-precipitation experiments with rabbit antireceptor serum or during velocity sedimentation in sucrose gradients and chromatography on 5M agarose. Most investigators have reported no difference in *d*-tubocurarine binding to junctional and extra-junctional acetylcholine receptors isolated from denervated and innervated adult rat muscles. However, differences in physiological effects of *d*-tubocurarine on cholinergic responses in junctional and extra-junctional regions of skeletal muscle fibers have been reported.[13,41] Fluctuation analysis of acetylcholine responses at neuromuscular junctions before and after denervation and at extra-junctional regions of normal and denervated frog muscle fibers reveals differences in unit conductance and in the mean open time of acetylcholine receptor ion channels.[57,116,149] The mean open times for junctional receptor channels are two to three times shorter than for extra-junctional receptor channels. These differences in conductance and mean ion channel open time may reflect intrinsic differences in receptor structure, may be the result of differences in the properties of the lipid bilayer surrounding the receptor molecules, or may result from differing interactions between receptors and other peripheral membrane proteins.[73]

Trophic Effects of Nerve on Muscle[93,94,97]

All of the events described above that follow denervation clearly establish the importance of innervation in maintaining the integrity and health of muscle fibers. There is still considerable controversy, however, regarding the nature of the trophic interaction between nerve and muscle. It is clear that muscle activity is essential in preventing the changes that follow denervation. It is still unclear whether some other factor is also involved. Some of the pertinent literature regarding the trophic effects of nerve on muscle will now be reviewed.

Fibrillations in denervated muscle were described over 100 years ago by Schiff,[174] who noticed spontaneous twitching on the surface of the tongue three days to six months after section of the hypoglossal nerve. It was not until after the turn of the century that Langley questioned whether denervation atrophy was due to loss of muscle activity, loss of nutritive effect of the nerve, or to some other factor.[127] Langley proposed that the fibrillatory activity observed in denervated muscle produced fatigue, which then led to atrophy. Experiments performed in the early 1940s, demonstrating that drugs that suppressed fibrillation had no effect on muscle atrophy, cast doubt on Langley's proposal.[180] Subsequently, two different groups showed that direct muscle stimulation was effective in retarding or even preventing denervation atrophy.[62,179] In 1960, Miledi observed that if only one of the endplates of a multiply innervated muscle was denervated, focal denervation hypersensitivity appeared despite continued activity of the muscle fiber through its other endplates.[142] This observation strengthened the idea that the nerve exerts an influence on muscle that is independent of impulse transmission and activity. The pendulum shifted in 1972 when Lomo and Rosenthal reported that anesthetic blockade of a motor nerve produced changes in a muscle similar to denervation, while direct stimulation of a denervated muscle reversed those changes.[138] Lomo and Westgaard later performed quantitative studies of stimulated denervated muscles, which led them to propose that the effects of denervation could be totally attributed to disuse.[139] In terms of maintaining the resting membrane potential of the muscle and in preventing the spread of extra-junctional acetylcholine receptors and acetylcholine hypersensitivity, electrical stimulation of denervated rat soleus muscle was an effective substitute for the presence of an intact nerve. The frequency and pattern of electrical stimulation were critically important, with the optimal result observed in response to brief trains, every 100 seconds, of 100 Hz stimuli rather than continuous stimulation. These experimental observations established the importance of muscle activity in maintaining muscle integrity. On the other hand, there was no evidence that muscle activity played a role in regulating the endplate structure or function.

Numerous experiments attempting to establish whether muscle disuse is sufficient to produce the changes of denervation have been ambiguous, and the question of whether a nerve provides a trophic influence on muscle that is independent of muscle activity has remained controversial. Muscle atrophy has been reported in conjunction with many models of disuse, such as bedrest and limb immobilization, spinal cord section in conjunction with dorsal root section, hibernation, and hysterical paralysis, but none of these models of disuse precisely reproduces the effects of denervation.[3,78,99,114,179] Further, in none of these instances is it certain that impulse transmission has been completely blocked. Another model of disuse involves anesthetic-impregnation of a rubber cuff around a nerve in order to produce prolonged conduction block. After 14 days of paralysis with this model, no fibrillations or denervation hypersensitivity were found in rabbits, whereas in rats, all of the changes of denervation were observed.[164] Unfortunately, tightly fitting cuffs, with or without local anesthetic, have been shown to block both axonal transport and nerve impulse propagation, presumably due to local anoxia.[151] Local anesthetics themselves can also block axonal transport as well as impulses.[17] With the use of diphtheria toxin to produce conduction block, changes mimicking denervation have been observed; however, it has been recently discovered that fast axonal transport is totally blocked by diphtheria toxin.[119]

Another approach to the study of neurotrophic influences has been to utilize botulinum toxin to interfere with neuromuscular transmission.[53] This toxin acts on the presynaptic nerve terminal to prevent the release of acetylcholine. Botulinum toxin produces a marked decrease in both spontaneous and impulse-mediated quantal release of acetylcholine, resulting in complete paralysis of muscle and a marked reduction to less than 10% of normal of the frequency of the miniature endplate potentials. Prolonged treatment with botulinum toxin produces muscular atrophy, fibrillations, increased extra-junctional acetylcholine receptor density, and slowing of muscle twitch contraction and relaxation time. Most recently, Brown and co-workers demonstrated that after 10 days there was no difference between denervated muscles and muscles paralyzed with botulinum toxin with regard to contractile properties and acetylcholine sensitivity.[32] These authors have argued against an activity-independent nerve trophic effect on extra-junctional acetylcholine sensitivity and contractile properties in mammalian muscle. However, acetylcholine sensitivity develops more rapidly in denervated muscle, presumably due to the added effect of nerve degeneration products.

Perhaps the best model of muscle disuse involves the local application of tetrodotoxin.[54] This toxin blocks voltage-dependent sodium channels and completely interrupts action potential conduction, but has no other effect on nerves. There is no change in axonal transport, no morphologic change in the nerves, and no change in spontaneously released acetylcholine from nerve terminals. In this experimental model, the changes of denervation are reproduced but with a lesser magnitude: the extra-junctional acetylcholine receptor levels peak at only 50% of the denervated level after 10 days before slowly declining. The resting membrane potentials fall much more slowly and reach only 50% of the decrease that occurs in denervated muscles.

A controlled study of another form of disuse was performed in the baboon using nerve compression by a pneumatic tourniquet. There was a prolonged conduction block at the site of compression due to local myelin damage, with modest amounts of Wallerian degeneration (in 10% to 30% of the large fibers).[84] The acetylcholine sensitivity of nerve-blocked muscle fibers developed later than in denervated muscle fibers (10 vs. 7 days) and remained at a lower level than that of denervated muscle fibers for 21 to 63 days. In limbs where mild compression produced virtually pure conduction block without axonal degeneration, no spontaneous fibrillations were seen, although extra-junctional acetylcholine sensitivity developed. The authors concluded that in the baboon both muscular activity and some other neural influence independent of muscular activity influenced muscle properties. In this model, the neural influence was more effective in preventing fibrillation than in preventing acetylcholine hypersensitivity of the extra-junctional muscle membrane.

All of the experimental data cited above provide evidence that impulse-dependent acetylcholine release and its associated muscle activity are not the only factors in regulating extra-junctional acetylcholine receptors and the resting membrane potential of skeletal muscles. Further evidence for the presence of some factor other than activity can be drawn from the direct effect of the length of the distal nerve stump upon the appearance of changes following denervation. The onset of fibrillations occurs later in muscles with longer nerve stumps compared with nerve section close to the muscle.[140] Other changes in the muscle following denervation are similarly delayed by increasing the length of the distal stump. As mentioned earlier, in studies of denervated rat soleus muscle, the resting membrane potential fell three hours later with 40 mm distal stumps compared with 2 mm stumps. The delay of 45 minutes per cm of nerve is comparable to the rate of fast axonal transport.[183] In this experimental setting, all of the denervated muscles were inactive, suggesting that some factor other than activity must account for the difference in timing. If, as suggested by the nerve stump experiments, a substance is transported down the nerve axon to affect the muscle, then a blockade of axonal transport should produce the changes of denervation. The application to a nerve of colchicine or vinblastine, which interfere with fast axonal transport, partially reproduces the effects of denervation despite continued muscle activity. However, the experiments are ambiguous because both these drugs, when applied directly to a muscle with intact innervation, may produce changes of denervation even when axonal transport has not been blocked.[37]

Methods have been developed for producing seven days of blockade of acetylcholine receptors by infusion of α-bungarotoxin into the soleus muscle of rats.[55] Complete blockade of acetylcholine transmission by α-bungarotoxin results in an increase in the number of extra-junctional acetylcholine receptors equivalent to and with the same time course as produced by surgical denervation. Similarly, the effect of α-bungarotoxin treatment on the muscle resting membrane potential was identical to that of surgical section of the soleus nerve at its point of attachment to the muscle. In both denervated and α-bungarotoxin-treated animals, the fall in resting membrane potential began at 18 to 24 hours and reached a maximum change of 15 mv at 36 to 42 hours. The authors were also unable to detect an effect of α-bungarotoxin on fast axonal transport, acetylcholine release or motor nerve terminal morphology in their controlled studies.[156] The authors postulated that since elimination of impulse-dependent release of acetylcholine by tetrodotoxin produced only partial denervation-like effects, whereas blockade of all acetylcholine transmission by α-bungarotoxin resulted in a complete effect, the difference may be attributable to the spontaneously released acetylcholine.[55]

A large amount of evidence has accumulated that suggests that disuse can produce some or all of the signs of denervation, but with marked differences between different muscles and different species. The role of fast axonal transport in trophic regulation of muscles is still uncertain. The precise contribution of spontaneously released acetylcholine in the neural regulation of muscle properties remains to be determined, since there is no means at present of selectively blocking spontaneous acetylcholine release.

Repair Processes in Peripheral Nerve

After denervation, reinnervation is brought about by (1) sprouting of undamaged axons in close physical proximity to the denervated muscle, or (2) by axonal regeneration from the site of nerve injury. In partial denervation, sprouting accomplishes reinnervation within a few days, whereas axonal regeneration requires weeks to months, depending upon the type of nerve injury and the distance between the site of nerve injury and the muscle. Regenerating axon nerve terminals displace endplates formed by sprouts from neighboring neurons to complete the process of reinnervation.

Sprouting of Motor Nerves[31,45,141]

Exner in 1884 made one of the first references to motor nerve sprouting.[71] He showed that individual muscle fibers were not permanently denervated after partial transection of the nerve, and he proposed that recovery of muscle function was due to intramuscular (collateral) growth by the remaining intact nerves. It was later demonstrated that partial denervation was followed after several weeks by complete recovery of muscle tension in the absence of reinnervation by severed axons. Edds[63] and Hoffman[104] identified fine nerve outgrowths from the nodes of Ranvier of remaining intact axons (nodal sprouts) in partially denervated muscle. Using a silver stain, Hoffman also demonstrated fine outgrowths from intact nerve terminals (terminal sprouts). These observations confirmed that sprouting was actually new growth from axons which already had functional contact with other muscle fibers and that activation of previously non-functional nerve branches was not involved. *Terminal* sprouts first appear as fine, irregular extensions of nerve terminal branches, best visualized with zinc iodide-osmium tetroxide.[1] These sprouts can arise from a single nerve terminal, as well as from the unmyelinated preterminal axonal segment.[104] *Nodal* sprouts arise from nodes of Ranvier within the intramuscular nerves. Not all of the nodes within a nerve of a partially denervated muscle produce visible sprouts.[104,177] Within four days after partial denervation, most fine nodal sprouts arise from nodes within 200 μm of the endplates they were innervating.[104] There appears to be a definite clustering of nodal sprouts near points from which denervated nerve sheaths were branched. Long lengths of intramuscular nerve without branch points contain no sprouts, even though they are in close proximity to denervated endplates. The shortest denervated perineural sheaths are the first to become innervated. The major determinant of nodal involvement in sprouting is apparently the distance of the node from a denervated endplate via a vacant perineural sheath.[177] Each nodal sprout finds a vacant perineural sheath leading to the nearest denervated endplate, although the guidance mechanism is unknown. Terminal sprouts are more erratic in their growth pattern, with some preference for alignment along the long axis of the muscle fiber. The factors which regulate terminal sprout growth have not been subjected to systematic study. Terminal sprouts seem to innervate any endplate encountered, although the most successful terminal sprouts are those which grow to vacated endplate sites.[34]

Several factors influence the rate of sprouting in motor nerves. Hoffman observed that electrical stimulation of undamaged nerves enhances their sprouting in response to partial denervation of rat muscle.[106] Although its significance is uncertain, a conditioning lesion placed within a two-week period before a test lesion markedly enhances the ensuing sprouting at the neuromuscular junction.[90]

The age of the animal is another factor in determining sprout growth rate. Aging endplates develop a complex morphology,[193] and longer and more numerous terminal sprouts and nodal sprouts have been found in aged rats compared to young animals.[72] Sprouting in rat soleus, following partial denervation, was significantly reduced in aged animals compared to young adults,[72] but it has also been observed that motor neurons of newborn rats sprout less vigorously. Following partial denervation there is only a twofold increase in the size of neonatal motor units instead of the normal fivefold increase noted in adult muscles.[33,191] This fivefold increase in motor unit size is independent of the original size and type of the motor unit, and probably represents the limit of the ability of the neuron to supply functional nerve terminals.

Both the rate of nerve terminal degeneration and the maturation of sprouts is different in fast- and slow-twitch muscles.[30,160] Significant recovery of tension in partially denervated fast-twitch muscles begins six to seven days after denervation, with nodal sprouting beginning some two to three days earlier.[34] In the slow muscle (mouse soleus), relatively little nodal sprouting occurs by the sixth day, in spite of the presence of numerous terminal sprouts. Recovery of tension in slow-twitch muscle takes nine to ten days.

Regeneration of several axons into partially denervated muscle may result in double innervation of muscle fibers with the sprout and the regenerated axon innervating the same fiber.[105] Both histological evidence and tension measurements confirm that both sprouts and regenerated axons innervate the same muscle fibers.[92] In amphibia[48] and mammals[15,34,190] the regenerating axon apparently can produce synaptic repression of the sprouts. Early reinnervation by regenerating axons produces more complete displacement of the sprouts, but after late reinnervation the sprouts are less easily displaced.[190] The mechanism by which synapses are eliminated is not well understood, but is probably similar to the elimination of multiple innervation of mammalian muscle fibers soon after birth[7] (see chapter 2).

Factors That Initiate Sprouting

The signal which initiates nerve sprouting has been the source of considerable experimental study. The major possibilities include: (1) spread of a signal from a motor neuron undergoing chromatolysis, (2) loss of afferent input to the spinal cord, (3) a factor released by degenerating products in the distal stump, (4) release of a factor from denervated muscle, and (5) blocked axonal transport.

Sprouting has been observed when nerve impulse activity is blocked, and sprouting can be inhibited by direct electrical activation of the muscle.[139] Induction of terminal sprouting has been documented with: (1) tetrodotoxin blockade of nerve impulse conduction,[25] (2) presynaptic blockade with botulinum toxin,[60] (3) blockade of descending impulses in the spinal cord,[30] (4) postsynaptic blockade by α-bungarotoxin,[107] and (5) spinal cord transection with dorsal root section.[66] While the first three of these procedures may affect axonal transport, it appears that α-bungarotoxin does not affect either axonal transport[14] or presynaptic release mechanisms.[38]

Rotshenker has shown that after muscles are denervated on one side of a frog, sprouting in contralateral muscles occurs.[166-169] The onset of sprouting is earlier the closer the muscle is to the spinal cord. This sprouting was interpreted as a response to a central signal spread from the axotomized motor neuron across the spinal cord. However, in mice the same experimental design resulted in no evidence of sprouting.[30] There is evidence that terminal sprouting occurs in muscles in which only sensory fibers are degenerating.[27] It is possible that the products of nerve degeneration produce the sprouting stimulus in this situation.[139]

Hoffman found that extracts from either degenerating or intact nerve caused terminal sprouting in the motor neurons of intact muscle. The substance that produced sprouting, named "neurocletin," was presumed to be an unsaturated fatty acid ester from myelin.[105] Lomo and Westgaard showed in innervated muscle fibers that products of nerve degeneration caused extra-junctional acetylcholine hypersensitivity.[139] Pestronk and Drachman reported a direct relationship between extra-junctional receptors and terminal sprouting.[155] Although products of degenerating nerve may induce extra-junctional receptor formation which then stimulates terminal sprouting, nerve degeneration products cannot be the only sprouting stimulus because they do not induce nodal sprouting.[27] Furthermore, sprouting has been demonstrated in the absence of nerve degeneration. It has been shown that the stimulus for sprouting has a very short range.[31,198] The possibility that extra-junctional receptors provide the stimulus for sprouting was proposed by Pestronk and Drachman.[155] They reported that the acetylcholine sensitivity of the muscle correlated with the amount of sprouting after denervation, and that α-bungarotoxin, by binding with receptors to block acetylcholine transmission, produced no sprouting. Sanes and co-workers have shown that innervating axons grow toward receptors which are imbedded in the basement membrane, suggesting a stimulus for sprout growth that is bound within the basal lamina.[173] In their experiments, myofibers were allowed to degenerate after denervation and then irradiated to prevent regeneration. The sheath of the basal lamina survived the treatment and the original synaptic sites on the basal lamina could still be identified. Within two weeks, axons regenerated into the region, contacting the surviving basal lamina almost exclusively at the original synaptic sites. Factors present at synaptic sites that apparently guided the axon growth were maintained even though the myofibers were absent.

The possibility that a diffusible substance is released by the muscle after denervation has also been studied.[15] When tetrodotoxin was used to block one of two nerves supplying rat foot muscles, nerve terminal sprouting was found in both blocked and unblocked nerves.[15] Sprouting was observed in nerve terminals close to active muscle fibers, which presumably would have developed no extra-junctional acetylcholine receptors. Hoffman could not produce significant amounts of sprouting by infusion of extracts of denervated muscle into normal muscle.[104] More recently, Tweedle and Kabara injected lipid extracts of denervated and normal muscle into rat tongues.[194] Increased nodal sprouting was associated with the denervated muscle extract, which had a higher lipid content. Unfortunately, Tweedle and Kabara did not evaluate the presence or absence of denervation or inflammation in the tongue muscles. It is possible that future experiments may demonstrate a substance comparable to *nerve growth factor* (important in the development and maintenance of the sympathetic nervous system[161]).

A possibility that a sprout-inhibiting factor released by normal nerves is deficient in denervation has been proposed by Vrbova and co-workers.[195] They have described proteolytic enzyme release at the neuromuscular junction in response to acetylcholine, and have proposed that normal nerve terminal growth is an ongoing process that is balanced by the action of the proteolytic enzymes; when the proteolytic enzymes are no longer released, nerve terminals start to grow, and when the muscle again becomes active, the sprouts are removed by subsequent release of these enzymes. However, in partially denervated muscle, nerve stimulation does not inhibit sprouting, even though the innervated muscle fibers are more active than normal.[29] While the existence of some inhibitory mechanism in normal muscle remains a possibility, evidence supporting this concept is scant.

While denervated muscle gives rise to both terminal and nodal sprouting, inactive muscles produce only terminal sprouts.[60,111] Nodal sprouting is unaffected by chronic electrical stimulation, but terminal sprouting is inhibited. In any given muscle, the amount of terminal sprouting correlates poorly with the amount of nodal sprouting, and different types of muscles (slow vs. fast) have different amounts of terminal and nodal sprouting.[30] In one recent study of partially denervated rat muscle, both light and electron microscopic analysis revealed no nodal sprouts in partially denervated nerve trunks.[177] However, in a study of young adult mice, nodal sprouts were found after either paralysis with botulinum toxin or partial denervation.[108] Compared to control muscle, botulinum toxin-paralyzed muscle showed a higher proportion of nerve profiles containing one or two unmyelinated axons beside a single myelinated axon. In partially denervated muscles, after eight days, there were significant increases in the proportion of unmyelinated axons in nerve profiles which contained five to ten myelinated axons.[108] Twenty-one days after partial denervation, similar increases had occurred, and after 63 days there were large increases in the proportion of unmyelinated axons in the extramuscular nerve and the main intramuscular nerve branches. Nodal sprouting in response to partial denervation was localized initially to the smaller, more distal nerve branches. Later, some sprouts slowly grew in a distoproximal direction along denervated Schwann cell pathways. The existence of nodal sprouts in paralyzed muscles and their restricted distribution in paralyzed and partially denervated muscles suggest that the nodal sprouting stimulus is produced by the muscle and acts only at distal nodes. There is a distinct possibility that the stimuli are different for nodal and terminal sprouting, but more work is needed to clarify this point.

There is also a close relationship between terminal sprouting and the ability of a mammalian muscle to accept foreign innervation. Foreign innervation outside the endplate region will not be accepted by a mammalian muscle, except under conditions of denervation,[68] or if the muscle is paralyzed with botulinum toxin.[76] However, the time course for development of both acetylcholine supersensitivity and foreign innervation is delayed by a factor of 2 to 3 in paralyzed compared to denervated muscles.[4] Electrical stimulation of a denervated muscle not only will inhibit sprouting, but also will inhibit its acceptance of another nerve.[79]

At the present time, no single mechanism is consistent with all reported experimental observations on sprouting. It may well turn out that more than one mechanism exists to stimulate and regulate sprouting in peripheral motor nerves.

There is, as yet, no therapy which will enhance the rate of recovery after nerve injury. However, in 1952 Hoffman made the interesting observation that administration of a 0.1% solution of the dye pyronin, in the drinking water of rats, produced a remarkable acceleration in axonal sprouting at nodes of Ranvier in partially denervated muscle. Because of the known affinity of pyronin for RNA, he proposed that this effect was mediated by an enhancement of neuronal protein synthesis. Recent studies in mice administered a 0.1% solution of pyronin G in the drinking water have confirmed the accelerated nodal sprouting and motor nerve regeneration in partially denervated gluteus maximus muscles following crush injury of its nerve.[118] However, sprouting from motor nerve terminals in response to botulinum toxin-induced paralysis was unaffected by the pyronin. Removal of degenerating axons following the nerve section was accelerated by the pyronin treatment, suggesting that the dye acts upon the process of Wallerian degeneration rather than directly upon the intact motor neurons. This interesting line of investigation bears further attention in the future.

Nerve Regeneration

The Nobel laureate Santiago Ramón y Cajal first showed that viable nerve fibers grow out of the proximal stump of an injured neuron.[36] He showed a latent period between injury and sprouting (about six hours) and a further delay (approximately 36 hours) before outgrowth of the axon tips. He showed that growth through the scarred (damaged) area of nerve was slow (approximately 0.25 mm per day) and that invasion of the distal stump of severed nerves may not occur until after 10 or 15 days. Subsequently, the rate of regeneration for most fibers was 2–3 mm per day. These observations have been confirmed by many other authors.[89,175,200] Two recent studies have shown that the earliest sprouts (formed during the first 24 hours) may later degenerate.[59,90] Following nerve injury in humans, information on the course of regeneration can be provided by serial clinical observations of the location at which Tinel's sign is elicited. Tinel's sign is produced by tapping the skin over a damaged nerve with either a reflex hammer or another blunt object such as a finger. This mechanical stimulation of regenerating sensory axons produces a tingling or shock-like sensation, either locally or in the distribution of the nerve.[192] In detailed studies of human peripheral nerve regeneration, Sunderland found that a severed nerve repaired by simple suture of the cut ends regenerated at a rate of 2.5 mm per day in the upper forearm, 2 mm per day in the lower forearm, and 1 mm per day in the wrist and hand, suggesting a relationship between the distance from the cell body to the lesion and the rate of regeneration. Rates of regeneration are more rapid after a crush injury of nerve (8.5 mm per day in the upper arm, 6 mm per day in the upper forearm, $1-2$ mm per day at the wrist and $1-1.5$ mm per day in the hand)[186] than after complete section of a nerve. This difference has been attributed to the lesser degree of distortion of endoneurial tubes in a crush injury.[203] Age affects the rate of nerve regeneration, which is slower in older animals.[20]

Ultrastructurally, the growth cone of regenerating axons is a region of axoplasmic enlargement, rich in smooth endoplasmic reticulum, microtubules, microfilaments, large mitochondria, and lysosomes, from which fine sprouts may extend.[175] Weiss suggested that the elongation of the growth tip may be caused by outward axoplasmic streaming and the direction of the growth tip may be influenced by mechanical factors in the pathway.[198,199] Whenever possible, axons regenerate within pre-existing endoneurial tubes, thereby speeding the process of regeneration.

Electrophysiological Observations in Nerve Regeneration

Following injury to the rabbit peroneal nerve, Cragg and Thomas found that conduction velocities proximal to the lesion were reduced by 10% after 25 days and by 20% after $50-100$ days.[47] Conduction velocities returned to normal after 150 days and remained so beyond 400 days. One study showed that after successful reinnervation in man, maximal motor conduction velocity proximal to the site of nerve section returns to normal.[10] However, the question of whether slowing of conduction velocity occurs proximal to a compressive nerve lesion in humans remains controversial (see recent review[84]). In both experimental and human studies of regenerating nerves distal to a lesion, persistent reduction of conduction velocity by 20%$-$40% has been reported.[47,103,112] However, in at least one study of experimental animals[172] and in long-term studies of human nerve injuries,[52] motor nerve conduction velocity recovered to greater than 90% of normal after periods in excess of two years. In a study of regenerating frog neuromuscular junctions, nerve terminal length reached 90% of normal by day 16 after nerve crush, but quantal content per unit terminal length recovered to only 67% of normal by $7-12$ days with no subsequent increase.[51] Spontaneous potentials recovered more slowly to only 18% of normal after 30 days, but with normal levels later. The mechanisms underlying the differences in time course for recovery of different parameters in regenerating junctions have yet to be determined.

Biochemical Changes Accompanying Regeneration

One of the earliest changes in the cell body of an injured neuron is a major increase in neuronal cell volume, and after the initial chromatolytic reaction, cellular RNA content increases dramatically. The RNA content first increases in the nucleolus and then in the cytoplasm.[197] The increased synthesis and turnover of RNA after axotomy results in increased protein synthesis.[136] After the first week, there is increased oxidative metabolism and increased levels of the tricarboxylic acid cycle enzymes.[175] At the same time, there is an increase in the number and density of critae in enlarged mitochondria.[136] The increased utilization of the hexose monophosphate pathway is presumed to increase cellular levels of the NADPH required for synthesis of fatty acids, a major constituent of lipid membranes. These changes are all expected of neurons synthesizing new axonal membrane. In association with the possible enhancement of axonal transport following axotomy, there is a proliferation of both neurofilaments and neurotubules during regeneration. Increased synthesis of tubulin, the constituent of neurofilaments and neurotubules, has been found in rat motor neurons following axotomy.[128] More detailed reviews of the biochemical aspects of nerve regeneration have recently been published.[6,175]

The changes in axoplasmic transport that accompany regeneration in mammalian nerves are still incompletely understood. The rate of fast transport is unchanged following axotomy,[18,152] and there is still controversy as to whether regeneration is accompanied by changes in the volume of fast transport.[18,91] Whether the rate and volume of slow axoplasmic transport is altered is also uncertain. Preferential incorporation of fast transported protein into the regenerating part of transected motor axons has been demonstrated; however, the effect of selective blockade of axonal transport proximal to a nerve lesion has not been studied in terms of its effect on axonal regeneration.[91] Although in goldfish optic nerves the volume of retrograde transport of proteins is increased after injury,[90] there is considerable variation, in different species, of the effect of nerve injury on retrograde transport.[80,96]

The exact nature of the signals between the degenerating nerve stump and the regenerating axon have yet to be elucidated. Peripheral nerve fiber regeneration *in vivo* seems to be directed by factors in distal stumps of transected nerves.[158] This effect is possibly mediated over distances of several millimeters by diffusible factors. In elegant experiments, transected rat sciatic or cat peroneal nerve proximal stumps were inserted into the single inlet end of a hollow, Y-shaped, silastic implant. Regenerating axons were allowed to grow into a (1) vacant arm or one occupied by a sciatic nerve graft (rat) or (2) a tibial or peroneal distal nerve stump (cat). Four to six weeks postoperatively both morphometric analysis and quantification of an axonally transported label were used to evaluate the number of regenerating axons in each fork of the implant. Rat sciatic nerve fibers exclusively regenerated toward the nerve graft, suggesting the existence of a "neurotropic lure." In some cases, the peroneal distal nerve stump was rendered metabolically inert by exposing it to dry ice and to inhibitors of DNA and RNA synthesis. In cats, morphometric analysis revealed a six- to tenfold greater number of axons growing toward the untreated tibial nerve distal stumps. Analysis of transported label confirmed the preferential growth of both motor and sensory axons toward the untreated tibial nerve. The preferential regeneration toward untreated stumps was observed if the distance between proximal and distal nerve stumps was equal to but not greater than four to five millimeters. The results of this experiment imply that the presence of a distal nerve stump has a direct effect upon the direction of nerve regeneration, but these experiments offer no information about the signal that initiates the process of axonal regeneration. Nor is it possible, on the basis of this evidence, to determine whether preferential growth of axons toward the distal nerve stump is mediated by factors acting directly upon the axon, or factors acting indirectly by attracting Schwann cells, which then bring the axons along. Further such work is needed to elucidate the mechanisms involved in regulating peripheral nerve regeneration.

Lack of Specificity in Mammalian Nerve Regeneration

This topic has been recently reviewed.[45,126,175] Following axotomy in a fish or salamander, axonal regeneration usually leads to complete functional recovery. However, in mammals there appears to be no selectivity or specificity in re-establishing connections between nerve and muscle. When inaccurately formed neuromuscular connections are made, the central nervous system is unable to reorganize its connections in order to compensate. This disordered peripheral reinnervation can be detected clinically during electromyography as disordered recruitment of motor units and distortion of the usual size of units.[148] Aberrant reinnervation producing synkinesis is common in patients who recover from a lesion of the facial nerve.[202]

Studies of nerve regeneration in rats have shown that the correct nerve can displace the incorrect nerve, resulting in morphologic retraction of the foreign neuromuscular junctions.[79] Competition between two nerves experimentally implanted close together leads to elimination of the neuromuscular junctions from one of the nerves in a large percentage of cases; however, when the two nerves are implanted at opposite poles of the muscle, dual innervation of muscle fibers may persist.[123] Intracellular recordings of endplate potentials in partially denervated muscles have demonstrated that only about 10% of muscle fibers will remain doubly innervated following regeneration of damaged axons.[34] Some of the initially denervated fibers remain innervated by foreign sprouts, while others are reinnervated by the regenerating axons. These changes during reinnervation are similar to the normal developmental sequence of a mammalian neuromuscular junction in which initially polyinnervated muscles[11] mature to mononeuronal innervation by retraction of redundant axon terminals.[122] The mechanisms that account for the competition between axon terminals for innervation of muscle fibers are not understood.

Although in mammals regenerating nerves lack the ability to seek out the correct target muscles when they are separated from the muscle by great distances, the regenerating motor axons show a remarkable tendency to innervate the precise postsynaptic grooves of the muscle endplate that were occupied previously.[131] Despite the precise ability of nerve terminals to seek the exact location on the basal lamina where endplates should become established, there is an apparent lack of selectivity in establishing the correct nerve-muscle connection.[12,45]

Dynamic Properties of Reinnervated Muscle

Six months after nerve transection and self-reinnervation of cat soleus and flexor digitorum longus muscles, there is a greater variation in both tetanic tension and twitch tension than in control muscle,[8] but the normal relationships between the axonal conduction velocity, motor unit tetanic tension, twitch time to peak, and ratio of twitch to tetanic tension are maintained.[8,88] In experiments with cross-reinnervation between fast-twitch (flexor digitorum longus) and slow-twitch (soleus) muscle in the cat, motor unit tetanic tensions were higher in cross-reinnervated soleus than in cross-reinnervated flexor digitorum longus (reversing the normal differences between these muscles).[9] The changes in contraction time of motor units were less complete in soleus than in flexor digitorum longus (time to peak of its fastest motor unit was twice as long as seen in the normal flexor digitorum longus). In neither of the cross-reinnervated muscles were the fast-contracting motor units larger than the slow-contracting ones. These observations confirmed that reinnervation of a fast-twitch muscle by a nerve which normally supplies a slow-twitch muscle results in a slowing of the contraction speed of the muscle, and the cross-reinnervation of a slow-twitch muscle results in speeding of contraction.[35] Three years after cross-reinnervation, more consistency in motor units was noted than after the shorter period of reinnervation.[135] Cross-reinnervation of the slow-twitch cat soleus with the nerve from a fast-twitch muscle resulted in two distinct groups of motor units (one group with fast-twitch and low tetanic tension and the other group with slow-twitch and high tetanic tension) which had the reverse relationship between twitch time and tetanic tension of normal muscle. As in normal muscle, motor unit twitch time to peak was directly proportional to axonal conduction velocity, but tetanic tension was also proportional to axonal conduction velocity, which is distinctly abnormal. More than 95% of the fibers in the cross-reinnervated soleus muscle were oxidative, with type I fibers predominating over type IIA fibers in the ratio of about two to one. The inability of fast nerve to completely convert the mechanical and histochemical properties of cat soleus muscle was not due to failure of conversion of individual fibers, but to the small tension of the abnormally small fast motor units.[135]

Reinnervation in Human Muscle

Clinical electromyographic techniques have been utilized to examine motor unit potentials during reinnervation following a complete nerve section and subsequent regeneration from the proximal stump of the severed axons. As pointed out by Kugelberg, such motor units have an extremely compact arrangement, with grouped orientation of the muscle fibers and a smaller territory as well as a higher muscle fiber density.[124] During an early stage of regaining voluntary activity, nascent potentials are seen, sometimes including as few as one or two muscle fibers. Motor unit potentials that are seen first during nerve regeneration may resemble fibrillations because they often represent the activity of only a single muscle fiber as the earliest manifestation of a nascent motor unit potential.[21]

Using single-fiber electromyography, it is possible to determine the variation in firing of one component of the motor unit with respect to another (jitter). The jitter in normal motor units rarely exceeds 30 microseconds,[65] whereas in nascent motor unit potentials the jitter may be of the order of several hundred microseconds, suggesting a precarious neuromuscular transmission safety factor at the newly formed synapse.[21] (Fig. 5.3) Blocking (neuromuscular transmission failure) may intermittently occur. Motor unit potential recruitment is also disturbed in patients recovering from a complete nerve transection. Milner-Brown and his colleagues studied patients recovering from a complete transection of the ulnar nerve 6 to 24 months after repair.[148] (Fig. 5.4) At both 6 months and 24 months, the recruitment of motor unit potentials was random with respect to the increased force of voluntary contraction. In keeping with the size principle, smaller motor units were recruited first in the control extremity. During the late phase of regeneration, motor unit potentials, twitch tensions, and overall muscle strength reached normal values. However, motor unit recruitment was still not linear with respect to the correlation between threshold force of voluntary contraction and motor unit twitch tension as found in normal extremities.

Figure 5.3. Nascent motor unit potential recorded by coherent EMG in the frontalis muscle nine weeks after a traumatic lesion of the facial nerve. The motor unit includes only two muscle fibers, and neuromuscular transmission is not consistently achieved for the second fiber. (A) Superimposed oscilloscope sweeps show marked jitter and blocking of the second spike. (B) Same motor unit potential recorded on film moving vertically to display the successive sweeps from above downward. The vertical separation between individual sweeps corresponds to the firing intervals. The sweeps are triggered by either the first component (left column) or second component (right column). Missing sweeps in the right column (Xs) correspond to blocking of the second component. Reprinted by permission from the *Annals of Neurology*.[21]

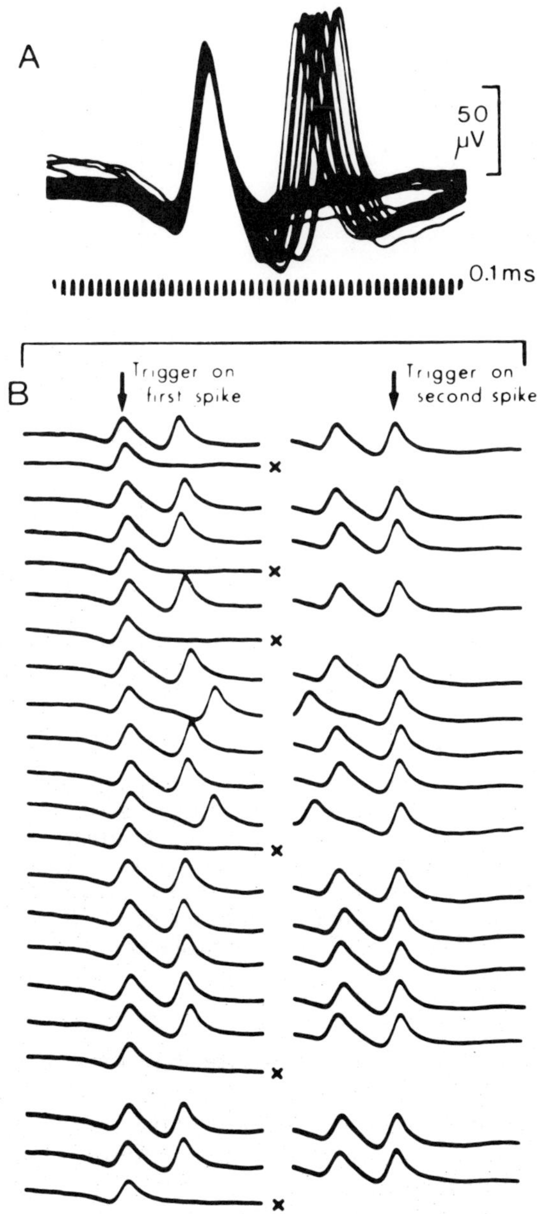
A
50
μV
0.1ms
B
Trigger on
first spike
Trigger on
second spike

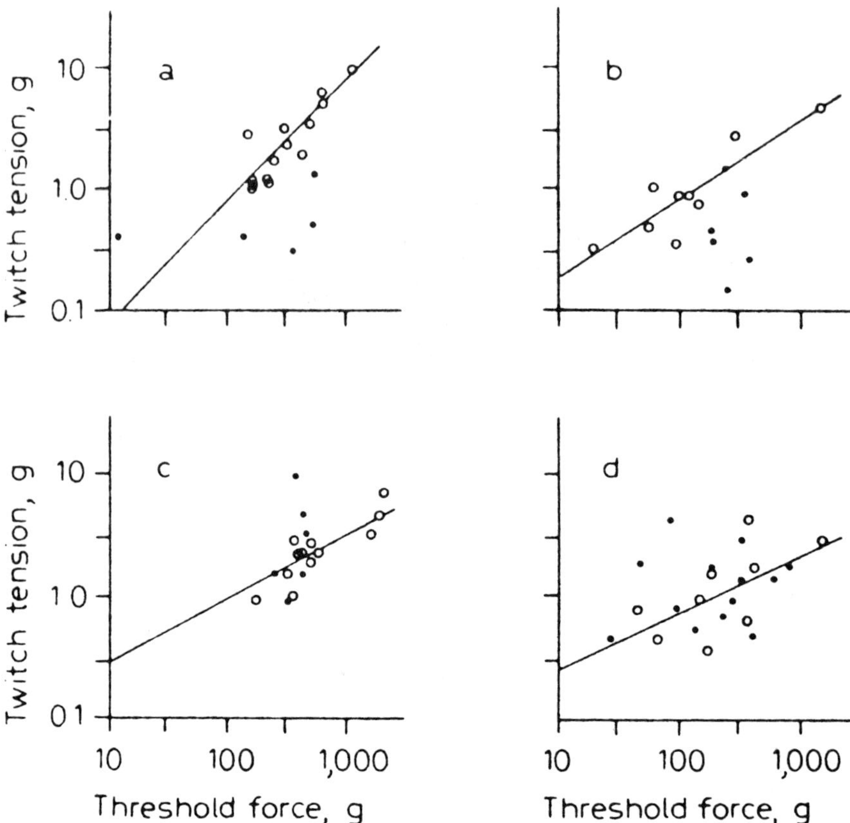

Figure 5.4. Twitch tensions produced by single motor units from 4 patients with previous complete severance of their ulnar nerves as a function of the threshold force at which the motor units were recruited. (*a,b*) Early stage of regeneration. (*c,d*) Advanced stage of regeneration. The computed best-fitting straight lines shown on these log-log plots are for the normal hands only. 0 = Clinically normal hand; ● = affected hand. Reprinted by permission from the text *Motor Unit Types, Recruitment and Plasticity in Health and Disease.*[148]

Non-traumatic Neurogenic Diseases

Despite the many studies of the neuromuscular junction in disuse and after nerve section, relatively little information is available concerning the effects of diseases of peripheral nerve on the structure and function of the neuromuscular junction. In one study of patients with peripheral neuropathies and anterior horn cell diseases, branching of intramuscular nerve fibers was carefully measured by staining the innervation zone of muscle biopsy specimens with methylene blue.[44] Axonal sprouts appeared as fine, beaded fibers ending in an axonal dilatation or growth cone which eventually reached a muscle fiber and formed a terminal arborization. The intramuscular nerve fibers were fine and beaded, ending in a plexiform network without forming a visible neuromuscular junction. The terminal innervation ratio was defined as the number of muscle fibers innervated by each intramuscular subterminal motor nerve. The diminished number of nerve fibers in some specimens prevented determination of a terminal innervation ratio. The terminal innervation ratio was higher than the upper limit of normal (1.26) in 97% of muscle biopsies from clinically weak muscles, and in 90% of muscles with atrophic changes. When grouped atrophy was found in the muscle biopsy, the terminal innervation ratio was increased in 100% of specimens. In patients with chronic peripheral neuropathy (including genetically determined neuropathy, diabetic neuropathy, and alcoholic neuropathy) without clinical weakness or histological evidence of atrophy, 74% of specimens exhibited a raised terminal innervation ratio. Only three patients with acute idiopathic polyneuritis were studied, and the findings were normal in two of the three. No information is given about the timing of the biopsy with regard to the evolution of the illness. In 25 patients with motor neuron disease, the mean terminal innervation ratio (2.01) was higher than the mean of the peripheral nerve disorders (1.64). In only one patient with amyotrophic lateral sclerosis was the terminal innervation ratio normal, while in the other 24 it was increased or could not be measured. An increased terminal innervation ratio provided a quantitative, sensitive indication of denervation and was found in a high proportion of clinically and histologically normal muscles in denervating diseases.[44]

Because of the substantial amount of sprouting observed in muscle biopsies from patients with amyotrophic lateral sclerosis and because of the clinical complaint of muscle fatigability, an electrophysiological study of neuromuscular transmission in patients with amyotrophic lateral sclerosis was reported.[49] Repetitive stimulation of the ulnar nerve at two impulses per second, while recording over the hypothenar muscles, disclosed an abnormal decremental response in 67% of 55 patients. The decrement was proportional to the amount of atrophy present in the muscle and was larger in muscles with the greatest degree of wasting. Frequent fasciculations were also found in muscles with the larger decrements, and the decrements were more pronounced with increased muscle temperatures. The defect was reversed or improved with the administration of edrophonium chloride, and post-tetanic exhaustion was observed several minutes after exercise. The basis for this decremental response is presumed to be the extensive terminal nerve sprouting that was first demonstrated by Wohlfart.[201] Morphological changes at the motor endplate in amyotrophic lateral sclerosis include enlargement of endplates and increased segmentation, as well as retraction of presynaptic terminals, all of which have been observed in muscle biopsy specimens of patients with amyotrophic lateral sclerosis.[19] These morphologic changes may produce a decrease in receptor density or excessive diffusion of acetylcholine in the enlarged synaptic cleft, which might contribute to neuromuscular transmission failure. Histograms showing abnormal miniature endplate potentials have been obtained from muscle biopsies of patients with amyotrophic lateral sclerosis and may be attributable to these same changes.[102]

Single-fiber electromyography has been utilized to study neuromuscular transmission in individual neuromuscular junctions of subjects with amyotrophic lateral sclerosis. Intermittent complete blockade of impulse transmission has been found in these patients and has been attributed to the presence of newly formed and immature sprouts. The firing rate of the motor neuron was important in that impulse blocking was observed more frequently at discharge frequencies in excess of ten per second and less frequently at low firing rates of four per second.[181]

Diabetic neuropathy is another neuropathic disorder, in which alterations of the neuromuscular junction have been found. Chokroverty studied eleven patients with proximal diabetic neuropathy who had clinical evidence of wasting and weakness of the quadriceps, hamstrings and glutei muscles, accompanied by diminished or absent quadriceps and hamstring tendon reflexes.[42] Biopsy specimens of the vastus medialis muscle in the region of the motor point were obtained for ultrastructural analysis of the motor endplates. Many degenerated or small nerve terminals were seen, and in some instances terminals were missing and the regions were occupied by Schwann cell processes (Fig. 5.5). Junctional folds underlying the degenerated or missing nerve terminals were atrophic and showed residual deposits of dense material and basement membrane remnants. (Fig. 5.5). Dystrophic axons were seen in several nerve terminal regions (Fig. 5.6). None of these changes were seen in control muscle endplates. Presynaptic membrane length was significantly reduced in the patients compared to controls, whereas postsynaptic membrane length, postsynaptic area, and nerve terminal area were not significantly different from controls.

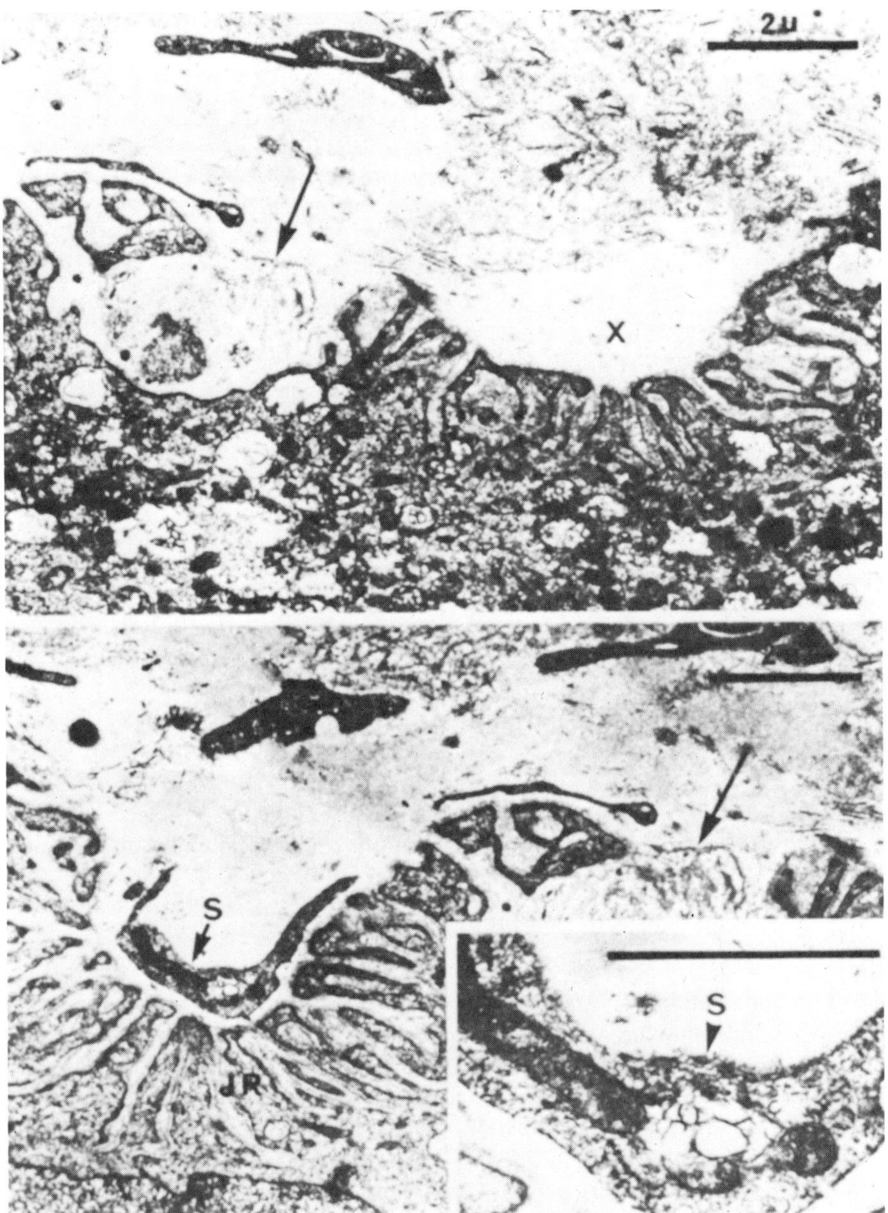

Figure 5.5. Motor endplate in right vastus medialis muscle showing three adjacent regions. Arrows indicate atrophic residues of junctional folds and basement membrane remnants in region denuded of nerve terminal. Top: Note that the nerve terminal is missing in another region (X). Scale indicates 2 μm. Bottom: S indicates Schwann cell process occupying another missing nerve terminal area; scale indicates 2 μm. Inset: Same as bottom in higher magnification; scale indicates 1 μm. Reprinted by permission from the *Archives of Neurology*.[42]

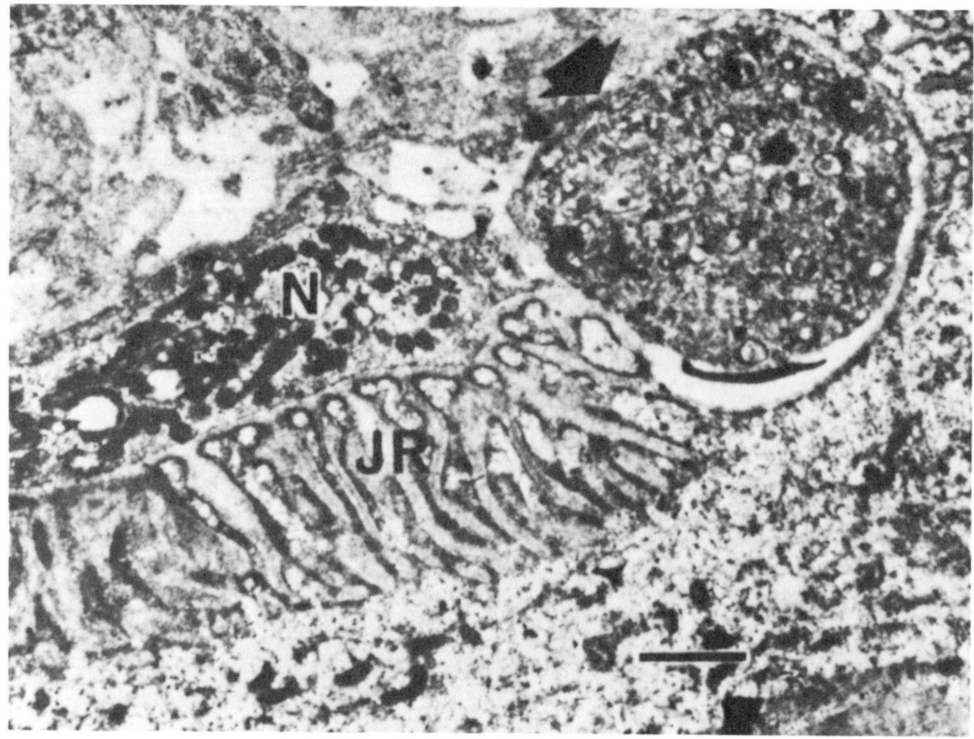

Figure 5.6. Portion of motor nerve endplate showing dystrophic axon (arrow) in nerve terminal area adjacent to apparently normal nerve terminal (N) and junctional region (JR) of folds and clefts. Scale indicates 1 μm. Reprinted by permission from the *Archives of Neurology*.[42]

The diseased intramuscular nerve filaments near the neuromuscular junctions showed axonal degeneration with dense axonal deposits and collections of glycogen granules within axons (Fig. 5.7). Focal collections of glycogen granules and dense deposits were also seen associated with Reich granules in Schwann cells. Intramuscular nerve filaments near the control neuromuscular junctions did not show these abnormalities. These morphologic observations indicated abnormal femoral nerve branches to the vastus medialis muscles and were consistent with a neurogenic disorder. It is interesting that diabetic distal polyneuropathy, which is a much more common entity, has not been studied from the point of view of morphometry of the motor endplate fine structure. The cause of proximal diabetic neuropathy is uncertain; but in some patients, when the onset of symptoms

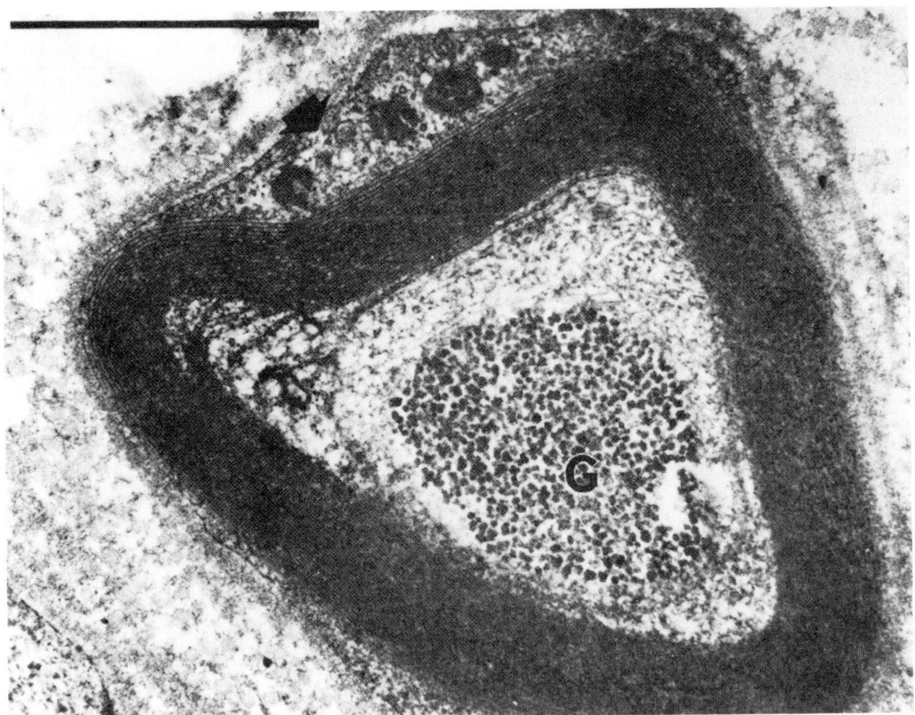

Figure 5.7. Aggregate of glycogen granules (G) in axis cylinder of intramuscular myelinated nerve fiber. Arrow indicates Schwann cell cytoplasm. Scale indicates 1 μm. Reprinted by permission from the *Archives of Neurology.*[42]

and signs is abrupt, a vascular or ischemic lesion has been postulated, while in other patients with a gradual and insidious onset, a metabolic disorder has been proposed.[5] In the latter condition, abnormalities of axonal transport may play a role in the development of peripheral nerve dysfunction.

A neuromuscular disorder of mice, murine muscular dystrophy (in 129/ReJ-dy strain mice), has been studied for its effect on the neuromuscular junction. There is a primary defect in the development of the peripheral nervous system, most prominent in dorsal and ventral spinal roots. Schwann cell development and myelinogenesis are arrested early, and the axolemma in dystrophic axons differs from normal myelinated axons.[67] Schwann cells fail to develop an adequate basement membrane, a step critical in the establishment of the complex relationship between Schwann cells and axons in mamma-

lian peripheral nerve.[173] Despite normal nerve fiber diameter, myelin thickness, internodal length and gross nodal morphology in peripheral axons, nerve conduction velocity is reduced by 25%–30%.
Axoplasmic transport is impaired. There is an increase in the low
molecular weight acetylcholinesterase and a decrease in the higher
molecular weight forms of the enzyme. Mechanisms for transmitter
release and acetylcholine production are normal, but quantal content
is increased. Utilizing freeze-fracture techniques, the nerve terminal
specializations associated with vesicle fusion and acetylcholine release appear normal. Electron micrographs reveal that the postsynaptic folding at the neuromuscular junction is reduced in complexity[67] (Fig. 5.8); in particular, there is a reduction of the infolding of
the postsynaptic membrane which forms the secondary synaptic cleft
at the motor endplate and is the site of acetylcholinesterase activity
(Figs. 5.9, 5.10). Despite decreased postjunctional folding, the particles on top of the junctional folds appeared normal, suggesting normal sensitivity to acetylcholine.

Abnormalities of Axonal Transport and Nerve Terminal Dysfunction

Axonal transport, the system whereby axons deliver materials
synthesized in the nerve cell body and provide essential constituents
for the maintenance of normal function to its distal regions, has been
the subject of several recent reviews.[23,150,157] Many questions still
remain about the mechanisms involved in axonal transport, but
there is general agreement that it is an active process which depends
upon divalent cations, ATP and contractile proteins such as myosin
and actin, possibly in association with microtubules. Slow axonal
transport carries major structural components of axoplasm at a rate

---

Figure 5.8. (A) Thin section of a dystrophic mouse neuromuscular junction
on extensor digitorum longus (EDL) muscle. The dark granules are a reaction
product of cholinesterase and label the synaptic cleft. Notice that there is a
reduction in both the regularity and depth of the postsynaptic infolding. The
nerve terminals (NT) appear normal with numerous mitochondria and synaptic vesicles (SV). ×25,000. (B) A normal mouse neuromuscular junction
from EDL muscle. Cholinesterase staining is evident in the primary synaptic cleft (SC[1]) and the secondary cleft infoldings (SC[2]) as well as in the
extracellular matrix (EM). ×30,000. Reprinted by permission from *Brain
Research*.[67]

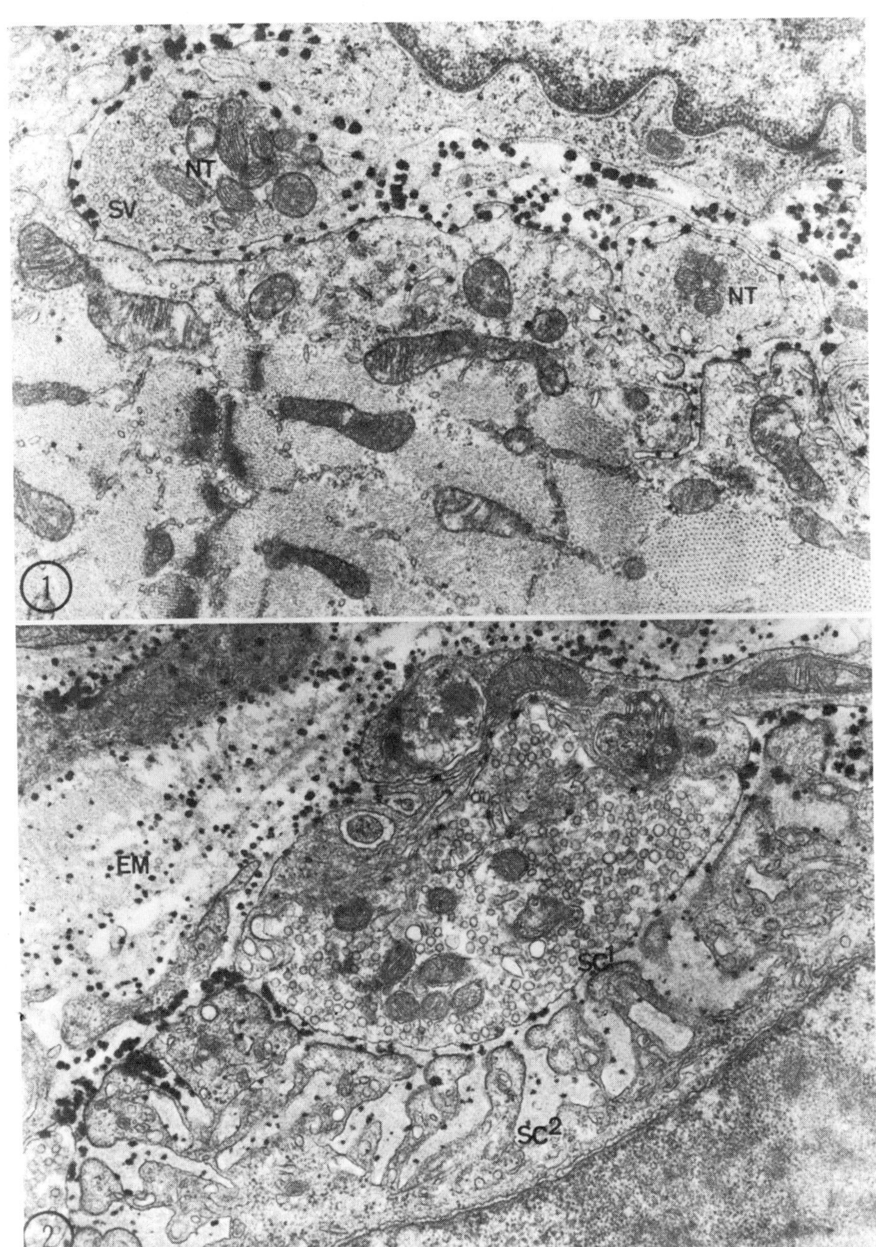
NT
SV
NT
1
EM
SC¹
SC²
2

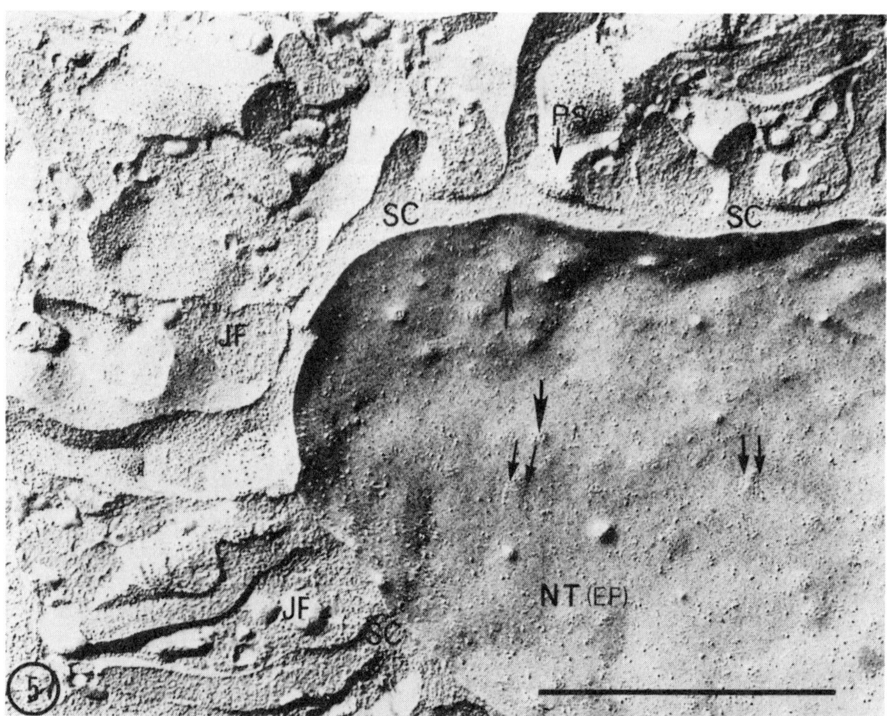

Figure 5.9. Normal neuromuscular junction in which the external fracture-face (EF) of the nerve terminal (NT) is surrounded by numerous regular junctional folds (JF) of the postsynaptic (PS) membrane. Note the double rows of pits in the nerve terminal membrane associated with transmitter release (small arrows) and the clumps of particles associated with endocytosis (larger arrows). ×45,000. Reprinted by permission from *Brain Research*.[67]

Figure 5.10. Fracture through a dystrophic neuromuscular junction in which the external fracture-face (EF) of the nerve terminal (NT) (upper right) as well as a cross-fractured nerve terminal (lower left) are exposed. Between and around these two nerve terminals are the synaptic cleft (SC) and numerous regions of postsynaptic membrane (PS) and protoplasmic fracture-faces (PF). Notice that here again the postsynaptic infolding is reduced while the postsynaptic membrane particles remain at high density (asterisk). Compare this figure to a similar fracture of a normal endplate (Fig. 5.9). ×50,000. Reprinted by permission from *Brain Research*.[67]

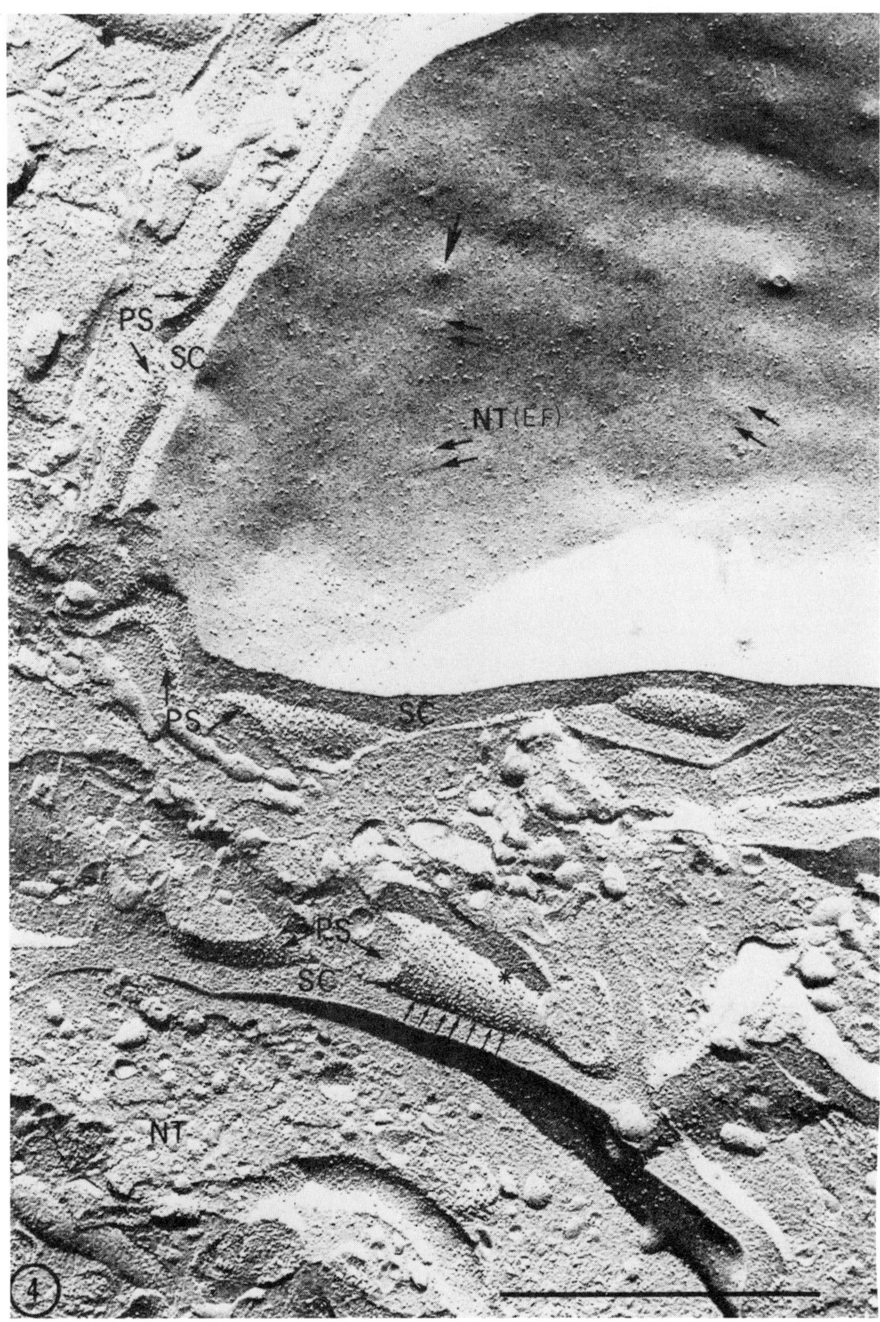
PS
SC
NT(EF)
PS
SC
SC
PS
NT
4

of one to two millimeters per day. Slow transport appears to be important in renewing structural constituents, although little is known about this process. Rapid axonal transport, with velocities in excess of 400 mm per day, involves elements of smooth endoplasmic reticulum with deposition of a substantial portion of the rapidly transported elements along the course of the axon, and subsequent insertion into the axolemma. Also, a large proportion of rapidly transported constituents reach the synaptic terminal, where they contribute to the formation of synaptic vesicles and terminal axolemma. Some of the material which reaches the synaptic ending subsequently reverses direction and returns in a retrograde fashion toward the cell body. It has been proposed that the retrograde axonal transport provides feedback about the milieu at the synaptic cleft.

Axonal transport is crucial for the survival of the axon, and following either transection or a focal blockade of axonal transport (reviewed above), Wallerian degeneration occurs distal to the injury. Reduced axonal transport has been documented in hereditary motor and sensory neuropathy and in diabetic neuropathy.[23] The reduced average velocity of axonal transport in both of these conditions cannot be attributed to nerve fiber loss. It is not certain whether the abnormalities of axonal transport are early steps in the development of the pathological changes or whether, as suggested by experimental neuropathies in animals, the breakdown of rapid axonal transport occurs late in the course of nerve degeneration.

In rats made diabetic with streptozotocin, hyperglycemia led to the slowing of nerve conduction velocity and the characteristic increased resistance of action potentials to ischemia typically found in human diabetic neuropathy.[109] Even though treated rats show no muscle weakness or sensory defect, reduced retrograde transport of pulse-labelled glycoprotein occurs within 24 hours after onset of hyperglycemia.[176] It is possible that the impaired turnaround of rapidly transported material in the distal axon could be an antecedent event in the development of diabetic neuropathy. It has recently been shown that the turnaround defect may be reversed by treating the diabetic rats with insulin, which would be consistent with this hypothesis.[113]

Acrylamide produces a dying-back, axonal neuropathy in which abnormalities appear first in the most distal part of the neuron with a gradual centripetal spread of dysfunction.[185] Both fast and slow anterograde axonal transport velocities are normal;[170] however, there is a reduced amount of retrogradely transported material consistent with a defect in turnaround at the nerve terminal. Electron microscopic autoradiographic studies have shown that the defective retro-grade transport stream is associated with distal accumulation of smooth endoplasmic reticulum.[43]

Despite these preliminary observations on axonal transport in peripheral nerve disease, the role of these abnormalities in the development of the pathological changes remains uncertain. Although it is unlikely that the breakdown of axonal transport is the cause of most peripheral neuropathies, abnormal axonal transport in certain dying-back neuropathies may contribute to the abnormalities which appear first in the most distal part of the nerve terminals.[23]

References

1. Akert K, Sandri C: An electromicroscopic study of zinc-iodide-osmium impregnation of neurons. I. Staining of synaptic vesicles of cholinergic junctions. *Brain Res* 7:286–295, 1968.
2. Albuquerque EX, Schuh FT, Kaufman FC: Early membrane depolarisation of the fast mammalian muscle after denervation. *Pfluegers Arch* 328:36–50, 1971.
3. Albuquerque EX, Deshpande SS, Guth L, Warnick JE: Trophic and nontrophic regulation of skeletal muscle and regeneration in the central nervous system. In Gorio A, Millesi H, Mingrino S (eds): *Posttraumatic Peripheral Nerve Regeneration, Experimental Basis and Clinical Implications*. New York, Raven Press, 1981, pp 360–395.
4. Antony MT, Tonge DA: Effects of denervation and botulinum toxin on muscle sensitivity to acetylcholine and acceptance of foreign innervation in the frog. *J Physiol* 303:23–31, 1980.
5. Asbury AK: Proximal diabetic neuropathy. *Ann Neurol* 2:179–180, 1977.
6. Austin L, Langford CJ: Nerve regeneration: A biochemical view. *Trends in Neurosci*, 131–132, May, 1980.
7. Bagust J, Lewis DM, Westerman RA: Polyneuronal innervation of kitten skeletal muscle. *J Physiol* (London) 229:241–255, 1973.
8. Bagust J, Lewis DM: Isometric contractions of motor units in self-reinnervated fast and slow twitch muscles of the cat. *J Physiol* 237: 91–102, 1974.
9. Bagust J, Lewis DM, Westerman RA: Motor units in cross-reinnervated fast and slow twitch muscles of the cat. *J Physiol* 313:223–235, 1981.
10. Ballantyne JP, Campbell MJ: Electrophysiological study after surgical repair of sectioned human peripheral nerves. *J Neurol Neurosurg Psychiat* 36:797–805, 1973.
11. Bennett MR, Pettigrew AG: The formation of synapses in striated muscle during development. *J Physiol* (London) 241:515, 1974.
12. Bennett MR, Pettigrew AG: The formation of neuromuscular synapses. *Cold Spring Harbor Symp Quant Biol* 40:409–424, 1976.

13. Beranek R, Vyskocil F: The action of tubocurarine and atropine on the normal and denervated rat diaphragm. *J Physiol* (London) 188:53–66, 1967.
14. Berg DK, Hall ZW: Increased extrajunctional acetyl-choline sensitivity produced by chronic post-synaptic neuromuscular blockade. *J Physiol* (London) 244:659–676, 1975.
15. Betz WJ, Caldwell JH, Ribchester RR: Sprouting of active nerve terminals in partially inactive muscles of the rat. *J Physiol* 303:281–297, 1980.
16. Birks R, Katz B, Miledi R: Physiological and structural changes at the amphibian myoneural junction, in the course of nerve degeneration. *J Physiol* 150:145–168, 1960.
17. Bisby MA: Inhibition of axonal transport in nerves chronically treated with local anesthetics. *Exp Neurol* 47:481–489, 1975.
18. Bisby MA: Fast axonal transport of labeled protein in sensory axons during regeneration. *Exp Neurol* 61:281, 1978.
19. Bjornskov EK, Dekker NP, Norris FH Jr, Stuart ME: Endplate morphology in amyotrophic lateral sclerosis. *Arch Neurol* 32:711–712, 1975.
20. Black MM, Lasek RJ: Slowing of the rate of axonal regeneration during growth and maturation. *Exp Neurol* 63:108, 1979.
21. Borenstein S, Desmedt JE: Range of variations in motor unit potentials during reinnervation after traumatic nerve lesions in humans. *Ann Neurol* 8:460–467, 1980.
22. Bray JJ, Hawken MJ, Hubbard JI, Pockett S, Wilson L: The membrane potential of rat diaphragm muscle fibers and the effect of denervation. *J Physiol* 255:651–667, 1976.
23. Brimijoin WS: Abnormalities of axonal transport. Are they a cause of peripheral nerve disease? *Mayo Clin Proc* 57:707–714, 1982.
24. Brockes JP, Hall ZW: Synthesis of acetylcholine receptor by denervated rat diaphragm muscle. *Proc Nat Acad Sci USA* 72:1368–1372, 1975.
25. Brown MC, Goodwin GM, Ironton R: Prevention of motor nerve sprouting in botulinum toxin poisoned mouse soleus muscles by direct stimulation of the muscle. *J Physiol* (London) 267:42–43, 1977.
26. Brown MC, Holland RL: A central role for denervated tissues in causing nerve sprouting. *Nature* 282:724–726, 1979.
27. Brown MC, Holland RL, Ironton R: Degenerating nerve products affect innervated muscle fibers. *Nature* 275:652–654, 1978a.
28. Brown MC, Holland RL, Ironton R: Variations in the amount and type of α-motoneurone sprouting following partial denervation of different mouse muscles. *J Physiol* (London) 284:177–178, 1978b.
29. Brown MC, Holland RL, Ironton R: Evidence against an intraspinal signal for motoneurone sprouting in mice. *J Physiol* (London) 291:35–36, 1979.
30. Brown MC, Holland RL, Ironton R: Nodal and terminal sprouting from motor nerves in fast and slow muscles of the mouse. *J Physiol* (London) 306:493–510, 1980.
31. Brown MC, Holland RL, Hopkins WG: Motor nerve sprouting. *Ann Rev Neurosci* 4:17–42, 1981.

Effects of Nerve Injury 247

32. Brown MC, Hopkins WG, Keynes RJ: Comparison of effects of denervation and botulinum toxin paralysis on muscle properties in mice. *J Physiol* 327:29–37, 1982.

33. Brown MC, Ironton R: The fate of motor axon sprouts in a partially denervated mouse muscle when regenerating nerve fibers return. *J Physiol* (London)263:181P–182P, 1976.

34. Brown MC, Ironton R: Sprouting and regression of neuromuscular synapses in partially denervated mammalian muscles. *J Physiol* (London) 278:325–348, 1978.

35. Buller AJ, Lewis DM: Further observations on mammalian cross-innervated skeletal muscle. *J Physiol* (London) 178:343–358, 1965.

36. Cajal S Ramón y: *Studies on Degeneration and Regeneration of the Nervous System* (translated and edited by RM May). London, Oxford University Press, 1928.

37. Cangiano A, Fried, JA: The production of denervation-like changes in rat muscle by colchicine, without interference with axonal transport or muscle activity. *J Physiol* 265:63–84, 1977.

38. Chang CC, Lee C-Y: Isolation of neurotoxins from the venom of *Bungarus multicinctus* and their modes of neuromuscular blocking action. *Arch Intern Pharmacodyn* 144:241–257, 1963.

39. Chang CC, Tung LH: Inhibition by actinomycin D of the generation of acetylcholine receptors induced by denervation in skeletal muscle. *Eur J Pharmacol* 26:386–388, 1974.

40. Chang CC, Chuang ST, Huang MC: Effects of chronic treatment with various neuromuscular blocking agents on the number and distribution of acetylcholine receptors in the rat diaphragm. *J Physiol* (London) 250:161–173, 1975.

41. Chiu TH, Lapa AJ, Barnard EA, Albuquerque EX: Binding of d-tubocurarine and α-bungarotoxin in normal and denervated mouse muscles. *Exp Neurol* 43:399–413, 1974.

42. Chokroverty S: Proximal nerve dysfunction in diabetic proximal amyotrophy. *Arch Neurol* 39:403–407, 1982.

43. Chretien M, Patey G, Souyri F, Droz B: Acrylamide-induced neuropathy and impairment of axonal transport of proteins. II. Abnormal accumulations of smooth endoplasmic reticulum at sites of focal retention of fast transported proteins: Electron microscope radiographic study. *Brain Res* 205:15–28, 1981.

44. Cöers C, Telerman-Toppet N, Gerard J-M: Terminal innervation ratio in neuromuscular disease. *Arch Neurol* 29:215–222, 1973.

45. Cotman CW, Nieto-Sampedro M, Harris EW: Synapse replacement in the nervous system of adult vertebrates. *Physiol Rev* 61:684–784, 1981.

46. Couteaux R, Pecot-Dechavassine M: Vesicules synaptiques et poches au niveau des zones actives de la jonction neuromusculaire. *C R Acad Sci Ser D* 271:2346–2349, 1970.

47. Cragg BG, Thomas PK: The conduction velocity of regenerated peripheral nerve fibers. *J Physiol* (London) 171:164, 1964.

48. Dennis MJ, Yip JW: Formation and elimination of foreign synapses on adult salamander muscle. *J Physiol* (London) 274: 299–310, 1978.

49. Denys EH, Norris FH: Amyotrophic lateral sclerosis: Impairment of neuromuscular transmission. *Arch Neurol* 36:202–205, 1979.

50. Devreotes PN, Fambrough DM: Synthesis of the acetylcholine receptor by cultured chick myotubes and denervated mouse extensor digitorum longus muscles. *Proc Nat Acad Sci USA* 73:161–164, 1976.

51. Ding R: Lack of correlation between physiological and morphological features of regenerating frog neuromuscular junctions. *Brain Res* 253: 47–55, 1982.

52. Donoso RS, Ballantyne JP, Hansen S: Regeneration of sutured human peripheral nerves: An electrophysiological study. *J Neurol Neurosurg Psychiatry* 42:97, 1979.

53. Drachman DB, Johnston DM: Neurotrophic regulation of dynamic properties of skeletal muscle: Effects of botulinum toxin and denervation. *J Physiol* 252:657–667, 1975.

54. Drachman DB, Pestronk A, Stanley EF: Neurotrophic interactions between nerves and muscles: Role of acetylcholine. In Schotland DL (ed): *Disorders of the Motor Unit*. New York, John Wiley & Sons, 1982, pp 107–117.

55. Drachman DB, Stanley EF, Pestronk A, Griffin JW, Price DL: Neurotrophic regulation of two properties of skeletal muscle by impulse-dependent and spontaneous acetylcholine transmission. *J Neurosci* 2:232–243, 1982.

56. Dreyer F, Peper K, Akert K, Sandri C, Moor H: Ultrastructure of the "active zone" in the frog neuromuscular junction. *Brain Res* 62: 373–380, 1973.

57. Dreyer F, Walther C, Peper K: Junctional and extrajunctional acetylcholine receptors in normal and denervated frog muscle fibers. Noise analysis experiments with different agonists. *Pfluegers Arch* 366:1–9, 1976.

58. Droz B: Synthetic machinery and axoplasmic transport: Maintenance of neuronal connectivity. In Brady RO (ed): *The Nervous System*, Vol 1. New York, Raven Press, 1975, pp 111–127.

59. Duce IR, Reeves JF, Keen P: Scanning electron microscope study of the development of free axonal sprouts at the cut ends of dorsal spinal nerve roots in the rat. *Cell Tissue Res* 170:507, 1976.

60. Duchen LW, Strich SJ: The effects of botulinum toxin on the pattern of innervation of skeletal muscle of the mouse. *Q J Exp Physiol* 53:84–89, 1968.

61. Eccles JC: Disuse atrophy of skeletal muscle. *Med J Aust* 2: 160–164, 1941.

62. Eccles JC: Investigations on muscle atrophies arising from disuse and tenotomy. *J Physiol* 103:253–266, 1944.

63. Edds MV: Experiments on partially deneurotized nerves. *J Exp Zool* 111:211–226, 1949.

64. Edwards C: The effects of innervation on the properties of acetylcholine receptors in muscle. *Neuroscience* 4:565–584, 1979.

65. Ekstedt J, Stalberg E: Single fiber electromyography for the study of the microphysiology of the human muscle. In Desmedt JE (ed): *New Developments in Electromyography and Clinical Neurophysiology*, Vol 1. Basel, Karger, 1973, pp 89–112.

66. Eldridge L, Liebhold M, Steinbach JH: Alterations in cat skeletal neuromuscular junctions following prolonged inactivity. *J Physiol* 313:529–545, 1981.

67. Ellisman MH: The membrane morphology of the neuromuscular junction, sarcolemma, sarcoplasmic reticulum and transverse tubule system in murine muscular dystrophy studied by freeze-fracture electron microscopy. *Brain Res* 214:261–273, 1981.
68. Elsberg CA: Experiments on motor nerve regeneration and the direct neurotization of paralyzed muscles by their own and by foreign nerves. *Science* 45:318–320, 1917.
69. Engel AG: Morphological effects of denervation of muscle. A quantitative ultrastructural study. *Ann NY Acad Sci* 228:68–88, 1974.
70. Erlanger J, Schoepfle GM: A study of nerve degeneration and regeneration. *Am J Physiol* 147:550–581, 1946.
71. Exner S: Die Innervation des Kehlkopfes. *S B Akad Wiss Wein* 89(3): 63–118, 1884.
72. Fagg GE, Scheff SW, Cotman CW: Axonal sprouting at the neuromuscular junction of adult and aged rats. *Exp Neurol* 74:847–854, 1981.
73. Fambrough DM: Control of acetylcholine receptors in skeletal muscle. *Physiol Rev* 59:165–225, 1979.
74. Fambrough DM: Specificity of nerve-muscle interaction. In Barondes S (ed): *Neuronal Recognition*. New York, Plenum, 1976, pp 25–67.
75. Fambrough DM: Acetylcholine sensitivity of muscle fiber membranes: Mechanism of regulation by motoneurones. *Science* 168:372–373, 1970.
76. Fex S, Sonesson B, Thesleff S, Zeleńa J: Nerve implants in botulinum poisoned mammalian muscle. *J Physiol* (London) 184:872–882, 1966.
77. Finol JH, Lewis DM, Ownes R: The effects of denervation on contractile properties of rat skeletal muscle. *J Physiol* 319: 81–92, 1981.
78. Fischbach GD, Robbins N: Changes in contractile properties of disused soleus muscles. *J Physiol* 201:305–320, 1969.
79. Frank E, Jansen JKS, Lømo T, Westgaard RH: The interaction between foreign and original nerves innervating the soleus muscle of rats. *J Physiol* (London) 247:725–743, 1975.
80. Frizell M, McLean WG, Sjostrand J: Retrograde axonal transport of rapidly migrating labelled proteins and glycoproteins in regenerating peripheral nerves. *J Neurochem* 27:191, 1976.
81. Gilliatt RW, Fowler TJ, Rudge P: Peripheral neuropathy in baboons. *Adv Neurol* 10:253–272, 1975.
82. Gilliatt RW, Hjorth RJ: Nerve conduction during Wallerian degeneration in the baboon. *J Neurol Neurosurg Psychiatry* 35:335–341, 1972.
83. Gilliatt RW, Taylor JC: Electrical changes following section of the facial nerve. *Proc R Soc Med* 52:1080–1083, 1959.
84. Gilliatt RW, Westgaard RH: Nerve-muscle interactions. Some clinical aspects. *Comtemp Clin Neurophysiol* 34:547–553, 1978.
85. Gilliatt RW, Westgaard RH, Williams IR: Extrajunctional acetylcholine sensitivity of inactive muscle fibers in the baboon during prolonged nerve pressure block. *J Physiol* (London) 280: 499–514, 1978.
86. Goldberg AL: Protein turnover in skeletal muscle. II. Effects of denervation and cortisone on protein catabolism in skeletal muscle. *J Biol Chem* 244:3223–3229, 1969.
87. Gordon T, Jones R, Vrobova G: Changes in chemosensitivity of skeletal muscles as related to endplate formation. *Progr Neurobiol Oxford* 6:103–136, 1976.

88. Gordon T, Stein RB: Time course and extent of recovery in reinnervated motor units of cat triceps surae muscles. *J Physiol* 323:307–323, 1982.
89. Gorio A, Carmignoto G: Reformation, maturation, and stabilization of neuromuscular junctions in peripheral nerve regeneration: The possible role of exogenous gangliosides on determining motoneuron sprouting. In Gorio A, Millesi H, Mingrino S (eds): *Posttraumatic Peripheral Nerve Regeneration, Experimental Basis and Clinical Implications.* New York, Raven Press, 1981, pp 481–493.
90. Grafstein B, McQuarrie IG: Role of the nerve cell body in axonal regeneration. In Cotman CW (ed): *Neuronal Plasticity.* New York, Raven Press, 1978, pp 155–195.
91. Griffin JW, Drachman DB, Price DL: Rapid axonal transport in motor nerve regeneration. *J Neurobiol* 7:355, 1976.
92. Guth L: Neuromuscular function after regeneration of interrupted nerve fibers into partially denervated muscle. *Exp Neurol* 6:129–141, 1962.
93. Guth L, Kemerer VF, Samaras TA, Warnick JE, Albuquerque EX: The roles of disuse and loss of neurotrophic function in denervation atrophy of skeletal muscle. *Exp Neurol* 73:20–36, 1981.
94. Gutmann E: Neurotrophic relations. *Ann Rev Physiol* 34: 177–216, 1976.
95. Gutmann E, Holubar J: The degeneration of peripheral nerve fibers. *J Neurol Neurosurg Psychiatry* 13:89–105, 1950.
96. Halperin JJ, LaVail JH: A study of the dynamics of retrograde transport and accumulation of horseradish peroxidase in injured neurons. *Brain Res* 100:253, 1975.
97. Harris AJ: Trophic effects of nerve on muscle. In Sumner AJ (ed): *The Physiology of Peripheral Nerve Disease.* Philadelphia, WB Saunders, 1980, pp 195–220.
98. Hartzell HC, Fambrough DM: Acetylcholine receptors. Distribution and extrajunctional density in rat diaphragm after denervation correlated with acetylcholine sensitivity. *J Gen Physiol* 60:248–262, 1972.
99. Harvey AM, Kuffler SW: Motor nerve function with lesions of the peripheral nerves. *Arch Neurol Psychiatry* (Chicago) 52:317–322, 1944.
100. Heuser JE, Reese TS, Dennis MJ, Jan Y, Jan L, Evans L: Synaptic vesicle exocytosis captured by quick freezing and correlated with quantal transmitter release. *J Cell Biol* 81:275–300, 1979.
101. Heuser JE, Reese TS, Landis DMD: Functional changes in frog neuromuscular junctions studied with freeze-fracture. *J Neurocytol* 3: 109–131, 1974.
102. Highstone HH, Colton RP, Norris FH: Amyotrophic lateral sclerosis: Changes in motor nerve terminal function. In *Recent Advances in Mycology; Proceedings of the Third International Congress on Muscle Diseases, Newcastle-upon-Tyne, England, Sept. 1974,* Amsterdam, Excerpta Medica International Congress Series No. 360, pp 542–545.
103. Hodes RMG, Larrabee MG, German W: The human electromyogram in response to nerve stimulation and the conduction velocity of motor axons. *Arch Neurol Psychiatry* 60:340, 1948.
104. Hoffman H: Local reinnervation in partially denervated muscle: A histophysiological study. *Aust J Exp Biol Med Sci* 28:383–397, 1950.

105. Hoffman H: Fate of interrupted nerve fibers regenerating into partially denervated muscles. *Aust J Exp Biol Med Sci* 29: 211−219, 1951.

106. Hoffman H: Acceleration and retardation of the process of axonsprouting in partially denervated muscles. *Aust J Exp Biol Med Sci* 30:541−566, 1952.

107. Holland RL, Brown MC: Post-synaptic transmission block can cause motor nerve terminal sprouting. *Science* 207:649−651, 1980.

108. Hopkins WG, Brown MC: The distribution of nodal sprouts in a paralysed or partly denervated mouse muscle. *Neuroscience* 7:37−44, 1982.

109. Horowitz SH, Ginsberg-Fellner F: Peripheral nerve responses during ischemia in the evaluation of diabetic neuropathy. *Muscle & Nerve* 1:388−391, 1978.

110. Hubbard AL, Cohn ZA: Externally disposed plasma membrane proteins. I. Enzymatic iodination of mouse L cells. *J Cell Biol* 64:438−460, 1975.

111. Ironton R, Brown MC, Holland RL: Stimuli to intramuscular nerve growth. *Brain Res* 156:351−354, 1978.

112. Jacobson S, Guth L: An electrophysiological study of the early stages of peripheral nerve regeneration. *Exp Neurol* 11:48, 1965.

113. Jakobsen J, Brimijoin S, Skau K, Sidenius P, Wells D: Retrograde axonal transport of transmitter enzymes, fucose-labeled protein, and nerve growth factor in streptozotocin-diabetic rats. *Diabetes* 30: 797−803, 1981.

114. Johns TR, Thesleff S: Effects of motor inactivation on the chemical sensitivity of skeletal muscle. *Acta Physiol Scand* 51:136−141, 1961.

115. Kaeser HE, Lambert EH: Nerve function studies in experimental polyneuritis. *Electroencephalogr Clin Neurophysiol Suppl* 22:29−35, 1962.

116. Katz B, Miledi R: The statistical nature of the acetylcholine potential and its molecular components. *J Physiol* (London) 224:665−699, 1972.

117. Kean CJC, Lewis DM, McGarrick JD: Dynamic properties of denervated fast and slow twitch muscle of the cat. *J Physiol* 237:103−113, 1974.

118. Keynes RJ: The effects of pyronin on sprouting and regeneration of mouse motor nerves. *Brain Res* 253:13−18, 1982.

119. Kidman AD, Dolan L, Sippe HJ: Blockade of fast axonal transport by diphtheritic demyelination in the chicken sciatic nerve. *J Neurochem* 30:57−62, 1978.

120. Kimura M, Kimura I: Increase of nascent protein synthesis in neuromuscular junction of rat diaphragm induced by denervation. *Nature New Biol* 241:114−115, 1973.

121. Ko CP: Electrophysiological and freeze-fracture studies of change following denervation at frog neuromuscular junctions. *J Physiol* 321: 627−639, 1981.

122. Korneliussen H, Jansen JKS: Morphological aspects of the elimination of polyneuronal innervation of skeletal muscle fibers in newborn rats. *J Neurocytol* 5:591, 1976.

123. Kuffler D, Thompson W, Jansen JKS: The elimination of synapses in multiply innervated skeletal muscle fibers of the rat: Dependence on distance between endplates. *Brain Res* 138:353, 1977.

124. Kugelberg E: The motor unit: Morphology and function. In Desmedt JE (ed): *Motor Unit Types, Recruitment and Plasticity in Health and Disease*, Vol 9. Basel, Karger, 1981, pp 1–16.

125. Landau WM: The duration of neuromuscular function after nerve section in man. *J Neurosurg* 10:64–68, 1953.

126. Landmesser LT: The generation of neuromuscular specificity. *Ann Rev Neurosci* 3:279–302, 1980.

127. Langley JN: Remarks on the cause and nature of the changes which occur in muscle after nerve section. *Lancet* 191:6–7, 1916.

128. Lasek RJ, Hoffman PN: The neuronal cytoskeleton, axonal transport, and axonal growth. In Goldman R, Pollard T, Rosenbaum J (eds): *Cell Motility, Book C, Microtubules and Related Proteins*. Cold Spring Harbor, NY, Cold Spring Harbor Laboratory, 1976, pp 1021–1051.

129. Lee JC: Electron miscroscopic observations on myogenic free cells of denervated skeletal muscle. *Exp Neurol* 12:123–135, 1965.

130. Lee CY, Tseng LF, Chiu TH: Influence of denervation on the localization of neurotoxins from elapid venoms in rat diaphragm. *Nature* 215:1177–1178, 1967.

131. Letinsky MS, Fischbeck KH, McMahon VJ: Precision of reinnervation of original postsynaptic sites in frog muscle after a nerve crush. *J Neurocytol* 5:691, 1976.

132. Levitt TA, Salpeter MM: Denervated endplates have a dual population of junctional acetylcholine receptors. *Nature* 291:239–241, 1981.

133. Lewis DM: The effect of denervation on the mechanical and electrical responses of fast and slow mammalian twitch muscle. *J Physiol* 222:51–75, 1972.

134. Lewis DM, Kean CJC, McGarrick JD: Dynamic properties of slow and fast muscle and their trophic regulation. *Ann NY Acad Sci* 228:105–120, 1974.

135. Lewis DM, Rowlerson A, Webb SN: Motor units and immunohistochemistry of cat soleus muscle after long periods of cross-reinnervation. *J Physiol* 325:403–418, 1982.

136. Lieberman AR: The axon reaction: A review of the principal features of perikarial responses to axon injury. *Int Rev Neurobiol* 14:49, 1971.

137. Linden DC, Fambrough DM: Biosynthesis and degradation of acetylcholine receptors in rat skeletal muscles. Effects of electrical stimulation. *Neurosci* 4:527–538, 1979.

138. Lømo T, Rosenthal J: Control of ACh sensitivity by muscle activity in the rat. *J Physiol* (London) 221:493–513, 1972.

139. Lømo T, Westgaard RH: Control of ACh sensitivity in rat muscle fibers *Cold Spring Harbor Symp Quant Biol* 40:263–274, 1975.

140. Luc JV, Eyzaguirre C: Fibrillation and hypersensitivity to ACh in denervated muscle: Effect of length of degenerating nerve fibers. *J Neurophysiol* 18:65–73, 1955.

141. Mark RF: Synaptic repression at neuromuscular junctions. *Physiol Rev* 60:355–395, 1980.

142. Miledi R: The acetylcholine sensitivity of frog muscle fibers after complete or partial denervation. *J Physiol* (London) 151:1–23, 1960.

143. Miledi R, Slater CR: On the degeneration of rat neuromuscular junctions after nerve section. *J Physiol* 207:507–528, 1970.

144. Miller RG: Different mechanisms for impaired neuromuscular efficiency and speed of tension development in neurogenic and myogenic weakness. *Neurology* 32:A68, 1982.
145. Miller RG: Dynamic properties of partially denervated muscle. *Ann Neurol* 6:51–55, 1979.
146. Miller RG, Sherratt M: Firing rates of human motor units in partially denervated muscle. *Neurology* (Minneap) 28:1241–1248, 1978.
147. Milner-Brown HS, Stein RB, Lee RG: Contractile and electrical properties of human motor units in neuropathies and motor neuron disease. *J Neurol Neurosurg Psychiatry* 6:670–676, 1974.
148. Milner-Brown HS, Stein RB, Lee RG, Brown WF: Motor unit recruitment in patients with neuromuscular disorders. In Desmedt JE (ed): *Motor Unit Types, Recruitment and Plasticity in Health and Disease*, Vol. 9. Basel, Karger, 1981, pp 305–318.
149. Neher E, Sakmann B: Single-channel currents recorded from membrane of denervated frog muscle fibers. *Nature* 260:799–802, 1976.
150. Ochs S: Calcium and the mechanism of axoplasmic transport. In Schotland DL (ed): *Disorders of the Motor Unit*. New York, John Wiley & Sons, 1982, pp 157–172.
151. Ochs S: Energy metabolism and supply of ~ P to the fast axoplasmic transport mechanism in nerve. *Fed Proc* 33:1049–1058, 1974.
152. Ochs S: Fast axoplasmic transport in the fibers of chromatolyzed neurones. *J Physiol* (London) 255:249, 1976.
153. Olek A, Younkin S, Slugg RM, Konieczkowski M, Robbins N: A transient increase in junctional acetylcholine receptors after denervation. *Brain Res* 214:429–432, 1981.
154. Peper K, Bradley RJ, Dreyer F: The acetylcholine receptor at the neuromuscular junction. *Physiol Rev* 62:1271–1340, 1982.
155. Pestronk A, Drachman DB: Motor nerve sprouting and acetylcholine receptors. *Science* 199:1223–1225, 1978.
156. Pestronk A, Drachman DB, Stanley EF, Price DL, Griffin JW: Cholinergic transmission regulates extrajunctional acetylcholine receptors. *Exp Neurol* 70:690–696, 1980.
157. Pleasure D: Axoplasmic transport. In Sumner AJ (ed): *The Physiology of Peripheral Nerve Disease*. Philadelphia, WB Saunders, 1980, pp 221–237.
158. Politis MJ, Ederle K, Spencer PS: Trophism in nerve regeneration in vivo. Attraction of regenerating axons by diffusible factors derived from cells in distal nerve stumps of transected peripheral nerves. *Brain Res* 253:1–12, 1982.
159. Porter CW, Barnard EA: Distribution and density of cholinergic receptors at the motor endplates of a denervated mouse muscle. *Exp Neurol* 48:542–556, 1975.
160. Pulliam DL, April EW: Degenerative changes at the neuromuscular junctions of red, white and intermediate muscle fibers. *J Neurol Sci* 43:205–222, 1979.
161. Purves D, Lichtman JW: Formation and maintenance of synaptic connections in autonomic ganglia. *Physiol Rev* 58:821–862, 1978.
162. Purves D, Sakmann B: The effect of contractile activity on fibrillation and extrajunctional acetylcholine sensitivity of rat muscle maintained in organ culture. *J Physiol* 337:157–182, 1974.

163. Redfern P, Thesleff S: Action potential generation in denervated rat skeletal muscle. II. The action of tetrodotoxin. *Acta Physiol Scand* 82:70−78, 1971.

164. Robert ED, Oester YT: Absence of supersensitivity to acetylcholine in innervated muscle subjected to a prolonged pharmacologic nerve block. *J Pharmacol Exp Ther* 174:133−140, 1970.

165. Rosenblueth A, Dempsey EW: A study of Wallerian degeneration. *Am J Physiol* 128:19−30, 1939.

166. Rotshenker S: Transneuronal and peripheral mechanisms for the induction of motor neuron sprouting. *J Neurosci* 2:1359−1368, 1982.

167. Rotshenker S: Sprouting and synapse formation by motor axons separated from their cell bodies. *Brain Res* 223:141−145, 1981.

168. Rotshenker S: Synapse formation in intact innervated cutaneous-pectoris muscles of the frog following denervation of the opposite muscle. *J Physiol* (London) 292:535−547, 1979.

169. Rotshenker S, McMahan UJ: Altered patterns of innervation in frog muscle after denervation. *J Neurocytol* 5:719−730, 1976.

170. Sahenk Z, Mendell JR: Acrylamide and 2,5-hexanedione neuropathies: Abnormal bidirectional transport rate in distal axons. *Brain Res* 219:397−405, 1981.

171. Salafsky B, Bell J, Prewitt M: Development of fibrillation potentials in denervated fast and slow skeletal muscles. *J Physiol* 215:637−643, 1968.

172. Sanders FK, Whitteridge D: Conduction velocity and myelin thickness in regenerating nerve fibers. *J Physiol* (London) 105:152, 1946.

173. Sanes JR, Marshall LM, McMahan UJ: Reinnervation of muscle fiber basal lamina after removal of myofibers. *J Cell Biol* 78:176−198, 1978.

174. Schiff M: Ueber motorische Laehmung der Zunge. *Tub Arch Phys Heilk* 10:579−593, 1851.

175. Selzer ME: Regeneration of peripheral nerve. In Sumner AJ (ed): *The Physiology of Peripheral Nerve Disease*. Philadelphia, WB Saunders, 1980, pp 358−431.

176. Sidenius P, Jakobsen J: Retrograde axonal transport: A possible role in the development of neuropathy. *Diabetologia* 20:110−112, 1981.

177. Slack JR, Williams MN: The absence of nodal sprouts from partially denervated nerve trunks. *Brain Res* 226:291−297, 1981.

178. Smith JW, Thesleff S: Spontaneous activity in denervated mouse diaphragm muscle. *J Physiol* 257:171−186, 1976.

179. Solandt DY, Delury DB, Hunter J: Effect of electrical stimulation on atrophy of denervated skeletal muscle. *Arch Neurol Psychiatry* 49:802−807, 1943.

180. Solandt DY, Magladery JW: The relation of atrophy to fibrillation in denervated muscle. *Brain* 63:255−263, 1940.

181. Stalberg E, Schwartz MS, Trontelj JU: Single fiber electromyography in various processes affecting the anterior horn cell. *J Neurol Sci* 24:403−415, 1975.

182. Stanley EF, Drachman DB: Denervation accelerates the degradation of junctional acetylcholine receptors. *Exp Neurol* 73:390−397, 1981.

183. Stanley EF, Drachman DB: Denervation and the time course of resting membrane potential changes in skeletal muscle in vivo. *Exp Neurol* 69:253−259, 1980.

184. Stewart DM, Sola OM, Martin AW: Hypertrophy as a response to denervation in skeletal muscle. *J Physiol* 76:146–167, 1972.

185. Sumner AJ: Axonal polyneuropathies. In Sumner AJ (ed): *The Physiology of Peripheral Nerve Disease.* Philadelphia, WB Saunders, 1980, pp 340–357.

186. Sunderland S: *Nerves and Nerve Injuries,* 2nd Ed. Edinburgh, Churchill Livingstone, 1978, pp 82–132.

187. Takamori M, Hazama R, Tsujihata M: Active state properties of denervated and immobilized muscle; Comparison with dystrophic muscle. *Neurology* (Minneap) 28:603–608, 1978.

188. Thesleff S, Sellin LC: Denervation supersensitivity. *Trends in Neurosci* 4:122–126, 1980.

189. Thesleff S, Ward MR: Studies on the mechanism of fibrillation potentials in denervated muscle. *J Physiol* 244:313–323, 1975.

190. Thompson W: Reinnervation of partially denervated rat soleus muscles. *Acta Physiol Scand* 103:81–91, 1978.

191. Thompson W, Jansen JKS: The extent of sprouting of remaining motor units in partly denervated immature and adult rat soleus muscles. *Neuroscience* 2:523–535, 1977.

192. Tinel J: Le signe du fourmillement dans les lesions des nerfs peripheriques. *Presse Med* 23:388, 1915.

193. Tuffery AR: Growth and degeneration of motor endplates in normal cat hindlimb muscles. *J Anat* 110:221–247, 1971.

194. Tweedle CD, Kabara JJ: Lipophilic nerve sprouting factor(s) isolated from denervated muscle. *Neuroscience Lett* 6:41–46, 1977.

195. Vrbova G, Gordon T, Jones R: *Nerve-Muscle Interaction.* London: Chapman & Hall, 1978.

196. Waller AV: Experiments on the section of the glossopharyngeal and hypoglossal nerves of the frog, and observation on the alterations produced thereby in the structure of their primitivefibers. *Philo Trans R Soc Lond* (Biol) 140–423, 1830.

197. Watson WE: Observations on the nucleolar and total cell body nucleic acid of injured nerve cells. *J Physiol* (London) 196:655, 1968.

198. Weiss P, Edds MV: Spontaneous recovery of muscle following partial denervation. *Am J Physiol* 145:587–607, 1946.

199. Weiss P, Hoag A: Competitive reinnervation of rat muscles by their own and foreign nerves. *J Neurophysiol* 9:413, 1946.

200. West JR: Early history of mammalian nerve regeneration. *Neurosci Behav Rev* 2:27, 1978.

201. Wohlfart G: Collateral regeneration from residual motor nerve fibers in amyotrophic lateral sclerosis. *Neurology* (Minneap) 7:124–134, 1957.

202. Wolf SM, Wagner JH Jr, Davidson S, Forsythe A: Treatment of Bell palsy with prednisone: A prospective, randomized study. *Neurology* 28:158–161, 1978.

203. Young JZ: The functional repair of nervous tissue. *Physiol Rev* 22:318, 1942.

204. Zak R, Grove D, Rabinowitz M: DNA synthesis in the rat diaphragm as an early response to denervation. *Am J Physiol* 216:647–654, 1969.

Chapter 6

Acquired Myasthenia Gravis

Donald B. Sanders, M.D.

The most common disease that affects primarily the neuromuscular junction is myasthenia gravis (MG). There are several rare congenital forms of myasthenia, and these are discussed in Chapter 7. The acquired form of MG has attracted much interest recently because of major advances in our understanding of its pathophysiology and immunopathology. Careful study of this disease reveals much about the normal function of the neuromuscular junction and can indicate the directions of future productive study of synaptic transmission in general.

Clinical Features

Acquired MG is estimated to have an incidence of from 20 to 100 per million and a prevalence of approximately 40 per million.[52,72,96,102,126] Thus, at any one time it affects at least 8000 patients in the US. The disease is frequently not recognized, however, and the true incidence is probably higher than this. The modal age of onset of symptoms is 20 years, with a second peak in the 40's. Among younger patients, women are affected more often, whereas when the disease begins after age 50 years, men are more often affected.[52]

The majority of patients have ocular symptoms initially and almost all will have double vision or ptosis within two years of onset of their disease.[52] Bulbar muscles also tend to be involved early on, producing difficulty in chewing, swallowing or talking.

The disease follows a variable course. In up to 16% of patients weakness remains restricted to the ocular muscles.[52] However, even in the majority of patients with purely ocular weakness, abnormalities of neuromuscular transmission can be demonstrated in extremity muscles by electromyographic (EMG) tests[53] (Table 6.1) or by administration of low doses of curare.[53] Most patients will experience a progression of disease, with ultimate weakness of extremity muscles. The symptoms usually fluctuate over relatively short periods of time and progress in severity and distribution for several years ("active stage").[125] In those patients who survive, a relatively stable state then ensues ("inactive stage") during which fluctuations in strength still occur but are usually attributable to fatigue, intercurrent illness or other identifiable factors. After 15 to 20 years, weakness tends to become fixed and atrophy is frequent in the most severely involved muscles ("burnt-out stage"). As the distribution and severity of weakness increase, even slight changes in strength can markedly affect function, including the vital functions of breathing and swallowing. Many factors can cause worsening of myasthenia: emotional upset, systemic illness (especially viral respiratory infections), thyroid dysfunction (hypo- and hyperthyroidism), pregnancy, the menstrual cycle and drugs whose neuromuscular blocking effects would not be noticeable in patients without neuromuscular disease. Defects of neuromuscular transmission are made worse by increased temperature and many patients will note clinical worsening in hot weather, with fever or following a hot bath.

Since many patients with MG have fluctuating weakness and symptoms that conform to no clear anatomical distribution, it is common for psychiatric diagnoses to be entertained early on. In others, eyelid ptosis and ocular muscle weakness may suggest an intracranial mass lesion; many patients will have had cranial CT scans or arteriography performed before the correct diagnosis is made.

The Diagnosis of Myasthenia Gravis

The diagnosis of myasthenia gravis (MG) is made on the basis of the following clinical features:

1.   Weakness that has a characteristic distribution, frequently affecting the ocular and bulbar muscles.

2.   Fluctuations in strength such that weakness is significantly greater following effort and less after brief rest. Since changes in symptomatic weakness are common in many diseases, and since accurate determinations of strength require full patient cooperation,

Table 6.1
Diagnostic Sensitivity of Initial Studies
in Myasthenia Gravis[a]

Test	Muscle	Disease Class[b]				
		1	*2*	*3*	*4/5*	*Total*
SF	EDC	18/31(58)	105/130(81)	38/40(95)	70/70(100)	231/271(85)[c]
	FRONTALIS	22/23(96)	28/32(88)	5/5(100)	4/4(100)	59/64(92)
RS	ADM	2/13(15)	24/71(34)	10/24(42)	36/58(62)	72/166(43)
	BICEPS	2/7(29)	17/43(40)	12/18(67)	13/19(68)	44/87(51)
AChR-AB[d]		10/16(62)	40/55(73)	20/22(91)	29/38(76)	99/131(76)

[a]Data are expressed as: number of abnormal studies/total number of studies (percentage of abnormal studies).

[b]Definitions of disease class: 1 - purely ocular weakness, 2 - mild generalized weakness, usually with ocular weakness, 3 - predominately bulbar weakness, with mild generalized weakness, 4 - moderately severe generalized weakness, 5 - severe generalized weakness.

[c]If the EDC was normal and another muscle was tested, selected on the basis of clinical weakness, an abnormality was found in 99% of patients.

[d]Performed in the laboratory of A. D. Roses, Duke University Medical Center.[81]

Abbreviations: SF = single-fiber EMG, EDC = extensor digitorum communis, RS = repetitive stimulation EMG, ADM = abductor digiti minimi, AChR-AB = anti-acetylcholine receptor antibody titer.

it is not uncommon to find fluctuations in observed performance on muscle tests in diseases other than MG. This is especially true if performance on these tests induces pain. Observations of ocular and bulbar muscle functions are less likely to be affected by extraneous factors and thus provide more convincing demonstrations of fluctuating strength in many patients.

3.   Improvement after the administration of cholinesterase inhibitors such as edrophonium (see Appendix). As with observations of fluctuations in strength, the most convincing demonstrations of response to cholinesterase inhibitors are usually made in the ocular and bulbar muscles. In an attempt to improve the objectivity of this test, many clinicians will administer the drug in a "blinded" or "double-blinded" fashion. One can question how truly effective such blinding procedures are, however, since cholinesterase inhibitors produce unique symptoms that most patients easily recognize and that are not mimicked by the agents commonly given as placebo. It should also be recognized that chance alone would allow one to correctly distinguish the cholinesterase inhibitor from a single placebo 50% of the time even if the blinding is effective.

It is sometimes difficult to demonstrate these clinical characteristics despite the presence of symptoms that strongly suggest the disease. This is especially true in the early stages of the disease when the weakness is mild or intermittent. Nevertheless, the diagnosis of MG can be made with considerable assurance in the majority of patients on the basis of these criteria.

It has been recognized recently that antibodies to the muscle acetylcholine receptor (AChR-Ab) are present in the serum of most patients with MG. These antibodies are virtually specific for MG, and confirm the diagnosis when present in patients with characteristic clinical findings. The patients most likely not to have detectable AChR-Ab, however, tend to be those in whom the clinical diagnosis is also most questionable, i.e., those with early, mild or purely ocular weakness. Objective measurements of neuromuscular function, as provided by various electromyographic and physiologic techniques, can add greatly to the diagnostic certainty in such situations.

Electromyography

When the nerve to a normal muscle is stimulated, the nerve terminal releases a large number of packages (quanta) of acetylcholine (ACh) which produce a depolarization of the endplate sufficient to trigger the process that ultimately leads to muscle contraction. Normally, the amount of ACh released is several times greater than is necessary to produce a depolarization that exceeds the muscle action potential threshold, and every nerve impulse is followed by a muscle contraction.

Measurement of the amount of ACh released from the motor nerve and determination of the response of the muscle to known amounts of this transmitter can be performed using biopsies of intercostal muscle. This is not practical as a diagnostic test but has provided much of our knowledge about the pathophysiology of MG. The intercostal muscle is used since small portions can be removed safely and the entire length of muscle fibers can be obtained undamaged. Glass microelectrodes are inserted into the muscle cells near the endplate. Single quanta of ACh are constantly being released spontaneously from the nerve terminals, producing transient depolarizations at the endplate called miniature endplate potentials (mepps). Their amplitude is a measure of the effective amount of ACh in each quantum. In MG, mepp amplitude is reduced.[39] This could result from changes in the amount of ACh per quantum, the amount that reaches the endplate or the sensitivity of the endplate area to ACh. It is difficult to measure accurately the amount of ACh released from the nerves but the sensitivity of the endplate can be assessed by applying known amounts of ACh via a micropipette and measuring the voltage changes thus produced. Using this technique, it has been shown that in MG the post-junctional membrane has a decreased sensitivity to applied ACh.[6] Not all nerve-muscle junctions in a given myasthenic muscle are equally involved, and there is a spectrum of severity among endplates.[116] The severity of clinical weakness depends on the proportion of involved fibers, as well as the severity of involvement of the individual fibers.

The number of quanta released from the nerve terminal after stimulation varies from impulse to impulse, especially during the first few impulses in a train. Thus, the first nerve impulse releases more quanta than the second, and so on, until about the fifth impulse, after which the amount of ACh released per impulse becomes relatively constant (Fig. 6.1). This phenomenon is a characteristic of normal neuromuscular transmission but has no clinical expression in normal muscle since even the latest impulses in a train release more than enough ACh to guarantee a muscle response. When neuromuscular transmission is impaired, only the first few impulses may exceed the action potential threshold with failure of transmission after the later impulses in some muscle fibers. With repetitive stimulation of

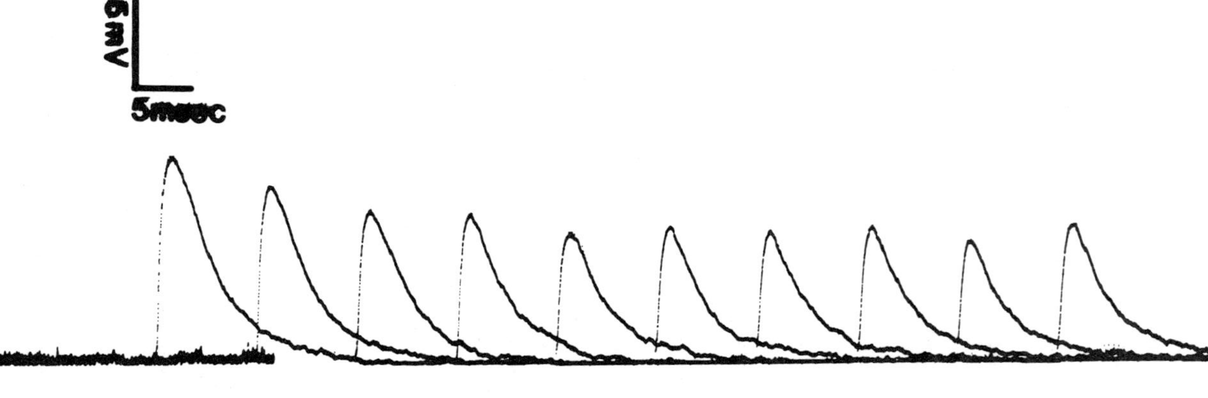

Figure 6.1.   Endplate potentials (epps) recorded with an intracellular electrode from a biopsied intercostal muscle fiber from a patient with MG. The intramuscular nerve was stimulated at 1 Hz. The amplitude decrement is most marked in the fifth response. The variations in amplitude thereafter result from fluctuations in the number of ACh quanta released from the nerve terminal (Reproduced by permission of the publishers, from Stalberg and Sanders.[130])

all the nerve fibers to a muscle, an increasing number of muscle fibers drop out and we see a decrementing muscle response. Progressive reduction or disappearance of visible muscle contraction during faradic stimulation in MG was described by Jolly in 1895.[64] He called this a "myasthenic reaction." The earliest reports of electromyographic abnormalities in MG were those of Lindsley in 1935 who reported variability in the motor unit potential amplitude with consecutive discharges.[76] Harvey and Masland (1941) confirmed these findings and also described a decrementing muscle response with repetitive nerve stimulation.[54,55] The first finding is still one of the major characteristics of conventional electromyography in MG but is not used for quantitative testing. The second observation is the basis of the electrodiagnostic method that is most commonly used in MG.

Repetitive Nerve Stimulation.   The electrical responses of a muscle are recorded while the corresponding nerve is stimulated electrically at a frequency of 1 to 5 Hz. The amplitudes of the muscle responses are measured and the change in amplitude between the first and fourth (or fifth) responses is calculated. The characteristic pattern in MG is a reduction of more than 10% in the amplitude thus measured ("decremental response") (Fig. 6.2). In some cases, stimulation frequencies up to 10 Hz are useful. For example, when no decrement is found with 5 Hz stimulation in children with MG, 10 Hz stimulation may reveal a decrement. The patient is then asked to activate the muscle by contracting it maximally for a brief period. The stimulation is repeated intermittently for several minutes thereafter. This procedure is designed to demonstrate any immediate improvement in the dec-

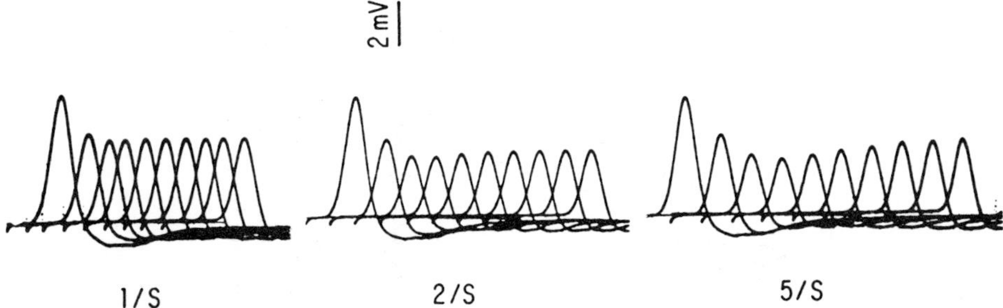

Figure 6.2.   Repetitive stimulation studies in the abductor digiti minimi muscle of a patient with MG. The decrement becomes greater as the stimulation frequency increases. At 2 Hz and 5 Hz stimulation there is a secondary increase in amplitude after the maximum decrement, a phenomenon frequently seen in MG.[97,98]

rement or increase in initial amplitude ("facilitation") to indicate a presynaptic abnormality, such as is found in Lambert-Eaton syndrome,[37,130] but may also be followed at a later time by development or worsening of the decrement ("exhaustion") (Fig. 6.3). A more quantitative method of activation involves tetanic nerve stimulation at 20 to 50 Hz for ten seconds.

In normal muscle the decrement to repetitive nerve stimulation is less than 5% before and after activation, and facilitation is less than 5%. In myasthenic muscle the amplitude of the initial muscle response is normal or slightly reduced, decrement is more than 5% and facilitation is usually seen when the initial amplitude is reduced from normal.

Repetitive stimulation may be performed in many muscles of the arm, leg or face. Hand muscles are usually tested first, since stimulation and recording are convenient and less uncomfortable for the patient. However, the myasthenic abnormality is more often present in proximal muscles, such as the biceps or deltoid.[97,98] A normal test in the hand muscles should always be followed by tests of proximal muscles. In patients with MG, we have found an abnormality in the abductor digiti minimi muscle in 47%, in the biceps in 53% and in the deltoid in 64% of studies (Table 6.1). It may be necessary to study facial muscles in patients with mainly ocular MG in order to demonstrate a decremental response.

Increased muscle temperature can be used to unmask abnormalities since the decrement to repetitive nerve stimulation increases with temperature elevation (Fig. 6.4). The temperature of the hand muscles is usually below 30°C, and should be raised to 35°C before testing. If serial tests are to be compared, they should be performed at

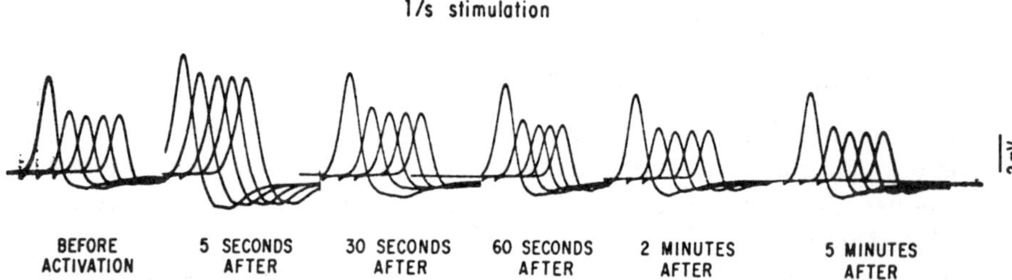

Figure 6.3. Repetitive stimulation studies before and at indicated intervals after maximum voluntary contraction ("activation") in a patient with MG. Five seconds after the end of activation, the amplitude of the initial response is greater and the decrement is less ("facilitation").

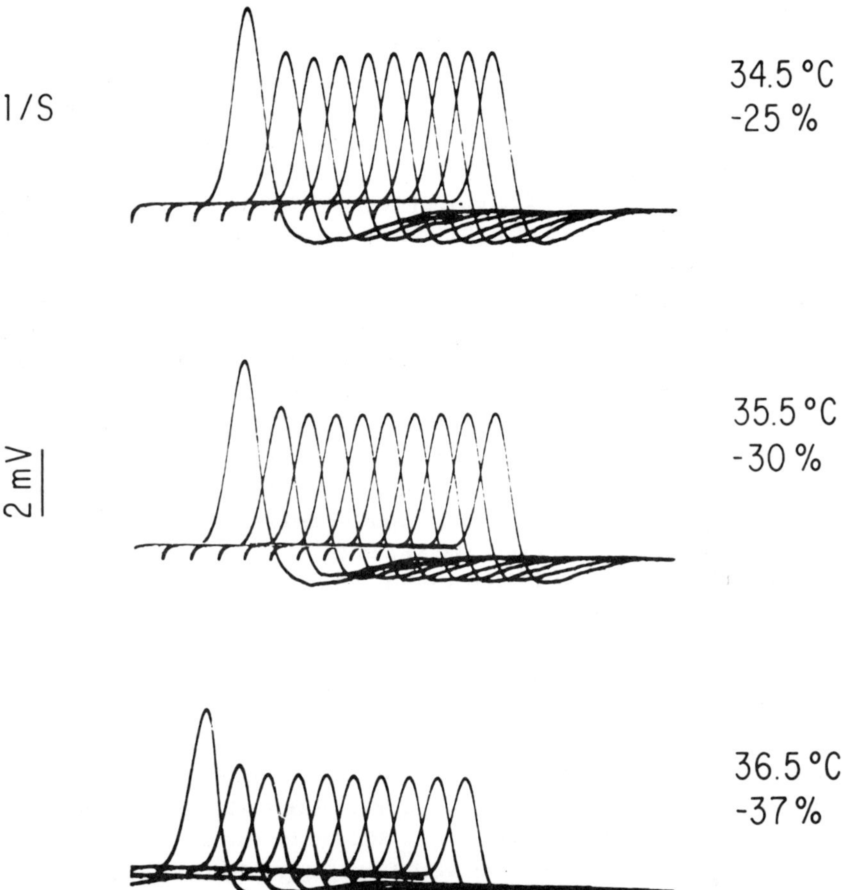

Figure 6.4. The effect of temperature on repetitive stimulation studies in the abductor digiti minimi muscle of a patient with MG. The intramuscular temperature and the percent change of amplitude of the fifth response relative to the first response of each train are noted.

the same intramuscular temperature. Ischemia has also been used by some investigators to bring out an otherwise inapparent decremental response. A blood pressure cuff is placed around the upper arm and inflated above systolic pressure. After three minutes of ischemia, repetitive nerve stimulation is performed. In some laboratories a small dose of curare is injected, usually as a regional curare test, and its effect on neuromuscular transmission is studied. This technique is not without hazard, however, since patients with MG may become significantly weaker when exposed to even very low doses of curare.

Another way of testing neuromuscular transmission is to measure the mechanical twitch during supramaximal nerve stimulation. This is technically more difficult than measuring the electrical responses. It should be noted that mechanical twitch measures the contractile characteristics of the muscle fibers as well as the neuromuscular transmission. With repetitive nerve stimulation the twitch tension typically decreases in MG in a pattern similar to that described for the electrical responses. Facilitation and postactivation exhaustion may also be seen with this technique.

Though these techniques are straightforward and easily performed, they are not without technical pitfalls for the unwary. Since they are the most commonly performed electrodiagnostic tests in MG, they are also the source of many erroneous diagnoses. The most common error results from movement of the recording electrode or the muscle being tested, or from variations in the stimulus applied to the nerve. These problems can usually be recognized if the shape of the muscle electrical response is monitored during the train of stimuli. Variations in the shape of the waveform would indicate the presence of a technical problem. Intramuscular needle electrodes should not be used to record the electrical response since their position within the muscle cannot be kept constant during nerve stimulation. Another potential error results from the use of rates of stimulation greater than 10 Hz.

Needle EMG.   Needle electrode EMG is performed in patients suspected of having MG for two reasons. The first, and most important, is to exclude other diseases that may resemble or occur concomitantly with MG, such as myositis or thyroid myopathy. The second reason is to confirm the diagnosis of MG. When neuromuscular transmission is impaired and there is intermittent impulse blocking to the individual muscle fibers, the motor unit potential (MUP) (which represents the temporal and spatial summation of action potentials from 5 to 15 muscle fibers) may show a variability in shape among consecutive discharges (Fig. 6.5). This explains the variations in MUP amplitude frequently seen in severely involved muscles in MG. The small motor unit potentials that result from neuromuscular block have sometimes been misinterpreted as a sign of myopathy. A superimposed myopathy is actually found occasionally and can be verified by biopsy. Normalizaton of the motor unit potential, after rest or administration of anticholinesterases such as edrophonium, is not seen when the abnormality is due to myopathy but may be seen when it is due solely to a defect in neuromuscular transmission. Differentiation is very difficult when myasthenia and myopathy coexist.

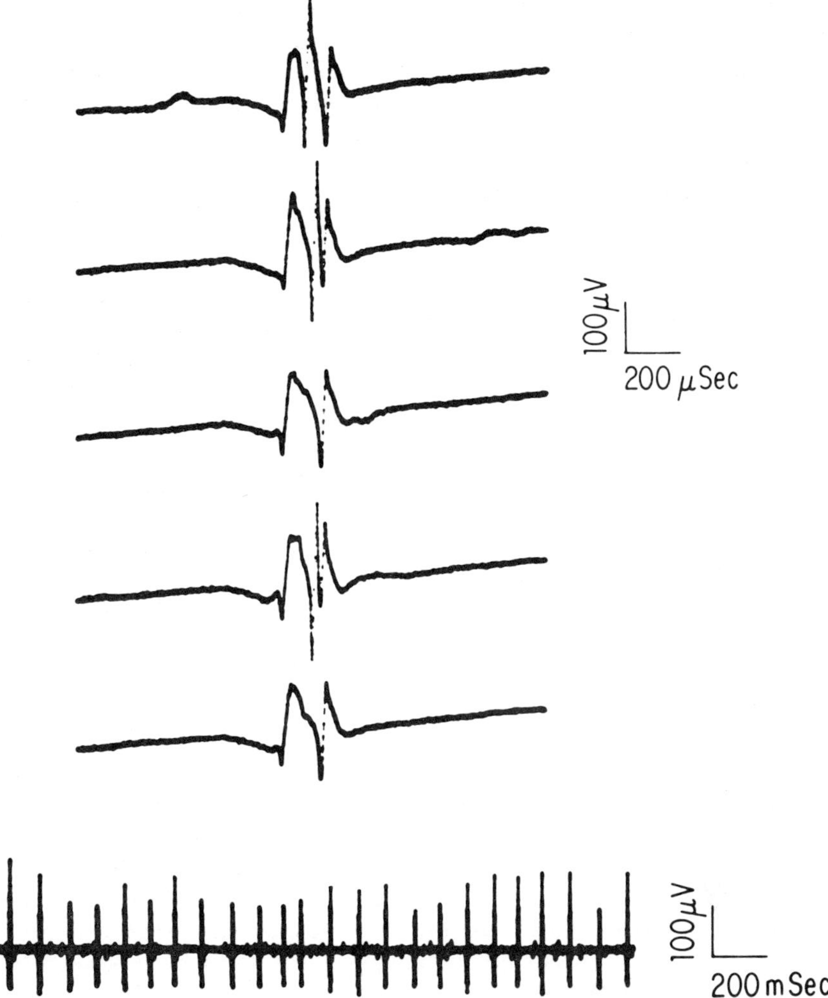

Figure 6.5. Potentials from a single motor unit recorded with a concentric needle electrode in the biceps brachii muscle of a patient with MG during voluntary activation. Fluctuations in the waveform are seen in the top traces. In the bottom trace, recorded at a slower oscilloscope sweep speed, these appear as variations in amplitude.

Single-Fiber EMG. By means of a selective EMG recording technique it is possible to study neuromuscular transmission quantitatively in individual endplates *in situ*. This is the basis of single-fiber EMG (SF-EMG).[131]

When action potentials are recorded from two muscle fibers in the
same motor unit, the time interval between them varies during
consecutive discharges, a phenomenon called neuromuscular jitter
(Fig. 6.6). This jitter is due mainly to variability in synaptic trans-

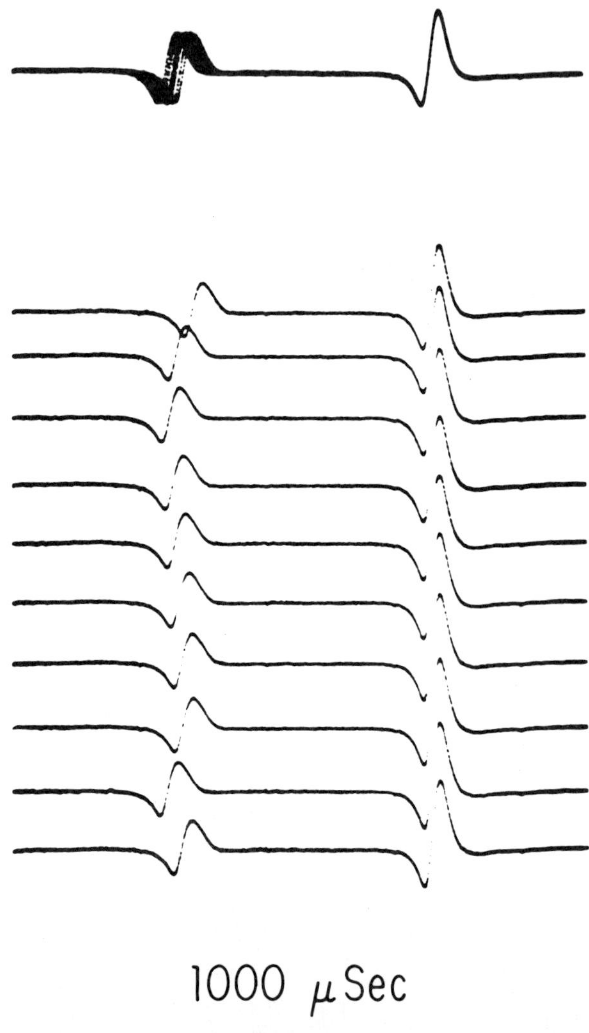

Figure 6.6.   Action potentials from two muscle fibers in the same motor
unit recorded with a single-fiber EMG electrode during voluntary muscle contraction. The potentials are delayed electronically and the oscilloscope is
triggered by the second potential. Ten oscilloscope traces are superimposed at
the top, and are displayed in rastered mode below. The variations in the interval between the two potentials represent the *neuromuscular jitter*.

mission time and is on the order of 10 to 50 microseconds (expressed as the mean value of the consecutive time interval difference—MCD) in normal human muscle. When neuromuscular transmission is disturbed, jitter is increased. With more severe involvement, impulses to individual muscle fibers may intermittently fail to occur (blocking of impulses). Only at this point is there clinical weakness or abnormality on other tests of neuromuscular transmission. With SF-EMG it is possible to detect abnormalities as increased jitter before any impulse blocking occurs.

The typical finding in a patient with MG is that within one muscle some motor endplates have normal jitter, some have increased jitter and others have increased jitter with intermittent blocking (Fig. 6.7). This spectrum of abnormality may be seen even within the muscle fibers of a single motor unit. In order to quantify the findings in a single muscle, a population of endplates must be studied. The results can be expressed as the mean jitter (MCD) of all fiber pairs studied, the percentage of fiber pairs in which blocking is seen and the percentage of pairs with normal jitter (Fig. 6.8).

In 271 patients with MG in whom the extensor digitorum communis muscle (EDC) was tested at the time of initial examination we found an abnormality in this muscle in 231 (85%) (Table 6.1). If, when this muscle was normal, another muscle, more likely to be affected clinically, was examined, an abnormality was found in all but three patients, giving an overall detection rate of 99% for this approach.

In MG the distribution of normal and abnormal endplates varies with the degree of clinical involvement and all three SF-EMG parameters listed above correlate with the clinical severity of disease.[114] In any single patient, weak muscles show more abnormalities than do muscles with normal strength. Even in clinically unaffected muscles jitter is usually abnormal in some fibers. For example, we have

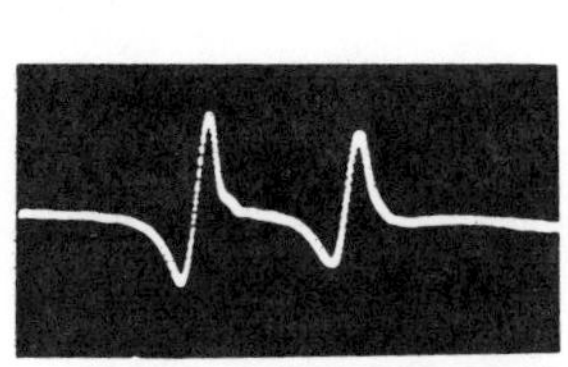
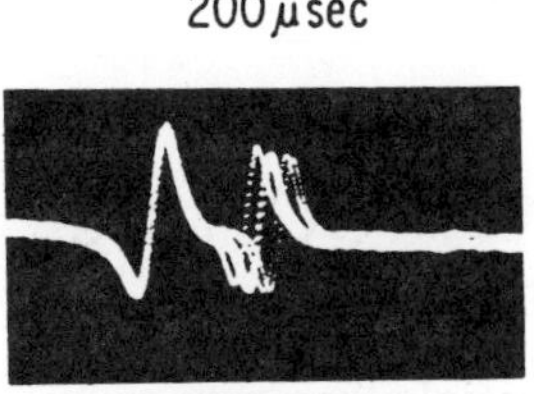
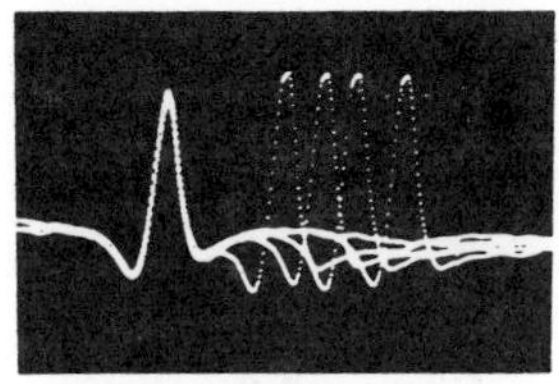

Figure 6.7. Single-fiber EMG recordings from three potential pairs in the extensor digitorum communis muscle of a patient with MG. The degree of abnormality can vary markedly among the endplates within a single muscle.

MEAN= 25.7 SD= 11.6 MIN= 12. MAX= 66.
*** 0- 5- 95 ***   N= 22
10
9
8
7
6
Counts 5
4
3
2
1
10 20 30 40 50 60 70 80 90 100 110 120 130 140 150 160 170   uSec

A.

MEAN= 49.1 SD= 19.4 MIN= 5. MAX=208.
*** 20- 30- 50 ***   N= 20
10
9
8
7
6
Counts 5
4
3
2
1
10 20 30 40 50 60 70 80 90 100 110 120 130 140 150 160 170   uSec

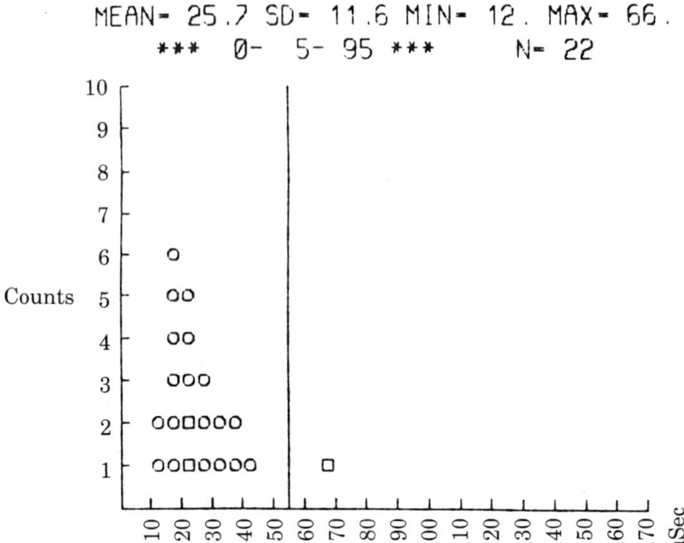

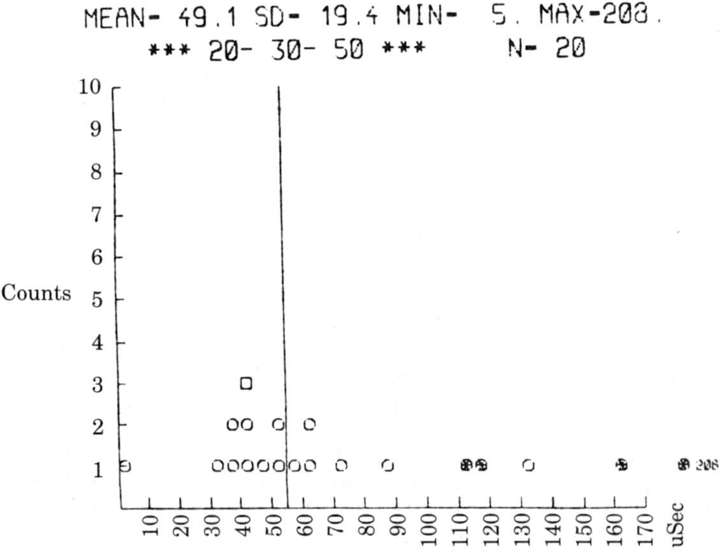

B.

found abnormalities on SF-EMG testing of the EDC in over 50% of patients whose clinical weakness was restricted to the ocular muscles (Table 6.1).

In patients who are not receiving cholinesterase inhibitors, jitter decreases after the administration of edrophonium.[132] The degree of blocking decreases as the jitter decreases toward normal. In patients receiving cholinesterase inhibitors, jitter may increase in some end-plates after injection of edrophonium, indicating a cholinergic overdose in those muscle fibers.[132]

Increased jitter is a sign of disturbed neuromuscular transmission and may be seen in many diseases of the motor unit.[112] When increased jitter is found, other electromyographic tests must be performed to exclude primary diseases of the nerve or muscle.

In our experience the diagnostic sensitivity of these electromyographic tests is not affected by ongoing treatment with cholinesterase inhibitors. Thus it is not necessary to withhold these drugs prior to testing. However, if quantitative comparisons of the physiologic abnormalities are to be made in the same patient over a period of time, the tests should be performed with the same time relationship to the previous drug administration.

Stapedial Reflex Fatigue

The stapedius muscle acts to change the tension on the ear drum and its action can be inferred from measurements of the acoustic impedance of the tympanic membrane. Reflex contraction of this muscle is induced by sound presented to either ear. Thus, stimulation of the stapedial reflex can be used to produce impedance changes that quantitatively reflect the tension of stapedial contraction.

Figure 6.8. Interval histograms of the results of two single-fiber EMG studies in the extensor digitorum communis muscle.[10] Study A is normal. Study B is from a patient with generalized MG. Each symbol represents the jitter (in microseconds) in a pair of potentials. If the jitter exceeds 170 microseconds, the value is printed beside the symbol. Filled symbols indicate blocking. The vertical lines indicate the upper limit of normal jitter for individual potential pairs. The top line of each figure contains the summary statistics for the jitter in all pairs measured. The second line lists the percentage of fiber pairs with blocking, the percentage of fiber pairs with increased jitter (without blocking), the percentage of fiber pairs with normal jitter and the number of fiber pairs measured.

During sustained contraction of the stapedius the acoustic impedance of the tympanic membrane progressively decreases in MG because of fatigue of this muscle.[18] For technical reasons, however, it is
difficult to make reliable measurements of steady impedance changes
for more than several seconds at a time. To overcome this problem,
pulsed sound stimulation has been used to produce rapid changes in
the acoustic impedance.[109] The amplitude of the excursions of these
impedance changes can be measured over prolonged periods. When
neuromuscular transmission is abnormal in the stapedius muscle,
there is a decrementing pattern to these excursions that can be
reversed by administering edrophonium.[109]

Using pulsed sound stimulation an abnormal degree of stapedial
reflex fatigue was demonstrated in 84 of 89 patients with MG.[71] Such
fatigue has also been found in other diseases of the motor unit,
however, and the full range of conditions that can produce this abnormality has yet to be defined.

The technique for measuring stapedial reflex fatigue is painless
and requires only minimal patient cooperation. Since experience
with the technique is still limited, it is necessary to establish local
normal and disease control values before using it in the clinical
diagnosis of neuromuscular disorders.

Oculography and Tonometry

It is frequently difficult to confirm defective neuromuscular transmission in patients with MG when the weakness is limited to the
extraocular muscles. Several techniques have been developed to demonstrate edrophonium responses in these muscles.

Ocular Muscle EMG.   Direct-needle EMG of ocular muscles in MG
may show a reduction in motor unit activity after sustained effort and
increased activity after administration of edrophonium.[22] This procedure is unpleasant and may not be tolerated by all patients. Quantitation of changes in motor unit activity is relatively crude and is
usually subjective. This technique has not been tested in large disease and control populations and has limited clinical applicability.

Tonometry.   Tonometric measurements demonstrate increases in
intraocular pressure after edrophonium administration in patients
with ocular myasthenia. In a study of 22 patients with MG there was
a significant tonometric response to edrophonium in all if cholines-

terase inhibitors were withheld for two days before study.[70] However, similar responses were seen in nonmyasthenic disease controls.[146] In another study of 17 patients with MG, tonometric responses were found in all patients except one whose ocular muscle weakness was fixed.[27]

Oculography. Electronystagmography has been used to measure the amplitude of optokinetic nystagmus (OKN) excursions before and after administration of edrophonium. This procedure demonstrated significant increases in OKN amplitude after edrophonium in 24 of 25 patients with MG reported in four papers,[13,19,85,133] but in only 6 of 12 patients reported in another study. When infrared measurements of OKN deflections were made, an increase after edrophonium was seen in 100% of 40 patients with MG, including 8 without demonstrable ophthalmoparesis.[129]

Lancaster red-green tests of ocular motility can also demonstrate and quantitate the neuromuscular abnormality and the response to edrophonium in MG. In a group of 16 patients with MG, 14 of whom had only ocular muscle weakness, 13 had a positive response to this test.[68]

Tests of ocular muscle function before and after administration of edrophonium may be quite sensitive in detecting the neuromuscular abnormality of MG if local control values are established in normal and non-myasthenic disease populations.

Comparison of Techniques

When several of these diagnostic techniques are available to the clinician, he has the luxury of deciding which are more valuable to him in a specific situation. Usually it suffices to demonstrate that an abnormality exists in any one of these studies in order to confirm the clinical diagnosis. Much more critical is the situation that arises when one or more of the tests does not demonstrate the abnormality.

Repetitive nerve stimulation tests for decrement are most commonly available in the clinical EMG laboratory and offer the advantage of relative simplicity. Studies of the hand muscles are well tolerated by most patients and offer few technical problems. The muscle tested must be warmed to at least 34°C and the decrement must be measured after exhaustion to obtain the maximum diagnostic yield. Even so, we have found that no more than 50% of patients with MG have an abnormality on this test (Table 6.1). Decrement studies in proximal muscles will detect abnormalities in a greater percentage of patients with MG, and in up to 70% of patients with moderate or severe weakness. Studies of proximal muscles are more painful, however, especially if stimulation is performed using surface electrodes, and are more subject to artifactual changes that can hamper interpretation by the non-critical electromyographer. Decrement studies of facial muscles are frequently not tolerated by patients and are also prone to artifactual changes. SF-EMG measurements require fairly elaborate equipment and extensive training and experience as well as patient cooperation. They have a very high diagnostic yield and can be especially valuable in demonstrating defective neuromuscular transmission in patients with the milder forms of MG and with purely ocular disease. If the EDC is tested first, it will demonstrate the abnormality in most patients with MG. If this test is normal, a muscle more likely to be clinically involved should then be examined. In most patients, the frontalis or facial muscles will be abnormal, though occasional patients with predominantly proximal muscle weakness will have more abnormalities in shoulder or thigh muscles. Most patients, including children older than seven, can cooperate well enough for adequate study, although a distal tremor may make recording from the EDC difficult. A more proximal muscle can usually then be studied successfully. Many patients find this test less uncomfortable than repetitive stimulation of the ulnar nerve for decrement studies. Because of its great sensitivity, SF-EMG can demonstrate defective neuromuscular transmission in diseases other than MG, which must be excluded by appropriate measures.

Tests of intraocular tension, ocular movements or stapedial reflex fatigue are painless and require minimal patient cooperation. The diagnostic specificity of these techniques has yet to be conclusively demonstrated. More widespread use of these tests will be necessary before their clinical applicability can be adequately assessed.

Anti-Acetylcholine Receptor Antibodies

Antireceptor antibody (AChR-Ab) titers are elevated in 75% to 90% of patients with MG, demonstrating conclusively the immunologic abnormality in these patients[30,73,80,90] (Table 6.1). The advantages of this test in confirming the diagnosis are clear. However, since antibody measurements are normal in some patients with MG, failure to demonstrate an elevated AChR-Ab titer does not exclude the disease. Elevated AChR-Ab has been seen only rarely in patients without MG.[14,89,90] Thus, although a negative test does not exclude the disease, a positive test is virtually diagnostic. At the present time, these determinations are not universally available, and they should be regarded as complementing the physiologic tests described.

The Pathophysiology of Myasthenia Gravis

The physiologic abnormality in acquired MG results from a reduction in the effective concentration of acetylcholine receptors (AChR) on the muscle endplate.[6,42,46] The overwhelming weight of current evidence indicates that this results from an immunologic attack directed against the AChR (Fig. 6.9). This was actually postulated over 20 years ago by Simpson, based on clinical observations.[122] The concept has been substantiated by observations made in the inter-

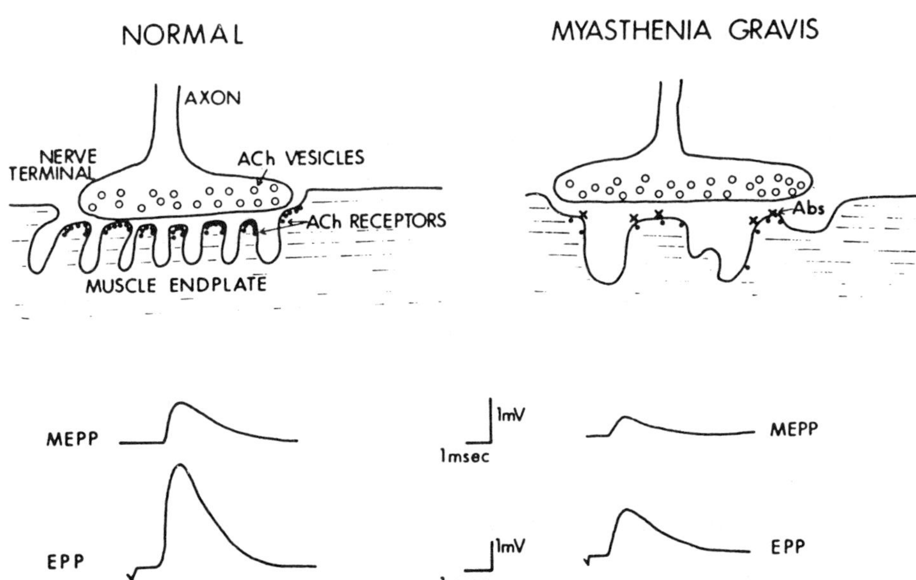

Figure 6.9. The pathophysiology of MG. The postsynaptic muscle endplate membrane is distorted and simplified, the concentration of ACh receptors is decreased and antibodies (Abs) are attached to the endplate. As a result of these changes, the amplitudes of miniature endplate potentials (mepps) and endplate potentials (epps) are reduced.

vening years. The following summarize the clinical evidence that an immunological abnormality is present in patients with MG:

1.　MG is frequently associated with other diseases that have a presumed or known immunological etiology.[122] The age and sex distribution of MG is similar to that of autoimmune diseases such as systemic lupus erythematosus.[122]

2.　Neonatal passage of a transient form of disease is seen in autoimmune diseases, as in MG.[120] The time course of this neonatal form of myasthenia correlates with the period during which maternal antibodies persist in the neonatal serum.[20]

3.　Most diseases that have been linked to a particular HLA tissue histocompatibility locus have a definite or suspected autoimmune pathogenesis. The HLA-B8 tissue haplotype is more common in patients with MG than in the general population.[47,48,102,103] This tissue marker has been associated with other autoimmune diseases.

4.　A number of diseases with an autoimmune etiology, occur in patients who receive D-penicillamine. The most common is a form of myasthenia gravis (See page 282).

Non-specific Immunologic Abnormalities in MG

A number of non-specific immunologic abnormalities have been described in MG:

1.　Serum antimuscle antibodies are found in 30% of patients with MG.[134] Fluorescent antibody staining localized to the A-band of muscle is virtually specific for the presence of a thymoma, though I-band staining is also seen in other diseases.[140]

2.　Many myasthenic patients have abnormal antibodies against thyroid and gastric parietal cells.[123] An antinuclear factor is also commonly present.[124]

3.　Serum complement activity is decreased with exacerbations or increased with remissions of the disease in some patients with MG.[93]

4.　Serum IgA levels may be low in some patients, especially when a thymoma is present.[127] These levels tend to increase slowly after thymectomy.[21]

5.　The histology of the thymus gland in MG resembles that of the thyroid in Hashimoto's disease.[28,128] The "germinal centers" that characterize the thymic histology in MG suggest lymphocytic activity.[122]

6.　"Lymphorrhages" (small collections of lymphocytes), frequently seen on muscle biopsy in MG, suggest an inflammatory or immunologic process.[122]

Specific Immunologic Abnormalities in MG

More recently, a number of observations have provided evidence for a specific immunologic abnormality in MG:

1. Treatment with ACTH, corticosteroids or other immunosuppressive drugs can produce marked improvement in up to 90% of patients.[60,115]

2. Myasthenic weakness improves following removal of lymph by thoracic duct drainage and recurs following re-infusion of a high molecular weight protein fraction from the lymph, probably IgG.[17,83] Plasma exchange, which removes noncellular blood components including circulating auto-antibodies, can produce a temporary improvement in most patients.[33,62]

3. Serum antibodies directed against the human AChR are found in 75% to 93% of patients with MG[30,73,80] and in neonates born to myasthenic mothers (See pages 280–281).

4. A globulin fraction in myasthenic serum blocks the binding of α-bungarotoxin to the AChR.[8]

5. Myasthenic serum or globulin produces a defect of neuromuscular transmission when injected into immunologically tolerant mice[137,138] or rats.[57] Myasthenic serum applied to myasthenic muscle *in vitro* produces reversible worsening of neuromuscular blockade.[116]

6. IgG and complement components are attached to the postsynaptic myasthenic endplate membrane and their concentration correlates with the degree of reduction in AChR content and the amplitude of miniature endplate potentials (mepps).[42]

7. Lymphocytes from many patients with MG are sensitized to AChR from eels and rays.[1,104]

The Thymus in Myasthenia Gravis

An association between the thymus and MG has been known since Weigert described a thymoma in a patient with MG in 1901[144] and Bell reported a high incidence of thymic hyperplasia in the disease in 1917.[15]

The thymus is necessary in early life for the development of the normal mechanisms of cellular immunity. Lymphocytes produced by the thymus (T-cells) migrate to other sites in the body and are thought to be the precursors of immunologically competent cells.[86] T-cells may persist in the periphery for many years. In addition to their role in cellular immunity, T-cells interact with lymphocytes produced in the bone marrow (B-cells) in the formation of circulating antibodies.[87] The role of the thymus in adult life is not known and the organ usually involutes and disappears with age.

Thymic abnormalities occur in about 80% of patients with MG. Ten to fifteen percent have true neoplasms of the thymus and the remainder have lymphoid hyperplasia of the medullary regions in the form of germinal center proliferation.[141] Thymomatous changes are seen most frequently in older patients. This has led to the speculation that these tumors develop as a result of chronic overactivity of the gland. This could not be the case in all patients, however, since the clinical manifestations of the myasthenia may develop years after removal of a thymoma.[69,106] The most compelling evidence against this hypothesis, though, is provided by the observation that MG with thymic hyperplasia is associated with the HLA-B8 histocompatibility locus while MG with thymoma is not.[110]

Improvement of MG following thymectomy was first reported by Schumacher and Roth in 1913[119] and has subsequently been described in many papers.[59] In many patients, improvement occurs only after a delay of two or more years. This observation has led to the hypothesis that MG is associated with abnormal clones of immuno-competent lymphocytes proliferating in the thymus. The delayed effect of thymectomy has been attributed to the long life-span of the peripherally distributed T-cells. In some patients, however, improvement can be seen very soon after thymectomy, implying that the same mechanism may not be operating in all patients.

Lymphocytes within the thymus as well as in peripheral blood have been shown to be sensitized to muscle tissue in patients with MG. Circulating antimuscle antibodies in MG cross-react with myoid cells in the thymus.[139] Also, cellular and humoral cross-reactivity between AChR and calf thymus has been demonstrated,[3] raising the possibility that both thymus and the neuromuscular junction are targets of an immunologic attack stimulated by an antigen common to both tissues.

An interesting relationship between muscle and the thymus observed in tissue culture may be relevant to this immunologic cross-reactivity. Skeletal muscle cells or myotubes containing AChR are found in cultures of thymic reticulum cells from normal rats or mice[145] and from patients with MG.[65] These muscle cells are thought to develop from primitive stem cells that are induced to differentiate *in vitro*. Hypothetically, differentiation could be induced to a less complete degree *in vivo*, producing cells with antigenically active AChR. Immunocompetent cells in the thymus could recognize this receptor as "non-self" and begin the reaction that results in MG.[145] The improvement in MG that follows thymectomy could thus result from the removal of a source of antigenic stimulation.

It has also been suggested that the post-thymectomy improvement in MG could result from a general, non-specific reduction in immunologic responsiveness.[3,88] However, Scadding et al[117] found no such reduction in non-specific immunologic function in myasthenics after thymectomy. It has also been hypothesized that the thymus produces a factor that blocks neuromuscular transmission directly[49,50] or that facilitates the immunologic reaction at the endplate.[95] Further knowledge about the function of the normal thymus is required before its peculiar relationship with MG can be explained.

Experimental Autoimmune Myasthenia Gravis

In 1971, Lennon and Carnegie speculated that MG could result from a break in immunological tolerance to the AChR.[74] Support for this concept was provided by Patrick and Lindstrom in 1973, who observed myasthenic weakness in rabbits immunized with AChR from the electric organ of the eel *Electrophorus*.[99] Since then an animal model of MG, called experimental autoimmune myasthenia gravis (EAMG), has been produced in many species and has been shown to be similar to MG in all essential characteristics. Much of our understanding of the mechanisms by which an autoimmune response to AChR can produce abnormal neuromuscular transmission has come from studies of EAMG in rats.

Following immunization with purified AChR from the electric eel (*Electrophorus*) or ray (*Torpedo*), rats develop an acute and transient period of weakness, during which there is a cellular inflammatory reaction at the neuromuscular junction.[44,45] The physiologic findings at this stage have characterisitics of denervation.[45] There is no well-recognized analogue to this stage of EAMG in the human disease, though rarely patients with MG will develop an acute transient period of worsening during which denervation changes are seen (D.B. Sanders and J.F. Howard, unpublished observations). Macrophagic invasion of the endplate as seen in the acute phase of EAMG has been described in one patient with MG who also had a thymoma.[43]

The chronic stage of EAMG in rats begins about 30 days after immunization and more closely resembles MG physiologically and by ultrastructural examination of the endplate.[44,45] In both conditions, the endplate membrane is simplified; with fewer α-bungarotoxin binding sites,[42,44,45] mepp amplitude is reduced[44] and less AChR can be extracted from muscle.[77-79]

Antibodies to AChR are found in the serum of rats with EAMG within several days after immunization and increase in concentration until after the acute phase has begun to resolve.[77,78] During the chronic phase of EAMG in rats, antibodies and complement component C3 are attached to the endplate.[111] Fragmentation of the terminal folds of the endplate to which IgG and C3 are attached implies that lysis of the endplate is mediated by complement.

The acute phase of EAMG can be reproduced in normal rats by injection of immunoglobulin from rats with chronic EAMG.[77] This passive transfer can be prevented by depletion of the C3 in the recipient animals by cobra venom factor.[75]

Further similarities between EAMG and MG have been demonstrated by the production of a neonatal form of EAMG.[113] Whereas human neonatal MG is transferred by the passage of antibodies *in utero*, in the rat model antibodies are transferred in the milk after birth.

The Role of the Antireceptor Antibody in Pathogenesis of MG

Antibodies directed against the acetylcholine receptor are found in the serum in the majority of patients with MG and are also attached to the postsynaptic muscle endplate membrane. It is intuitively attractive to assume that they play a significant role in the pathogenesis of the physiologic abnormality in MG. Several observations provide substantiation for this concept:

1. Removal of circulating factors, including antibodies, by thoracic duct drainage or plasma exchange can produce marked and relatively rapid improvement in many patients with MG.[18] Reinfusion of high molecular weight lymph components, probably IgG, can produce reversal of this improvement within 30 minutes.[83]

2. Passive transfer of the neuromuscular block of MG can be accomplished by injecting recipient animals with myasthenic IgG[137,138] or serum[57] or by bathing myasthenic muscle in myasthenic serum.[116] Nature provides us with an example of passive transfer in the form of neonatal MG, which occurs in ten to fifteen percent of infants born to myasthenic mothers.[92] Antibodies to AChR are found in the serum of neonates of myasthenic mothers in titers that correlate with the maternal levels.[66,73,94] Symptoms of weakness seem more likely to occur in neonates whose mothers have the

highest titers of AChR.[66,67,94] The AChR antibodies disappear from the neonatal serum with a half-life of two to three weeks,[94] reaching normal levels before five months.[66,67,73,91] This time course is consistent with the known rate of clearance of maternal antibodies from the neonatal circulation[20] and with the duration of clinical weakness in the neonates.[136] It should be emphasized that few infants develop clinical weakness though all receive antibodies at the maternal level. Conversely, neonates who receive maternal AChR antibodies may develop clinical weakness even when the mother is without myasthenic symptoms.[38] Thus, though passage of maternal antibodies to the neonate may be necessary for the production of neonatal myasthenia, it does not appear to be sufficient. It is possible that the antibodies measured in the serum are not the ones responsible for producing the neuromuscular abnormality or that the serum titer does not accurately reflect the concentration of antibody at the endplate. It has recently been reported that α-fetoprotein inhibits antibody binding *in vitro* and thus may protect neonates from the effects of the maternal AChR to a certain degree.[2,23]

3. Anti-acetylcholine receptor antibodies (AChR-Ab) can increase the degradation of surface AChR in rat myotubes in tissue culture and in isolated rat diaphragm.[11,16] The effect of antibodies from myasthenic patients in accelerating the degradation of AChR is attributed to their ability to cross-link the receptors.[36]

4. In most patients treated with corticosteroids or other immunosuppressive drugs, antibody titers decrease and clinical improvement occurs. In individual patients the antibody titer usually changes little if the disease severity remains constant. In these individual patients there is thus a correlation between the AChR-Ab titers and the clinical state.[73,121] In a series of 32 patients, most of whom were treated with steroids, Seybold and Lindstrom[121] found a relationship between the clinical improvement and the degree to which the AChR-Ab titer could be suppressed by therapy. The rapid and sustained decreases in AChR-Ab seen with clinical improvement after beginning prednisone implies that steroids may work, at least in part, by decreasing the synthesis of antibody. Other possible mechanisms of action include a direct effect to increase net AChR synthesis, an increase in immune tolerance to AChR or some protective effect against AChR-Ab or other immunologic insult.[40]

In patients treated with thymectomy alone, the changes in antibody titer are much less consistent.[105,107,121,136,143] A correlation between post-thymectomy clinical improvement and the reduction in antibody titer after surgery has been reported.[90,107] In other reports, however, improvement following thymectomy was seen before there was any reduction in AChR-Ab.[105] The reduction in antibody titer after thymectomy is rarely as marked as that seen following treatment with steroids or plasma exchange,[121] although the clinical improvement may be as great.

The relationship between antibody titer and disease severity in MG is not clear (Table 6.1). This discrepancy between the serum antibody titer and clinical severity makes it difficult to understand the role of the antibody in producing the disease. There are a number of possible explanations. The most likely is that the antibody responsible for the neuromuscular abnormality is not necessarily the one measured in the serum. It is also possible that the amount of antibody attached to the endplate is not necessarily reflected by the serum titer. This could be analogous to the situation in autoimmune thrombocytopenia, where serum antibody titers do not reflect the amount of immune complexes bound to the target organ.[29] Alternatively, the AChR-Ab may be produced as a result of the damage to the neuromuscular junction, rather than causing it. Some evidence for this was provided by observations made by Lefvert et al[73] that three patients with MG of short duration had no IgG AChR-Ab on initial testing, but developed them later. Two of these patients had IgM AChR-Ab initially which disappeared when the IgG antibodies appeared. This sequence can be interpreted as demonstrating that the synthesis of AChR-Ab was stimulated by damage to the endplate and that antibodies were not the primary cause of the physiologic abnormality.

In some patients with MG, circulating factors can significantly affect neuromuscular transmission. Evidence for this is provided by the rapid improvement in strength that may be seen following thoracic duct drainage or plasma exchange which is reversed within 30 minutes after re-infusion of cell-free lymph and by the rapidly reversible worsening of neuromuscular block that can be produced *in vitro* by applying myasthenic serum to myasthenic muscle.

Penicillamine-Induced Myasthenia Gravis

D-penicillamine is used in the treatment of rheumatoid arthritis, Wilson's disease and cystinuria. A number of diseases with an autoimmune etiology have occurred in patients receiving D-penicillamine, including systemic lupus erythematosus,[9] pemphigus,[56] immune complex nephritis,[35] polymyositis,[31,101,118] and, most frequently, myasthenia gravis.[12,24,25,32]

The myasthenia induced by D-penicillamine is usually relatively mild and may be restricted to the ocular muscles. In many patients the symptoms are not recognized and the mild weakness of the extremities may be difficult to demonstrate in the presence of severe arthritis. The diagnosis can be confirmed by the response to cholinesterase inhibitors, the characteristic electromyographic abnormalities and the presence of AChR-Ab.[82,108,142] The presence of these antibodies is not absolutely specific for MG, however, since they have been seen in a few patients receiving D-penicillamine who have had no clinical evidence of MG.[14]

When clinical MG is present in these patients, electromyographic studies reveal abnormalities of neuromuscular transmission, especially on single-fiber EMG measurements of jitter. In the author's experience, repetitive stimulation studies are abnormal less often, reflecting the relatively mild degree of neuromuscular abnormality present in most of these patients. Intercostal muscle biopsy studies have shown reduced miniature endplate potential amplitude as seen in acquired MG.[142]

It is not unusual for MG and rheumatoid arthritis to occur together.[122] However, when myasthenia begins while the patient is receiving D-penicillamine, it will remit in 70% of patients within a year after the drug is discontinued.[5] As the myasthenia improves, the AChR-Ab titer falls,[5,108,142] and the electromyographic abnormalities improve[5] or disappear altogether (D.B. Sanders, unpublished observation). If the neuromuscular abnormalities do not improve after the drug is discontinued, one must then entertain the possibility that the two diseases occurred coincidentally.

In patients with rheumatoid arthritis who are receiving D-penicillamine and who have no clinical evidence of MG, single-fiber EMG measurements of jitter have failed to demonstrate abnormalities of neuromuscular transmission that can be attributed to the D-penicillamine.[4] Attempts have been made to produce neuromuscular blockade in animals by administering D-penicillamine *in vivo* and *in vitro*. In normal rats, no significant effects were seen with levels of D-penicillamine equivalent to the human therapeutic dose.[7] In guinea pigs, chronic administration of doses more than ten times the therapeutic level produced a mild degree of neuromuscular blockade, which was probably too little to produce any clinical manifestations.[26] There is thus little reason to infer from these studies that D-penicillamine produces a direct, clinically significant effect on neuromuscular transmission. Other evidence against this is the long time period between beginning D-penicillamine administration and the onset of MG in most patients, and the relatively low incidence of MG in patients receiving D-penicillamine for Wilson's disease compared to those receiving it for rheumatoid arthritis.[32,34,82]

It is thus probable that D-penicillamine induces MG by stimulating or enhancing an immunologic reaction against the neuromuscular junction. Further definition of the way in which this occurs could increase our knowledge of the immunogenesis of acquired MG and other autoimmune diseases.

The Treatment of Acquired Myasthenia Gravis

The therapy of MG must be determined for the individual patient based on that patient's prognosis and potential response to various forms of treatment. There is considerable disagreement in the literature about the value and disadvantages of all therapeutic approaches. It will not be the purpose of this presentation to resolve these issues but to present the options available to the clinician.

Cholinesterase inhibitors can provide symptomatic improvement for variable periods of time in most patients with MG. Details of use are available in standard references[58] (see appendix). Pyridostigmine (Mestinon) works well for most patients, though occasionally patients will tolerate or respond better to neostigmine (Prostigmin) or ambenonium (Mytelase). In relatively few patients will these agents produce complete symptomatic relief. Usually they become less effective as the disease progresses. The dose and frequency of administration must be determined for each patient and must be reassessed frequently. The patient and the physician must be familiar with the side effects and signs of overdose of these drugs. There is some experimental evidence that chronic administration of cholinesterase inhibitors can damage the neuromuscular junction and thus actually worsen the clinical weakness.[41,63,100] However, clinical observations have not demonstrated that the use of these drugs adversely affects the course of disease[52] or response to corticosteroid therapy.[115]

Thymectomy is followed by clinical improvement in the majority of patients so treated, though the improvement may not be seen for many months or years in some cases.[59] There is probably little reason to consider thymectomy in purely ocular MG or when the disease has reached the "burnt-out" stage. Most reports indicate that thymectomy is most effective when performed early in the illness. It is not possible to predict accurately the response to this surgery in the individual patient and there is still a question as to whether it alters the natural history of the disease. When a thymoma is present it should be removed, regardless of the distribution or duration of MG.

Corticosteroid treatment can produce marked improvement in most patients with acquired MG.[60] The most consistent responses will be seen when high daily doses of prednisone are given until improvement occurs.[115] A temporary initial worsening occurs within three weeks after beginning such treatment in ⅓ to ½ of patients. The side-effects of chronic steroid administration accompany this form of therapy but can be reduced by using alternate-day doses after improvement has become established and by reducing the dose to the minimal level necessary to maintain improvement. Care must be taken in reducing the dose of prednisone, slow tapering of the dose over many months being necessary to avoid recurrence of weakness. Although most patients retain their improvement after prednisone is reduced to relatively modest doses, most will require chronic administration of the drug. In patients with mild or ocular disease, some clinicians prefer to begin treatment with low doses of prednisone on alternate days, gradually increasing the dose until improvement is seen.

Antimetabolites have been used in MG with some success in Europe, but the experience in the U.S. is limited.[61,84] The most extensive experience has been with azathioprine, given in low doses (150 to 200 mg/day). Improvement has been reported in most patients after 2 to 12 months, with maximal responses several months later. With close monitoring, side-effects have been mild and can usually be reversed by temporarily discontinuing the drug.

Plasma exchange (or plasmapheresis) therapy involves the removal of circulating non-cellular blood constituents and their replacement with balanced saline solutions. Almost all patients will improve temporarily following an adequate course of plasma exchange, even when other forms of therapy have failed.[62] Thus, plasma exchange can be used to great advantage when the patient requires relatively rapid improvement, e.g., before thymectomy or to avoid respiratory assistance during a crisis. Its use in other situations is limited by expense and complexity and by the temporary nature of the improvement that occurs in most patients.

The following is a synthesis of the considerations listed above:

After the diagnosis of MG is confirmed, patients with generalized disease are candidates for thymectomy. In those patients who have persistent generalized weakness despite optimal doses of cholinesterase inhibitors, some physicians would recommend treatment with prednisone or plasma exchange to produce improvement before thymectomy. Another approach is to proceed to thymectomy and use corticosteroids thereafter if there is persistent postoperative weakness. Disabling ocular muscle weakness may also be treated with prednisone. If corticosteroids are contraindicated in a given patient, azathioprine can be used instead, though improvement may not be seen for several months after beginning treatment with this drug. When side effects preclude chronic prednisone administration, azathioprine may be added and prednisone withdrawn after several months. *Note:* There is no definite relationship between antireceptor antibody titer and the prognosis or response to treatment. This assay should not be used to determine therapy nor to assess the clinical response to treatment.

Summary

Acquired myasthenia gravis results from an immunologic attack on the neuromuscular junction. The initial event probably involves a break in immunologic tolerance to the muscle endplate acetylcholine receptor, with subsequent production of humoral antibodies and complement-mediated lysis of the endplate. Degradation of the endplate receptor is increased by the attachment of antibodies, which results in a reduced concentration of receptor. Lysis and a possible cellular attack partially destroy the endplate, leaving it distorted and simplified. At the abnormal endplate, antibodies attached to the receptor further impair neuromuscular transmission by blocking access of acetylcholine.

The mechanism by which immunologic tolerance is broken is not known. There may be several mechanisms operating under different conditions, explaining the different clinical presentations and courses seen in this disease. The special relationship of the thymus to MG has yet to be specifically defined, but this gland may contribute to the induction and maintenance of the immunologic reaction against the neuromuscular junction.

References

1. Abramsky O, Aharonov A, Teitelbaum D, Fuchs S: Myasthenia gravis and acetylcholine receptor. Effects of steroids in clinical course and cellular immune response to acetylcholine receptor. *Arch Neurol* 32: 684–687, 1975.

2. Abramsky O, Brenner T, Lisak RP, et al: Significance in neonatal myasthenia gravis of inhibitory effect of amniotic fluid of binding of antibodies to acetylcholine receptor. *Lancet* 2:1333–1335, 1979.
3. Aharonov A, Tarrab-Hazdai R, Abramsky O, Fuchs S: Immunological relationship between acetylcholine receptor and thymus: A possible significance in myasthenia gravis. *Proc Nat Acad Sci USA* 72:1456–1459, 1975.
4. Albers JW, Belas CA, Levine SP: Neuromuscular transmission in rheumatoid arthritis, with and without penicillamine. *Neurology* 31:1562–1564, 1981.
5. Albers JW, Hodach RJ, Kimmel DW, Treacy WL: Penicillamine-associated myasthenia gravis. *Neurology* 30:1246–1250, 1980.
6. Albuquerque EX, Rash JE, Mayer RF, Satterfield JR: An electrophysiological and morphological study of the neuromuscular junctions in patients with myasthenia gravis. *Exp Neurol* 51:1–26, 1976.
7. Aldrich MS, Kim YI, Sanders DB: Effects of D-penicillamine on neuromuscular transmission in rats. *Muscle and Nerve* 2:180–185, 1979.
8. Almon RR, Andrew CG, Appel SH: Serum globulin in myasthenia gravis: Inhibition of α-bungarotoxin binding to acetylcholine receptors. *Science* 186:55–57, 1974.
9. Ansell BM: Other case reports and discussion of adverse reactions to penicillamine. *Postgrad Med J* 50:78–80, 1974.
10. Antoni L, Stalberg E, Sanders DB: Automated analysis of neuromuscular jitter. *Comput Programs Med*, in press.
11. Appel SH, Anwyl R, McAdams MW, Elias S: Accelerated degradation of acetylcholine receptor from cultured rat myotubes with myasthenia gravis sera and globulins. *Proc Nat Acad Sci USA* 74:2130–2134, 1977.
12. Bálint G, Szobor A, Temesvári P, et al: Myasthenia gravis developed under D-penicillamine treatment. *Scand J Rheumatol* 21–12, 1975. (abstract)
13. Baloh RW, Keesey JC: Saccade fatigue and response to edrophonium for the diagnosis of myasthenia gravis. *Ann N Y Acad Sci* 274:631–641, 1976.
14. Barada FA, Sanders DB: Unpublished observations.
15. Bell ET: Tumors of the thymus in myasthenia gravis. *Journal of Nervous and Mental Diseases* 45:130, 1917.
16. Beran S, Kullberg RW, Heinemann SF: Human myasthenic sera reduce AChR sensitivity of human muscle cells in tissue culture. *Nature* 267:263–265, 1977.
17. Bergstrom K, Frankson C, Matell G, von Reis G: The effect of thoracic duct lymph drainage in myasthenia gravis. *Eur Neurol* 9:157–167, 1973.
18. Blom S, Zakrisson JE: The stapedius reflex in the diagnosis of myasthenia gravis. *J Neurol Sci* 21:71–76, 1974.
19. Blomberg LH, Persson T: A new test for myasthenia gravis. *Acta Neurol Scand Suppl* 13:363–364, 1965.
20. Brambell FWR: The transmission of passive immunity from mother to young. In Neuberger A, Tatum EL (eds): *Frontiers of Biology*. New York, Elsevier, 1970, pp 80–141, 271.

21. Bramis J, Sloane C, Papatestas AE, et al: Serum IgA in myasthenia gravis. *Lancet* 1:1243–1244, 1976.
22. Breinin GM: Electromyography—a tool in ocular and neurological diagnosis. I. Myasthenia Gravis. *Arch Ophthalmol* 57:161–175, 1957.
23. Brenner T, Abramsky O: Suppression of clinical and experimental myasthenia gravis by alpha-fetoprotein. *Neurology* 30:380–381, 1980.
24. Bucknall RC: Myasthenia associated with D-penicillamine therapy in rheumatoid arthritis. *Pro R Soc Med* 70:114–117, 1977.
25. Bucknall RC, Dixon ASJ, Glick EN, et al: Myasthenia gravis associated with penicillamine treatment for rheumatoid arthritis. *Br Med J* 1:600–602, 1975.
26. Burres SA, Richman DP, Crayton JW, Arnason BGW: Penicillamine-induced myasthenic responses in the guinea pig. *Muscle and Nerve* 2:186–190, 1979.
27. Campbell MJ, Simpson E, Crombie AL, et al: Ocular myasthenia: Evaluation of Tensilon tonography and electronystagmography as diagnostic tests. *J Neurol Neurosurg Psychiatry* 33:639–646, 1970.
28. Castleman B: Tumors of the thymus gland. In *Atlas of Tumor Pathology*. Washington, Armed Forces Institute of Pathology, pp 7–62, 1955.
29. Cines DB, Schreiber AD: Immune thrombocytopenia. *N Engl J Med* 300:106–111, 1979.
30. Compston DAS, Vincent A, Newsom-Davis J, Batchelor JR: Clinical, pathological, HLA antigen and immunological evidence for disease heterogeneity in myasthenia gravis. *Brain* 103:579–601, 1980.
31. Cucher BG, Goldman AL; D-penicillamine-induced polymyositis in rheumatoid arthritis. *Ann Intern Med* 85:615–616, 1976.
32. Czlonskowska A: Myasthenia syndrome during penicillamine treatment. *Br Med J* 2:726–727, 1975.
33. Dau PC (ed): *Plasmapheresis and the Immunobiology of Myasthenia Gravis*. Boston, Houghton Mifflin, 1979.
34. Dawkins RL, Zilko PJ, Owen ET: Penicillamine therapy, antistriational antibody, and myasthenia gravis. *Br Med J* 2:759–760, 1975.
35. Dische FE, Swinson DR, Hamilton EBD, Parsons V: Immunopathology of penicillamine-induced glomerular disease. *J. Rheumatol* 3:145–154, 1976.
36. Drachman DB, Angus CW, Adams RN, et al: Myasthenic antibodies cross-link acetylcholine receptors to accelerate degradation. *N Engl J Med* 298:1116–1122, 1978.
37. Eaton LM, Lambert EH: Electromyography and electric stimulation of nerves in diseases of motor unit: observations on the myasthenic syndrome associated with malignant tumors. *JAMA* 163:1117–1124, 1957.
38. Elias SB, Butler I, Appel SH: Neonatal myasthenia gravis in the infant of a myasthenic mother in remission. *Ann Neurol* 6:72–75, 1979.
39. Elmqvist D, Hofmann WW, Kugelberg J, et al: An electrophysiological investigation of neuromuscular transmission in myasthenia gravis. *J Physiol* (London) 174:417–434, 1964.
40. Engel AG: Myasthenia gravis. In Vinken PJ, Bruyn GW, Ringel S (eds): *Handbook of Clinical Neurology,* Vol. 41. New York, North-Holland Publishing Co., 1979, pp 95–145.

41. Engel AG, Lambert EH, Santa T: Study of anticholinesterase therapy effects on neuro-muscular transmission and on motor end plate fine structure. *Neurology* 23:1273–1281, 1973.
42. Engel AG, Lindstrom JM, Lambert EH, Lennon VA: Ultrastructural localization of the acetylcholine receptor in myasthenia gravis and its experimental autoimmune model. *Neurology* 27:307–315, 1977.
43. Engel AG, Sakakibara H, Sahashi K, et al: Passively transferred experimental autoimmune myasthenia gravis. Sequential and quantitative study of the end-plate localization of immune complexes (IgG and C3) and of the acetylcholine receptor. *Neurology* 29:179–188, 1979.
44. Engel AG, Tsujihata M, Lambert EH, et al: Experimental autoimmune myasthenia gravis: A sequential and quantitative study of the neuromuscular junction ultrastructure and electrophysiologic correlation. *J Neuropathol Exp Neurol* 35:569–587, 1976.
45. Engel AG, Tsujihata M, Lindstrom J, Lennon VA: The motor end plate in myasthenia gravis and in experimental autoimmune myasthenia gravis. *Ann NY Acad Sci* 274:60–79, 1976.
46. Fambrough DM, Drachman DB and Satyamurti S: Neuromuscular junction in myasthenia gravis: Decreased acetylcholine receptors. *Science* 182:293–295, 1973.
47. Feltkamp TEW, van den Berg-Loonen PM, Nijenhuis LE, et al: Myasthenia gravis, autoantibodies and HL-A antigens. *Br Med J* 1:131–133, 1974.
48. Fritze D, Herrmann C, Smith GS, et al: HL-A types in myasthenia gravis. *Lancet* 2:211, 1973.
49. Goldstein G, Manganaro A: Thymin, a thymic polypeptide causing the neuromuscular block of myasthenia gravis. *Ann NY Acad Sci* 183:230–240, 1966.
50. Goldstein G, Whittingham S: Experimental autoimmune thymitis—an animal model of human myasthenia gravis. *Lancet* 2:215–318, 1966.
51. Grob D: Clinical manifestations of myasthenia gravis. In Albuquerque EX, Eldefrawi AT (eds): *Myasthenia Gravis.* London, Chapman and Hall, 1983, pp 319–345.
52. Grob D, Brunner NG, Namba T: The natural course of myasthenia gravis and effect of therapeutic measures. *Ann NY Acad Sci* 377:652–669, 1981.
53. Grob D, Johns RJ, Harvey AM: Studies in neuromuscular function in normal subjects and patients with myasthenia gravis. *Bull Johns Hopkins Hosp* 99:115–238, 1956.
54. Harvey AM, Masland RL: The electromyogram in myasthenia gravis. *Bull Johns Hopkins Hosp* 69:1–13, 1941.
55. Harvey AM, Masland RL: A method for the study of neuromuscular transmission in human subjects. *Bull Johns Hopkins Hosp* 68:81–93, 1941.
56. Hewitt J, Benveniste M, Lessana-Leibowitch M: Pemphigus induced by D-penicillamine. *Br Med J* 3:371, 1975.
57. Howard JF, Sanders DB: Passive transfer of human myasthenia gravis to rats: 1. Electrophysiology of the developing neuromuscular block. *Neurology* 30:760–764, 1980.

58. Howard JF, Sanders DB: The management of patients with myasthenia gravis. In Albuquerque EX, Eldefrawi AT (eds): *Myasthenia Gravis*. London, Chapman and Hall. (In press) pp. 462–465.
59. Ibid., pp. 465–470.
60. Ibid., pp. 470–473.
61. Ibid., pp. 474–476.
62. Ibid., pp. 477–482.
63. Hudson CS, Rash JE, Tiedt TN, Albuquerque EX: Neostigmine-induced alterations at the mammalian neuromuscular junction. *J Pharmacol Exp Ther* 250:340–356, 1978.
64. Jolly F: Ueber myasthenia gravis pseudoparalytica. *Berl Klin Wochenschr* 32:1–7, 1895.
65. Kao I, Drachman DB: Thymic muscle cells bear acetylcholine receptors: Possible relation to myasthenia gravis. *Science* 195:74–75, 1977.
66. Keesey J, Lindstrom J, Cokeley H, Herrmann C: Anti-acetylcholine receptor antibody in neonatal myasthenia gravis. *N Engl J Med* 296:55, 1977.
67. Keesey J, Lindstrom J, Littman B, Herrmann C: Antireceptor antibody in neonatal myasthenia. *Excerpta Medica* 427:242, 1977 (abstract).
68. Kelly JJ, Daube JR, Lennon VA, Howard FM, Younge BR: The laboratory diagnosis of mild myasthenia gravis. *Ann Neurol* 12:238–242, 1982.
69. Kimura J, Van Allen MW: Post-thymomectomy myasthenia gravis. Report of a case of ocular myasthenia gravis after total removal of a thymoma and review of literature. *Neurology* 17:413–420, 1967.
70. Kornbleuth W, Jampolsky A, Tamler E, Elwin M: Contraction of the oculorotatory muscles and intraocular pressure. A tonographic and electromyographic study of the effect of edrophonium chloride (Tensilon) and succinylcholine (Anectine) on the intraocular pressure. *Am J Ophthalmol* 49:1381–1387, 1960.
71. Kramer LD, Ruth RA, Johns ME, Sanders DB: A comparison of stapedial reflex fatigue with repetitive stimulation and single-fiber EMG in myasthenia gravis. *Ann Neurol.* 9:531–536, 1981.
72. Kurtzke J: Epidemiology of myasthenia gravis. In Schoenberg BS (ed): *Neurological Epidemiology: Principles and Clinical Applications.* (Advances in Neurology, 19) New York, Raven Press, 1979, pp 545–564.
73. Lefvert AK, Bergstrom K, Matell G, Osterman PO, Pirskanen R: Determination of acetylcholine receptor antibody in myasthenia gravis: Clinical usefulness and pathogenetic implications. *J Neurol Neurosurg Psychiatry* 41:394–403, 1978.
74. Lennon VA, Carnegie PR: Immunopharmacological disease: A break in tolerance to receptor sites. *Lancet* 1:630–633, 1971.
75. Lennon VA, Seybold ME, Lindstrom JM, et al: Role of complement in the pathogenesis of experimental autoimmune myasthenia gravis. *J Exp Med* 147:973–983, 1978.
76. Lindsley DB: Electrical activity of human motor units during voluntary contraction. *Am J Physiol* 114:90–99, 1935.
77. Lindstrom JM, Einarson B, Lennon VA, Seybold ME: Pathological mechanisms in EAMG. I: Immunogenicity of syngeneic muscle acetylcholine receptor and quantitative extraction of receptor and antibody:

Receptor complexes from muscles of rats with experimental autoimmune myasthenia gravis. *J Exp Med* 144:726–738, 1976.
78. Lindstrom JM, Engel AG, Seybold ME, et al: Pathological mechanisms in EAMG II: Passive transfer of experimental autoimmune myasthenia gravis in rats with acetylcholine receptor antibodies. *J Exp Med* 144: 739–753, 1976.
79. Lindstrom JM, Lambert EH: Content of acetylcholine receptor and antibodies bound to receptor in myasthenia gravis, experimental autoimmune myasthenia gravis and Eaton-Lambert syndrome. *Neurology* 28:130–138, 1978.
80. Lindstrom JM, Seybold ME, Lennon VA, et al: Antibody to acetylcholine receptor in myasthenia gravis. *Neurology* 26:1054–1058, 1976.
81. McAdams MW, Roses AD: Comparison of antigenic sources for acetylcholine receptor antibody assays in myasthenia gravis. *Ann Neurol* 8:61–66, 1980.
82. Masters CL, Dawkins RL, Zilko PJ, et al: Penicillamine-associated myasthenia gravis, antiacetylcholine receptor and antistriational antibodies. *Am J Med* 63:689–694, 1977.
83. Matell G, Bergstrom K, Franksson C, et al: Effects of some immunosuppressive procedures on myasthenia gravis. *Ann NY Acad Sci* 274: 659–676, 1976.
84. Mertens HG, Hertel G, Reuther P, Ricker K: Effect of immunosuppressive drugs. *Ann NY Acad Sci* 377:691–699, 1981.
85. Metz HS, Scott AB, O'Meara DM: Saccadic eye movements in myasthenia gravis. *Arch Ophthalmol* 88:9–11, 1972.
86. Miller JFAP: Effect of neonatal thymectomy on the immunological responsiveness of the mouse. *Proc R Soc London Ser B* 156:415–428, 1962.
87. Miller JFAP, Mitchell GF: Thymus and antigen reactive cells. *Transplant Rev* 1:3–42, 1969.
88. Miller JFAP, Mitchell GF, Weiss NS: Cellular basis of the immunological defect of thymectomized mice. *Nature* 214:992–997, 1967.
89. Mittag TW, Caroscio J: False-positive immunoassay for acetylcholine receptor antibody in amyotrophic lateral sclerosis (letter). *N Engl J Med* 302:868, 1980.
90. Morel E, Raimond F, Goulon-Goeau C, Berrih S, Vernet-Der-Garabedian B, Harb J, Bach J-F: Assay of acetylcholine receptor antibodies in myasthenia gravis. A study of 329 sera. *Nouv Presse Med* 11: 1849–1854, 1982.
91. Nakao K, Nishitani H, Suzuki M et al: Anti-acetylcholine receptor IgG in neonatal myasthenia gravis. *N Engl J Med* 297:169, 1977.
92. Namba T, Brown SB, Grob D: Neonatal myasthenia gravis: report of two cases and review of the literature. *Pediatrics* 45:488–504, 1970.
93. Nastuk WL, Plescia OJ, Osserman KE: Changes in serum complement activity in patients with myasthenia gravis. *Proc Soc Exp Biol Med* 105:177–184, 1960.
94. Ohta M, Matsubara F, Hayashi K, et al: Acetylcholine receptor antibodies in infants of mothers with myasthenia gravis. *Neurology* 31: 1019–1022, 1981.

95. Olanow CW, Roses AD: The pathogenesis of myasthenia gravis. A hypothesis. *Medical Hypotheses* 7:957–958, 1981.
96. Oosterhuis HJGH: Epidemiologie der myasthenia in Amsterdam. In Hertel G. Mertens HG (eds): *Myasthenia Gravis.* Stuttgart, Georg Thieme Verlag, 1977, pp 103–108.
97. Ozdemir C, Young RR: Electrical testing in myasthenia gravis. *Ann NY Acad Sci* 183:287–302, 1971.
98. Ozdemir C, Young RR: The results to be expected from electrical testing in the diagnosis of myasthenia gravis. *Ann NY Acad Sci* 274:203–222,1976.
99. Patrick J, Lindstrom J: Autoimmune response to acetylcholine receptor. *Science* 180:871–872, 1973.
100. Patten BM, Oliver KL, Engel WK: Adverse interaction between steroid hormones and anticholinesterase drugs. *Neurology* 24: 442–449, 1974.
101. Petersen J, Halberg P, Hojgaard K, et al: Penicillamine-induced polymyositis-dermatomyositis. *Scand J Rheumatol* 7:113–117, 1978.
102. Pirskanen R: Genetic associations between myasthenia gravis and the HL-A system. *J Neurol Neurosurg Psychiatry* 39:23–33, 1976.
103. Pirskanen R, Tiilikainen A, Hokkanen E: Histocompatibility (HL-A) antigens associated with myasthenia gravis. *Ann Clin Res* 4:304–306, 1972.
104. Richman DP, Patrick J, Arnason BGW: Cellular immunity in myasthenia gravis. Response to purified acetylcholine receptor and autologous thymocytes. *N Engl J Med* 294: 694–698, 1976.
105. Roses AD, Olanow CW, McAdams MW, Lane RJM: There is no direct correlation between serum anti-acetylcholine receptor antibody levels and the clinical status of individual patients with myasthenia gravis. *Neurology* 31:220–224, 1981.
106. Rowland LP, Aranow H, Hoefer PFA: Myasthenia gravis appearing after the removal of thymoma. *Neurology* 7:584–588, 1957.
107. Rubin JW, Ellison RG, Moore HV, Pai GP: Factors affecting the response to thymectomy for myasthenia gravis. *J Thorac Cardiovasc Surg* 82:720–728, 1981.
108. Russell AS, Lindstrom JM: Penicillamine-induced myasthenia gravis associated with antibodies to acetylcholine receptor. *Neurology* 28: 847–849, 1978.
109. Ruth RA, Johns ME, Kramer LD, Sanders DB, Cantrell RW: Evaluation of the stapedius muscle in neuromuscular disorders. In Penha R, Pizzaro P (eds): *Proceedings of the IVth International Symposium on Acoustic Impedance Measurements.* Lisbon, University of New Lisbon, 1981.
110. Sachs JA: The relevance of HLA antigens in some neurological diseases. In Rose FC (ed): *Clinical Neuroimmunology.* Oxford, Blackwell Scientific Publishers, 1979, pp 42–52.
111. Sahashi K, Engel AG, Lindstrom JM, et al: Ultrastructural localization of immune complexes (IgG and C3) at the end-plate in experimental autoimmune myasthenia gravis. *J Neuropathol Exp Neurol* 37:212–223, 1978.
112. Sanders DB: Electrodiagnosis of myasthenia gravis: Recent techniques. In Albuquerque EX, Eldefrawi AT (eds): *Myasthenia Gravis.* London, Chapman and Hall, 1983, pp 290–291.

113. Sanders DB, Cobb EE, Winfield JB: Neonatal experimental autoimmune myasthenia gravis. *Muscle and Nerve* 1:146–150, 1978.
114. Sanders DB, Howard JF, Johns TR: Single-fiber electromyography in myasthenia gravis. *Neurology* 29:68–76, 1979.
115. Sanders DB, Howard JF, Johns TR, Campa JF: High-dose prednisone in the treatment of myasthenia gravis. In Dau PC (ed): *Plasmapheresis and the Immunobiology of Myasthenia Gravis.* Boston, Houghton Mifflin, 1979, pp 289–306.
116. Sanders DB, Kim YI, Howard JF, et al: Intercostal muscle biopsy studies in myasthenia gravis: Clinical correlations and the direct effects of drugs and myasthenic serum. *Ann NY Acad Sci* 377:544–566, 1981.
117. Scadding GK, Webster ADB, Ross M, et al: Humoral immunity before and after thymectomy in myasthenia gravis. *Neurology* 29:502–506, 1979.
118. Schraeder PL, Peters HA, Dahl DS: Polymyositis and penicillamine. *Arch Neurol* 27:456–457, 1972.
119. Schumacher DR, Roth D: Thymektomie bei einen Fall von Morbus Basedowi mit Myasthenia. *Mitt Grenzgeb Med Chir* 25:746–765, 1913.
120. Scott JS: Pregnancy: Nature's experimental system. *Lancet* 1:78–80, 1976.
121. Seybold ME, Lindstrom JM: Patterns of acetylcholine receptor antibody fluctuation in myasthenia gravis. *Ann NY Acad Sci* 377:292–306, 1981.
122. Simpson JA: Myasthenia gravis: a new hypothesis. *Scott Med J* 5:419–436, 1960.
123. Simpson JA: Immunological disturbances in myasthenia gravis: with a report of Hashimoto's disease developing after thymectomy. *J Neurol Neurosurg Psychiatry* 27:485–492, 1964.
124. Simpson JA: Myasthenia gravis as an autoimmune disease: clinical aspects. *Ann N Y Acad Sci* 135:506–516, 1966.
125. Simpson JA: Myasthenia gravis. In Walton JN, Canal N, Scarlato G (eds): *Muscle Diseases.* Amsterdam, Excerpta Medica, 1969, pp 14–22.
126. Simpson JA: Myasthenia gravis and myasthenic syndromes. In Walton J. (ed): *Disorders of Voluntary Muscle.* London, Churchill Livingstone, 1981, p 585.
127. Simpson JA, Behan PO, Dick HM: Studies on the nature of autoimmunity in myasthenia gravis. Evidence for an immunodeficiency type. *Ann NY Acad Sci* 274:382–389, 1976.
128. Smithers DW: Tumours of the thyroid gland in relation to some general concepts of neoplasia. *J Fac Radiol* (London) 10:3–16, 1959.
129. Spector RH, Daroff RB: Edrophonium infrared optokinetic nystagmography in the diagnosis of myasthenia gravis. *Ann NY Acad Sci* 274:642–651, 1976.
130. Stalberg E, Sanders DB: Electrophysiological tests of neuromuscular transmission. In Stalberg E, Young RR (eds): *Clinical Neurophysiology.* Sevenoaks, Kent, Butterworth and Co., 1981, pp 88–116.
131. Stalberg E, Trontelj J: *Single Fibre Electromyography.* Old Woking, Surrey, Mirvalle Press, 1979.
132. Ibid., p 124.
133. Stella S: Optokinetic nystagmus in patients with ocular myasthenia. *Invest Ophthalmol* 6:668, 1967.

134. Strauss AJL, Seegal BC, Hsu KC, et al: Immunofluorescence demonstration of a muscle-binding, complement-fixing serum globulin fraction in myasthenia gravis. *Proc Soc Exp Biol Med* 105:184–191, 1960.

135. Teng P, Osserman KE: Studies in myasthenia gravis: Neonatal and juvenile types. *J Mt Sinai Hosp* 23:711–727, 1956.

136. Tindall, RSA: Humoral immunity in myasthenia gravis: Biochemical characterization of acquired antireceptor antibodies and clinical correlations. *Ann Neurol* 10:427–447, 1980.

137. Toyka KV, Drachman DB, Griffin DE, Pestronk A, et al: Myasthenia gravis. Study of humoral immune mechanisms by passive transfer to mice. *N Engl J Med* 296:125–131, 1977.

138. Toyka KV, Drachman DB, Pestronk A, et al: Myasthenia gravis: Passive transfer from man to mouse. *Science* 190:397–399, 1975.

139. van der Geld HWR, Strauss AJL: Myasthenia gravis. Immunological relationship between striated muscle and thymus. *Lancet* 1:57–60, 1966.

140. Vetters JM: Immunofluorescence staining patterns in skeletal muscle using serum of myasthenic patients and normal controls. *Immunology* 9:93–95, 1965.

141. Viets HR, Schwab RS: *Thymectomy for Myasthenia Gravis.* Springfield, Ill., Charles C. Thomas, 1960.

142. Vincent A. Newsom-Davis J, Martin V: Anti-acetylcholine receptor antibodies in D-penicillamine-associated myasthenia gravis. *Lancet* 1:1254, 1978.

143. Vincent A, Scadding GK, Clarke C, Newsom-Davis J: Anti-acetylcholine receptor antibody synthesis in culture. In Dau PC (ed): *Plasmapheresis and the Immunobiology of Myasthenia Gravis.* Boston, Houghton-Mifflin, 1979, pp 59–71.

144. Weigert C: Pathologisch-anatomischer Beitrag zur Erbsch'en Krankheit (Myasthenia Gravis). *Neurol Zentralblatt* 20:597–601, 1901.

145. Wekerle H, Ketelsen U-P: Intrathymic pathogenesis and dual genetic control of myasthenia gravis. *Lancet* 1:678–680, 1977.

146. Wray SH, Pavan-Langston D: A re-evaluation of edrophonium chloride (Tensilon) tonography in the diagnosis of myasthenia gravis. *Neurology* 21:586–593, 1971.

Chapter 7

Miscellaneous Neuromuscular Transmission Disorders

Thomas R. Swift, M.D. and
Michael K. Greenberg, M.D.

The complexity of events in neuromuscular transmission makes the junction a vulnerable site for the development of many clinical disorders.[258] Every event from nerve terminal action potential to transmitter-receptor interaction may be affected, leading to a large and heterogeneous group of clinically defined diseases (Table 7.1). As may be seen from the Table, some agents may affect more than one event in the sequence, and often it is not clear which is the more important. For the purposes of this discussion the clinical diseases of neuromuscular transmission will be arbitrarily classified as endogenous (either primary or secondary to other conditions) or exogenous (caused by biological toxins or pharmacologic agents). Progress in understanding the pathophysiology and treatment of these disorders is occurring rapidly, and when dealing with patients one should consult current references.

Primary Endogenous Disorders

Myasthenic Syndrome

A disorder of neuromuscular transmission characterized by generalized muscle weakness and fatigability was described by Eaton and Lambert in 1957.[75] This disorder is strikingly different from myasthenia gravis in distribution of weakness, predilection for males, age of onset and association with malignant tumors. A presynaptic defect

Table 7.1
Steps in Neuromuscular Transmission

Event	*Condition affecting event*
Nerve terminal action potential	Beta-adrenergic blocking drugs
	Chloroquine
	Congenital syndrome
	Hormonal agents
Calcium entry	Azathioprine
	Snake venoms
Acetylcholine release	Antiarrhythmic drugs
	Antibiotic drugs
	Botulinum and tetanus toxins
	Insect venoms
	Lithium
	Magnesium ion
	Myasthenic syndrome
	Snake venoms
	Spider venoms
Acetylcholine-receptor interaction	Antiarrhythmic drugs
	Antibiotic drugs
	Anticonvulsant drugs
	Beta-adrenergic blocking drugs
	Chloroquine
	Congenital syndrome
	D-penicillamine
	Ganglionic blocking drugs
	Hormonal agents
	Magnesium ion
	Phenothiazines
	Snake venoms
Hydrolysis of acetylcholine	Anticholinesterases
	Congenital syndrome
	Ganglionic blocking drugs
	Phenothiazines
Choline re-uptake	Hormonal agents
Acetylcholine synthesis	Anticonvulsant drugs
	Congenital syndrome
Vesicle packaging	Acrylamide
	Botulinum and tetanus toxins
	Insect venoms
	Snake venoms
	Spider venoms

in acetylcholine release underlies the defect in neuromuscular transmission found in the myasthenic syndrome.[149]

The initial symptoms are tiredness and weakness first noted on arising from a chair or climbing stairs. Improvement in strength may occur temporarily after voluntary contraction,[117] but prolonged effort results in fatigue. The weakness affects all muscle groups, especially proximal extremity and girdle muscles. Unlike myasthenia gravis, the extraocular muscles are rarely involved.[27] Non-specific leg, thigh and back pain and paresthesias occur. Disturbances of autonomic dysfunction produce dry mouth, constipation, impotence and dysuria.[117,222]

The syndrome is almost five times more common in men than in women,[151] and is associated with a malignant tumor in 70% of patients, most often oat-cell carcinoma of the lung.[151] The disease may precede discovery of the tumor by many months. The incidence of carcinoma in women with this syndrome approaches 20%.[199] Most cases occur in patients over the age of 40 years, but this syndrome has been described in children.[45,234] The disease has been reported in association with pernicious anemia,[102] thyroid disease,[143,193] and Sjögren syndrome.[29] Patients with this syndrome have been shown by Lennon and co-workers to have organ-specific autoimmunity and share with myasthenia gravis patients an increased incidence of HLA antigens B8 and DR3.[259] Cases with features of both myasthenia gravis and myasthenic syndrome have been reported.[28,54,230,238,262] A case has been reported in a 52-year-old woman with a malignant thymoma.[154]

Examination will show varying degrees of weakness, most notable in proximal upper and lower extremity muscles. Careful study may disclose an improvement in strength following a brief voluntary contraction. Muscle stretch reflexes are usually depressed, but may also improve following exercise.

The most useful laboratory examination for the diagnosis of myasthenic syndrome is repetitive stimulation of nerve while recording muscle action potentials (Fig. 7.1). The amplitude of the initial evoked compound muscle action potential is small, often as low as 2% to 20% of normal. The evoked potential amplitude declines at low rates of repetitive stimulation. At high rates of stimulation, augmentation of the amplitude up to ten- to twentyfold occurs.[45,152] Marked facilitation also occurs following exercise. Needle electromyography reveals variation in amplitude and shape of motor unit potentials. Using single-fiber electromyography (see chapter 6), increased jitter and blocking are found which improve as units fire at higher frequen-

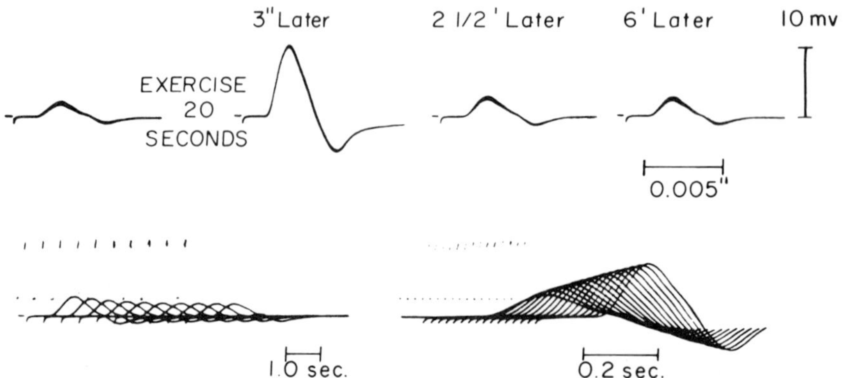

Figure 7.1. Repetitive ulnar nerve stimulation recording hypothenar muscles in myasthenic syndrome. Top: Each trace represents three muscle action potentials at 2 Hz. The initially low amplitude muscle action potentials facilitate greatly after exercise. Bottom: There is progressive decline in amplitude at 2 Hz (left) and progressive increase in amplitude at 50 Hz (right).

cies.[229,230] The defect in neuromuscular transmission worsens at higher temperatures[261,286] (Fig. 7.2).

Patients with myasthenic syndrome experience weakness due to impaired release of acetylcholine from the nerve terminal.[149] Acetylcholine synthesis and mobilization and the amplitude of miniature endplate potentials are all normal.[142,149] The impairment of quantal release results in a neurally evoked endplate potential which is too small to produce a muscle action potential.[142] The number of quanta released declines further with low rates of nerve stimulation, while at rates above 10 Hz, augmentation of release occurs, resulting in larger endplate potentials and improvement in neuromuscular transmission.[149] Elevation of calcium concentration or addition of guanidine will also augment transmitter release.[148,149,264]

Ultrastructural studies of the neuromuscular junction reveal overdeveloped postjunctional regions with an increase in surface area and

Figure 7.2. Effect of temperature in myasthenic syndrome. Top: At higher temperature the first and fourth hypothenar muscle action potential (bottom two lines) are reduced and the percent decrement is increased compared to those at lower temperature (top two lines). Bottom: At higher temperature the first and fourth hypothenar muscle twitch tension responses (bottom two lines) are reduced and the percent decrement increased compared to those at lower temperature (top two lines).

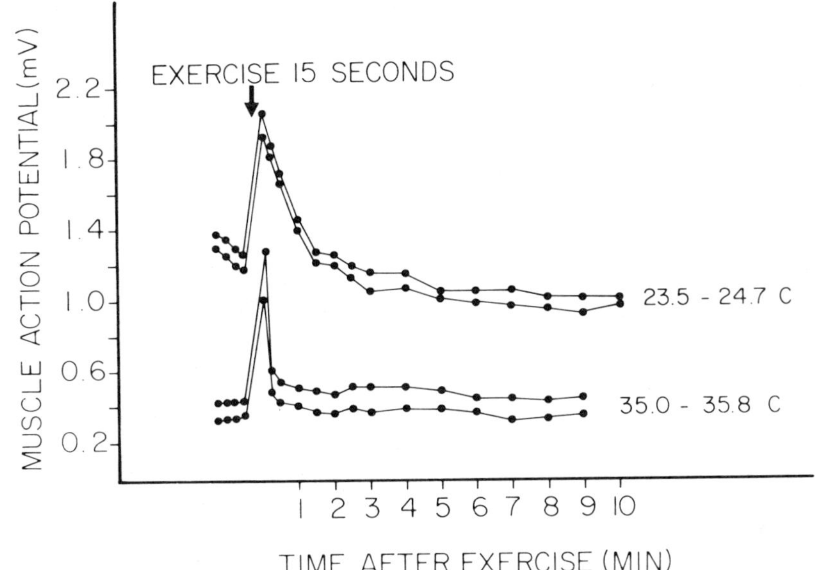
MUSCLE ACTION POTENTIAL (mV)
EXERCISE 15 SECONDS
2.2
1.8
1.4
1.0
0.6
0.2
23.5 - 24.7 C
35.0 - 35.8 C
1 2 3 4 5 6 7 8 9 10
TIME AFTER EXERCISE (MIN)

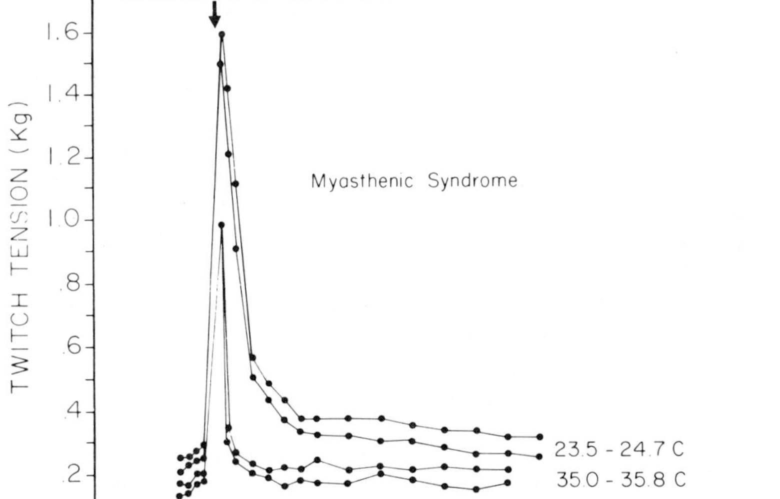
EXERCISE 15 SECONDS
TWITCH TENSION (Kg)
1.6
1.4
1.2
1.0
.8
.6
.4
.2
Myasthenic Syndrome
23.5 - 24.7 C
35.0 - 35.8 C
1 2 3 4 5 6 7 8 9 10
TIME AFTER EXERCISE (MIN)

highly complex clefts and folds.[78,83] The total number of presynaptic vesicles are normal, but the arrangement of vesicles at release zones is highly disorganized.[83,91]

The pathogenesis of this disorder is unknown. Tissue extract from an oat-cell carcinoma was shown to produce the characteristic electrophysiologic abnormalities in nerve-muscle preparation.[130] A serum IgG fraction from patients with myasthenic syndrome injected into mice reduced the initial evoked compound muscle action potential.[153] Likewise, these animals demonstrated a reduction in the quantal content of the endplate potential which increases at high rates of stimulation.[153,190] The experiments suggest a humoral factor, possibly an auto-antibody binding to a presynaptic site, resulting in impaired transmitter release.[190]

Treatment by anticholinesterase drugs may produce a limited improvement in strength.[75,117,148,152] Since poor release of transmitter is the cause of the weakness, drugs which increase transmitter release are of more value. The drug of choice at this time is guanidine, which has been shown to increase transmitter release in this syndrome.[149] Hazardous effects which limit the usefulness of guanidine include bone marrow depression,[194] renal and hepatic toxicity,[47] pancreatitis[117] and paresthesias. Guanidine is administered orally at a dose of 20–30 mg per kg body weight in three or four equally divided doses, with improvement noted within 24 hours of initiating treatment.[199] Substituted pyridines have been shown to increase the content of cyclic AMP in the nerve terminal and augment release of transmitter in this syndrome.[264] Both 4-aminopyridine and 3,4-diaminopyridine are drugs which enhance nerve-impulse-evoked transmitter release,[3,142,165,268] and have been shown clinically and electrophysiologically to improve weakness.[186] Newer substituted pyridines may be more effective and have less central nervous system effects.[259] The dosage of 4-aminopyridine is between 40–200 mg per day. Side effects include circumoral paresthesias, restlessness and anxiety, and nausea and vomiting.[186,268] Major adverse effects include seizures and acute confusional state.[186] Autonomic effects include exaggerated vagal response, moderate rise in systolic blood pressure, and decrease in cerebral blood flow (10%–20%).[268] Although the beneficial properties of substituted pyridines are well documented, serious adverse effects greatly limit their usefulness. In animal studies, 3,4-diaminopyridine has a more potent effect on cholinergic transmission but less convulsant side effects.[268]

Corticosteroids, which have well-proven beneficial effects in myasthenia gravis, have been less studied in the myasthenic syndrome.

Vroom and Engel[283] reported a young woman with the myasthenic syndrome who was improved for eleven years while on corticosteroids. This patient's weakness worsened with steroid withdrawal and was improved with re-institution of steroid therapy. Experimentally, corticosteroids have been shown to improve the potentiation induced by guanidine.[108] Streib and Rothner[254] reported three patients treated with prednisone, all of whom demonstrated an increase in muscle strength over three to four months. Deterioration occurred in all three with dosage reduction and improved with re-institution of the higher dose. Plasma exchange has produced transient improvement peaking at two to three weeks. Improvement was prolonged with immunosuppressive and steroid drug therapy.[56,64,153,230] Although 90% of the reported patients have shown improvement with this combined form of immunotherapy, further study will be necessary to determine the exact role of corticosteroids, plasma exchange or immunosuppression in treatment.

Congenital Myasthenia

Presynaptic Congenital Myasthenia

A group of disorders designated as congenital myasthenia syndromes share many common features including onset in the neonatal period or infancy and presentation with ptosis, poor feeding, or fatigue. Antiacetylcholine receptor antibodies as found in typical myasthenia gravis are lacking in these patients. This is in contrast to the transplacental transfer of maternal antiacetylcholine receptor antibodies found in neonatal myasthenia gravis (see chapter 6). In many cases siblings are affected,[183,161,293] but the mother usually is not.[36] Thymectomy is probably of no value.[140]

A clinical syndrome referred to as familial infantile myasthenia is characterized by respiratory depression at birth, episodic weakness, and recurrent episodes of apnea.[25,39,49,86,93, 98,187,220,266,289] These patients have a good response to anticholinesterase drugs and no detectable antireceptor antibodies.[220] A tendency for improvement with age has been noted. A detailed electrophysiological study of one such patient demonstrated normal miniature endplate potential amplitude at rest, and reduced miniature endplate potential amplitude following 10 Hz nerve stimulation for a few minutes.[111] These data were interpreted to reflect a defect in acetylcholine resynthesis due to impaired choline reuptake,[111] acetylcholine assembly by choline ace-

tyl transferase, or vesicle packaging.[78,81] Junctional ultrastructure
showed increased numbers of synaptic vesicles.

A patient who presented with respiratory difficulty at birth was
reported by Vincent et al.[277] Ptosis and limb weakness were responsive to edrophonium. A decrement of the compound muscle action
potential at 5 Hz stimulation was found. Miniature endplate potential amplitude was markedly reduced, but quantal content of endplate potentials was increased by a factor of 5 to 6. No postsynaptic
defects were found, and transmission improved with 4-aminopyri-
dine. From this data, the authors suggest a presynaptic defect, possibly in the releasable store of acetylcholine quanta.

Postsynaptic Congenital Myasthenia

A 14-year-old Hindu boy who developed fatigable weakness of
extraocular, bulbar, trunk, and extremity muscles has been described
by Engel et al.[80] Minimal improvement occurred with corticosteroid
treatment, but there was no response to anticholinesterase agents or
guanidine. The authors demonstrated changes in postsynaptic junctional architecture and complete absence of acetylcholinesterase.
Miniature endplate potential duration was prolonged, and there was
a reduction in the size of the releasable store of acetylcholine quanta.
Nerve terminals at the neuromuscular junctions were small or absent. A single stimulus to a motor nerve produced repetitive muscle
action potentials. This is the same phenomenon seen in anticholinesterase poisoning and is believed to be due to persistence of acetylcholine at the receptor surface.

An autosomal dominant disorder described by the same group of
workers is characterized by severe weakness of scapular and forearm muscles and variable weakness of face, jaw, and ocular muscles.[78,81,82] Weakness may begin in childhood or adulthood. A decrement in muscle action potential occurs with repetitive nerve stimulation. A prolonged acetylcholine effect is suggested by repetitive
muscle responses to single nerve stimuli. Endplate potentials are
further prolonged by addition of cholinesterase inhibitors. However,
in this syndrome, acetylcholinesterase levels are normal. Myopathic
changes present in the endplate zone are presumed to be secondary to
an abnormality of the acetylcholine receptor leading to prolonged
ion-channel open time.

Four additional cases of congenital myasthenia were described by
Vincent et al.[277] Three of these patients demonstrated neonatal hypo-

tonia, ptosis and extraocular muscle weakness followed by progressive facial, neck, and generalized weakness and fatigue. Strength improved with edrophonium. A decremental response to repetitive nerve stimulation was found in only one patient, but single-fiber electromyography was abnormal in all three. Miniature endplate potential amplitude was reduced as was α-bungarotoxin binding. Normal acetylcholine content in muscle was found. The authors consider the syndrome a defect in acetylcholine receptor.

The fourth patient in this series[277] showed a somewhat different course, in which poor feeding and ptosis in the neonatal period was replaced by generalized fatigue at age three and total ophthalmoplegia at age 13. Single-fiber electromyography was abnormal and a progressive decrement occurred with repetitive nerve stimulation. Miniature endplate potential amplitude was reduced. Although α-bungarotoxin binding sites were not greatly reduced with short wash times, binding was low at long wash times. Extrajunctional receptors were found. The authors postulated a defect in the acetylcholine receptor itself, possibly at or near the site of acetylcholine attachment. Morgan-Hughes et al studied two patients with congenital myasthenia and found a change in acetylcholine receptor affinity for *d*-tubocurarine and suggested an abnormal acetylcholine receptor macromolecule.[180] In a myopathy with tubular aggregates these same authors found alterations in the number and affinity of acetylcholine receptors.[181]

Secondary Endogenous Disorders

Neurologic Diseases

Amyotrophic lateral sclerosis,[184,236] polymyositis,[34,122] and syringomyelia[146] are all motor neuron diseases which have been associated with neuromuscular transmission disturbances. Some of the reported cases have shown symptomatic fatigue,[184] but most have had no symptoms attributable to disturbed neuromuscular transmission, the condition being discovered when repetitive stimulation of nerve revealed a decrement in the muscle action potential.[21] In some reports, the defects appeared only at rates of stimulation above 10 Hz and were not accompanied by postactivation facilitation or exhaustion. The decrement may be more prominent in weak muscles[184] or in patients with rapidly progressive disease.[21] Sensitivity to curare and improvement with anticholinesterase drugs have been shown in some of these disorders,[122,184] making it likely that they are due to disturbances at the neuromuscular junction. Neuromuscular transmission failure could occur in diseases of lower motor neurons if acetylcholine synthesis, mobilization, or release were impaired. Nerve terminals in amyotrophic lateral sclerosis have been reported to be abnormal and the endplate surface area increased.[298] However, the amount and distribution of acetylcholine receptors at the endplate has been shown to be well preserved. It is possible that transmission failures or impulse blocking could occur in newly formed axonal sprouts which occur in this disease[296] and which have been reported to release smaller amounts of acetylcholine.[63,267] A false-positive radio-immunoassay for anticholinesterase antibody[179] may occur in patients who have received modified neurotoxin therapy, but here the antibody is probably directed against α-bungarotoxin polypeptide rather than receptor.[179]

Patients with uremic,[269] diabetic,[235,269] alcohol-nutritional,[269] vitamin-deficient,[19,120] drug-induced,[175] and post-herpetic[239] peripheral neuropathies have been reported to have neuromuscular transmission disorders. Like anterior horn cell diseases, most reported patients did not experience unusual fatigue. Decremental muscle responses to repetitive stimulation of nerve occur at high frequencies,[235, 239] and postactivation facilitation is not prominent.[239] A polyneuropathy due to carbon disulphide has been associated with distal muscle fatigue in 35% of patients.[275] Repetitive stimulation at slow rates of stimulation (3–6 Hz) demonstrates a decremental response in these patients.

Impaired neuromuscular transmission has been reported in experimental neuropathies. Decremental muscle action potential response and abnormal nerve terminals have been reported in experimental isoniazid neuropathy in rats. Swift and Lambert (unpublished observations, 1973) found reductions in both miniature endplate potential frequency and size of the releasable store of transmitter in acrylamide-poisoned rats, which became greater the longer the rats were kept on the acrylamide-containing diet (Figs. 7.3 and 7.4). Decreased concentration and abnormal distribution of synaptic vesicles were seen in the reduced number of nerve terminals at endplates.[271]

A single-fiber electromyographic study of human neuropathies (uremic, diabetic, and alcoholic-nutritional) found increased fiber density, jitter, and blocking of nerve transmission, all typical of active reinnervation and believed to be due to impaired impulse conduction in newly formed reinnervation sprouts rather than neuromuscular transmission failure.[269]

There have been case reports of multiple sclerosis coexisting with myasthenia gravis.[2,6,42,138,147,166,200,225] It is not clear whether these cases represent a chance association, or whether they share common immunopathogenetic mechanisms. Some of the reported cases appear convincing, but in others the diagnosis of myasthenia gravis is uncertain or made only after repetitive stimulation revealed decrements. Many of the decrements appeared only at high rates of stimulation, suggesting that the disorder was not classical myasthenia gravis. Antireceptor antibody determinations have not been performed in most of these patients. However, a reduced neuromuscular transmission safety factor in multiple sclerosis has been demonstrated,[76] and sera from patients with multiple sclerosis have been found to contain neural blocking activity.[57] Recently, single-fiber EMG studies of patients with multiple sclerosis who had fatigue revealed increased jitter in 15 of 16 patients and impulse blocking in 9 of 16 patients, which improved with increased effort, suggesting a presynaptic defect. All of these patients had negative antireceptor antibody titers.[260]

Patients with inflammatory myopathy have been described who have demonstrated a decremental response to low-frequency repetitive stimulation, transient facilitation following tetanic stimulation, and post-tetanic exhaustion.[274] Improvement was observed in response to corticosteroids, immunosuppression and guanidine. A mixed pre- and postsynaptic mechanism has been presumed. Pestronk and Drachman have reported a reduction in the number of acetylcholine receptors per neuromuscular junction in patients with polymyositis.[202] In an associated study, they demonstrated reduced total acetylcholine receptors and increased rate of receptor degradation in cultures of mammalian skeletal muscle exposed to sera of patients with polymyositis.[202] Lymphocytes from patients with polymyositis show slight stimulation to acetylcholine receptor.[50] A short-lived syndrome of impaired neuromuscular transmission occurred in a young man 18 months following a bout of mononucleosis and an intervening episode of polymyositis.[204]

Complete understanding of the nature of the neuromuscular transmission disturbances in this heterogeneous group of disorders awaits further investigation.

Exogenous Disorders Induced by Biological Toxins

Botulism

Botulism is caused by a powerful polypeptide toxin produced by the organism *Clostridium botulinum.*[127,255] Contaminated food that is insufficiently heated to denature the toxin produces symptoms when ingested.[66] For reasons unknown, not all patients who consume toxin-contaminated food develop the clinical disorder.[145] In wound botulism, organisms contaminating a wound produce the toxin.[174] In infantile botulism, it is believed that organisms in the gut produce toxin which is systemically absorbed.[13,14,15,132,206]

Of the eight types of botulinum toxin recognized (A, B, C_α, C_β, D, E, F, G),[127,255] types A and B most commonly cause clinical botulism in the United States. Ingestion of marine products usually results in type E botulism.[66] A high index of suspicion is necessary, supported by epidemiologic, clinical and electrophysiologic findings. Confirmation of the diagnosis depends on the identification of the toxin and/or organism in food, stool or wound.[114]

Symptoms of botulism include nausea, vomiting, blurred vision, dysphagia, and increased oropharyngeal secretions, followed by generalized weakness more proximally in the upper extremities, and diplopia.[66] Central nervous system effects may be encountered.[209] Interestingly, behavioral testing in patients with peripheral botulism blockade demonstrate no impairment of immediate or recent memory.[105] Neurologic examination varies, frequently revealing dilated, poorly reactive pupils, but pupillary abnormality may be absent.[46,131] The patient may have extraocular palsies with ptosis, and facial, pharyngeal, and generalized proximal weakness.[66] Urinary retention and hypoactive bowel sounds are common findings.[131] Respiratory failure is the usual cause of death.[255] Symptoms of infantile botulism are constipation, weak sucking and cry, regurgitation and generalized weakness.[13,14,15,132,206] Sudden apnea may occur in some affected infants,[14] but studies of children suffering sudden infant death syndrome (SIDS or near SIDS) have failed to demonstrate significant bacteriologic or toxicologic evidence to suggest botulism as a major cause.[101] However, epidemiologic studies of infant botulism and SIDS have demonstrated a very similar age distribution.[13]

The electromyographic findings are helpful in confirming the diagnosis,[46,59,103,206] but changes may not be apparent early in the disease.[46] Motor and sensory nerve conduction velocities are normal.[59,103] The evoked muscle action potential may be normal but is usually reduced in amplitude.[59,103,212] There may be no decrement at low rates of stimulation.[59,103] Following exercise or at high stimulus frequencies, facilitation may be present.[59,103] Moderate paralysis may yield a greater facilitation with high stimulus frequency than when paralysis is severe.[46] Single-fiber electromyographic studies show increased jitter and blocking which improves at higher firing frequencies.[227] Needle EMG examination may show fibrillations in affected muscle fibers beginning at two weeks; these fibers show extrajunctional acetylcholine receptors similar to those seen in denervation.[203,231,255]

Botulinum toxin impairs neuromuscular transmission by interfering with the release of acetylcholine from the nerve terminal.[99,150,240,255] There is no effect on nerve terminal impulse conduction and no change in sensitivity of the muscle to directly applied acetylcholine.[99,251,255] Quantal release of acetylcholine is reduced in response to nerve stimulation.[127] Spontaneous quantal release also is reduced and may be absent at some junctions. In addition to decreased frequency, decreased amplitude of miniature endplate potentials is observed.[99,127,150,240,251] The reason for the reduction in miniature endplate potential amplitude is not known. Slower than normal miniature endplate potential rise times have been recorded.[251] The ability to release quanta of acetylcholine becomes reduced until endplate potentials in response to single nerve stimulation are abolished.[127,251,255] The nonquantal release of acetylcholine from the nerve terminal also is reduced.[99] The toxin does not act by affecting synthesis of acetylcholine (limiting availability of choline or acetyl CoA),[99,127,255] and the storage of acetylcholine in vesicles is not significantly affected.[99,127,135,240,241,255] Tetanic stimulation leads to an increase in the frequency of miniature endplate potentials with a normalization of miniature endplate potential amplitude distribution.[227] No effect on nerve terminal calcium influx has been directly shown,[127,135,241,255] although mitochondrial calcium influx in response to nerve stimulation is reduced.[121] The blockade appears to involve the acetylcholine release process.[135,241] The effect may be through a reduced sensitivity of the release site to Ca^{++} or through interference with exocytosis at the release site.[127,135] The action of the toxin at the nerve terminal occurs in steps which include binding of botulinum toxin to the terminal, translocation of the toxin into the nerve terminal and blockade of acetylcholine output.[99,240,241,242,255] Binding of the toxin to the nerve terminal is rapid, and not dependent on calcium, temperature or nerve activity. At this step antitoxin is effective.[242,255] Translocation and blockade exhibit a latent period which is inversely related to the nerve activity and is dependent on calcium concentration and temperature.[242] At this point, antitoxin is no longer effective.[242,255] Recovery from blockade is by terminal sprouting and establishment of new neuromuscular junctions.[73,255]

Treatment consists of the administration of bivalent (A and B) or trivalent (A, B, and E) antitoxin 20,000–40,000 units two to three times per day, in addition to removal of stomach and intestinal

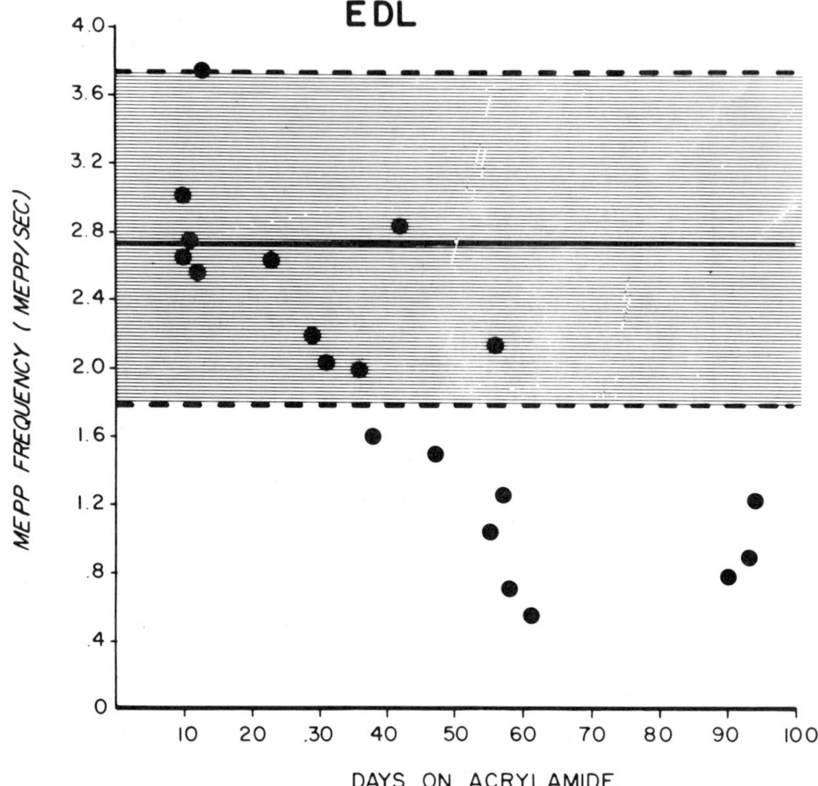

Figure 7.3. Experimental acrylamide neuropathy in rats. There is a progressive decrease in miniature endplate potential (mepp) frequency in extensor digitorum longus muscle the longer the animals are kept on the acrylamide-containing diet.

contents.[66] Treatment with oral penicillin to destroy organisms in the gut has not been proven to be beneficial.[132] Regardless of the apparent severity of the disease when first seen, full respiratory support must be readily available and endotrachial intubation should be performed when necessary.[66]

Guanidine in doses of 35 mg/kg may reverse the electrical defect and increase the muscle action potential.[46,103,196,212] It has been reported to be of benefit in some patients with botulism, but is not uniformly successful.[85,136] 4-Aminopyridine has also been used with some success,[20] including improvement of the electromyographic changes.[268] Neither of these agents significantly improve respiratory function.[46,212] There is little response to anticholinesterase agents.

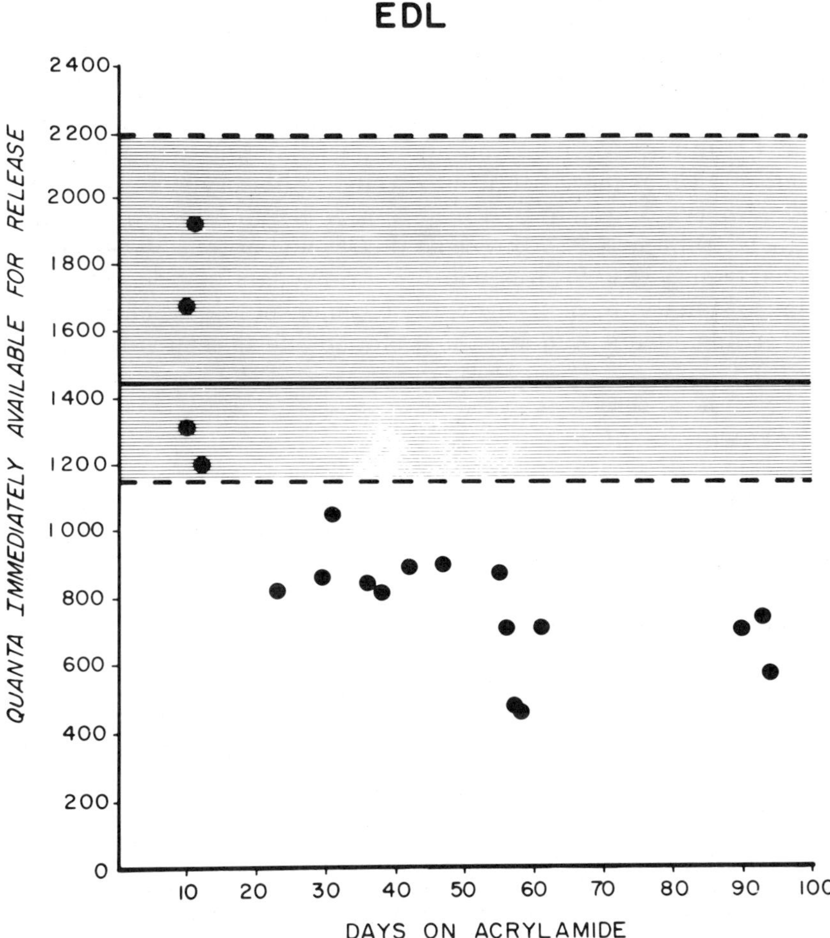

Figure 7.4. Experimental acrylamide neuropathy in rats. There is a progressive decrease in numbers of acetylcholine quanta available for release the longer the animals are kept on the acrylamide-containing diet.

Tetanus

Tetanus is caused by a closely related organism, *Clostridium tetani*, which produces an exotoxin inhibiting transmission at the neuromuscular junction.[127,211,255] A nerve-muscle preparation blocked by tetanus toxin generates miniature endplate potentials of reduced amplitude and frequency.[127,255] As with botulism, the steps which lead to tetanus neuromuscular blockade include binding (which is irreversible, independent of transmitter release and temperature, and prevented by antitoxin), translocation (which requires transmitter release, is dependent upon frequency of nerve stimulation and shows no effect from antitoxin), and paralysis (which is temperature dependent).[228] Tetanus toxin is 1000 times less potent than botulinum toxin at the neuromuscular junction, while it is about 500 times more potent at glycine inhibitory synapses in the central nervous system.[106] In contrast to botulinum toxin, tetanus toxin is transported to the central nervous system by retrograde axonal transport and subsequently by transynaptic retrograde movement to spinal interneurons where blockade of release of inhibitory neurotransmitters produces the profound effects seen clinically.[106]

Snake Envenomation

Envenomation by certain species of poisonous snakes may produce a clinical picture resembling myasthenic crisis.[40] Study of the compounds making up the crude venom has provided many investigational tools for the understanding of neuromuscular disorders in humans, yet most practicing physicians are unfamiliar with the clinical picture produced by envenomation.

Poisonous snakes belong to four families: Elapidae (cobras, coral snakes, mambas, kraits), Hydrophiidae (sea snakes), Viperidae (Old World vipers) and Crotalidae (rattlesnakes and related species). Neuromuscular blocking toxins are primarily those of the Elapidae and Hydrophiidae.[40,157,279] With Viperidae and Crotalidae toxins, death usually occurs through action on the cardiovascular system; the exception is the South American rattlesnake (*Crotalus durissus terrificus*) which produces a venom with potent neuromuscular toxicity.[40,115,127] In all four families of snakes, the venom is produced in specialized salivary glands analogous to the parotid glands and inoculated by modified premaxillary teeth or fangs.[40] The amount of venom injected is usually unknown, but in practice, the case fatality rate is low (estimated to be less than 5% from cobra bites). Even with this small number of deaths, every occurrence must be considered potentially lethal.

A preparalytic stage of envenomation occurs in 90% of victims who subsequently become paralyzed, particularly with krait, mamba and coral snakes, and less commonly with cobra bites.[40] The onset of symptoms may occur within 30 minutes or be delayed up to 12 hours.[40] The most common symptoms during this stage are headache and vomiting. Other symptoms include visual disturbances, parasthesias, drowsiness and hypotension.[40] Although the occurrence of these symptoms indicates venom injection, they are not necessarily followed by paralysis.

The paralytic stage will occur within one-half to twenty-three hours following the bite.[40] The first signs of paralysis appear in muscles supplied by cranial nerves with bilateral ptosis and extra-ocular muscle weakness or ophthalmoplegia. Tongue, laryngeal and pharyngeal weakness develops later.[5,40,219] Careful observation of victims is necessary because paralysis may continue to spread for up to 60 hours and tracheostomy may not be required until 24 to 48 hours following exposure.[40] Paralysis gradually reverses over the ensuing 3 to 10 days. Paralytic symptoms may show improvement with anticholinesterases;[188] however, antivenom[5,217,219] and ventilatory and cardiovascular support are the most effective forms of treatment.[173]

Case History

A 37-year-old Filipino was working in a field when he was bitten on the left ankle by a cobra (*Naja naja philippinesis*). Antivenom was administered at a local hospital, but he began progressively to lose strength. Four hours after the envenomation he required endotracheal intubation with assisted ventilation. He was transferred to the USAF Regional Medical Center at Clark Air Force Base where he was found by one of the authors (MKG) to have complete flaccid paralysis, complete external ophthalmoplegia, briskly reactive pupils, and absent muscle stretch reflexes. A repetitive stimulation study of the left ulnar nerve demonstrated an initial compound muscle action potential of 500 μV and a decrement of 70%. Partial repair of the decrement was evident after ten seconds of tetanizing stimulation. An electroencephalogram the following day was normal.

Two days following admission, the patient was found to have minimal voluntary movement, absent muscle stretch reflexes and complete external ophthalmoplegia. A repeat of the ulnar repetitive stimulation study demonstrated an initial compound muscle action potention of 5,000 μV and a decrement of 60%. The decrement disappeared following tetanization. At this time, a trial of neostigmine (1 mg I.V.) produced a reversal of his ophthalmoplegia and marked improvement in extremity strength. He was placed on pyridostigmine via nasogastric tube with gradual improvement in strength until he was extubated on the sixth hospital day. Pyridostigmine was discontinued on the eighth hospital day. Recovery was complicated by skin and tissue necrosis around the bite, necessitating skin grafting. He was discharged from the hospital in good condition 40 days following the cobra bite.

Venoms from cobras (*Naja* sp.), kraits (*Bungarus* sp.) and coral snakes (*Micrurus* sp.) are complex mixtures of proteins and polypeptides, some having enzymatic or mild digestive activity.[33,40,53,127,156,157,279] The purified neurotoxic components of venoms which act postsynaptically are all devoid of enzymatic activity.[40,127] Along with the neurotoxin, cobra venom contains a cardiotoxin that produces muscle contracture leading to necrosis[40,127,279] followed by paralysis which fails to respond to direct or indirect stimulation.[40] However, the principal lethal component in cobra venom for most animals is the neurotoxin.

The action of purified venom neurotoxins from these three species fall into three groups: (1) irreversible postsynaptic acetylcholine receptor blockade (e.g., α-bungarotoxin), (2) partially reversible postsynaptic acetylcholine receptor blockade (e.g. cobra neurotoxin) and (3) presynaptic neurotoxin, inhibiting release of acetycholine (e.g. β-bungarotoxin).[40,43,156] The postsynaptic effect of cobra neurotoxin and α-bungarotoxin are characterized by a non-depolarizing blockade due to occupation of acetylcholine receptors on the postjunctional membrane of the muscle fiber.[33,44,156,157,159] In contrast to α-bungarotoxin, cobra neurotoxin may be partially antagonized by anticholinesterase drugs[33,40,156,219,279] and can be removed by repeated washing *in vitro*. These neurotoxins show synergism with curare in inhibiting the effect of topically applied acetylcholine,[44,159] while pretreatment of the muscle-nerve preparation with curare will prevent permanent toxin fixation.[40] Miniature endplate potentials are of reduced amplitude but normal number. There are no effects on terminal nerve conduction, muscle membrane properties or acetylcholine release.[44,156,159] When administered to experimental animals, the purified toxins (both α-bungarotoxin and cobra neurotoxin) produce signs and symptoms resembling myasthenia gravis, including decreasing amplitude of evoked muscle action potential on repetitive nerve stimulation and postactivation exhaustion.[226,265]

The affinity and specificity of α-bungarotoxin for the nicotinic acetylcholine receptor is such that it has been used in the purification of receptor protein[198] and in the identification of receptor complexes in tissue sections.[10,272] The toxin is also used in the radioimmunoassay of antireceptor antibodies present in patients with myasthenia gravis.[163]

The presynaptic neurotoxins (β-bungarotoxin, notoxin, taipoxin) all are enzymatically active with phospholipase activity.[89,100,109,127] These toxins inhibit release of acetylcholine and may serve to potentiate the neuromuscular transmission defect. The reduction in acetylcholine release is usually preceded by an increased frequency of miniature endplate potentials.[156] The toxins have no effect on miniature endplate potential amplitude, acetylcholine response, or the terminal nerve spike.[40] Following toxin administration, quantum content of endplate potentials progressively decreases to the level of miniature endplate potentials. Complete failure of impulse-induced transmitter release then occurs. Finally, miniature endplate potentials disappear.[158] The mechanism of action of these toxins is not fully understood. They may depress transmitter release by interference with endocytosis of the vesicle membrane, block choline transport, or alter acetylcholine compartmentalization.[67,100,127]

Sea snakes are a specialized group of snakes adapted for marine life and are recognized by their vertically flattened tails. They are found in Southeast Asia, the Indian and Southwest Pacific Oceans and the western coast of tropical America.[250] One species inhabits a freshwater lake in the Philippines.[250] The snakes are generally found in shallow coastal waters, and fishermen are the usual human victims.[217,250] Symptoms from the bite of sea snakes may have a latent period from a few minutes to several hours. This is followed by myalgias, muscle stiffness with increased passive resistance, and trismus progressing to widespread rhabdomyolysis and myoglobinuria.[218,250] Other symptoms include parotid swelling, diaphoresis, nausea and vomiting. Death results from respiratory paralysis, hyperkalemia or acute renal failure. The toxin has been shown to have irreversible nondepolarizing neuromuscular blocking activity.[41,127,139,250] Antivenin therapy is available and may be helpful.[217,250]

The South American rattlesnake (*Crotalus durissus terrificus*) produces a clinical picture similar to that of Elapidae envenomation. The two major toxins are crotamine and crotoxin. Certain subspecies of this snake produce a venom which lacks crotamine. Crotamine produces repetitive muscle action potentials by a direct depolarizing effect on the muscle membrane and has no effect at the motor endplate.[156,250,280] The principal action of crotoxin is thought to be a nondepolarizing neuromuscular blockade; however, presynaptic inhibition of acetylcholine release has also been found.[115,127] The toxin may have more presynaptic activity in amphibian muscles, while in mammalian muscles the postsynaptic effects may be most prominent.[156]

Arthropod Envenomation

The arthropod neurotoxins affect release of transmitter at the neuromuscular junction. The mechanisms of action include:[207]

(1) increase in transmitter release followed by transmitter depletion (black widow spider venom, brown widow spider venom); (2) increase in transmitter release without transmitter depletion (funnel-web spider, some species of scorpion); (3) decrease in transmitter release without transmitter depletion (solitary wasps). No efficient or specific antagonism of transmitter-receptor interaction occurs with arthropod venoms; however, certain scorpion and solitary wasp venoms affect the postsynaptic ionophore without transmitter-receptor antagonism.[207]

Envenomation by the female black widow spider (*Latrodectus mactans*) causes diffuse central and peripheral nervous system stimulation with vasoconstriction, hypertension, and autonomic hyperactivity.[96] The effects on muscle and neuromuscular junction begin 15–60 minutes after envenomation, with muscle cramps involving the trunk and extremities. The abdomen may develop board-like rigidity, and pain may be extreme.[96]

Black widow spider venom has a presynaptic site of action when tested in nerve-muscle preparations. The purified toxin (α-latrotoxin) increases the release of acetylcholine quanta at vertebrate neuromuscular junctions to the point where vesicles are depleted from the nerve terminal and release stops.[90,127,207] A separate toxin (Fraction E) is responsible for venom effect studied in certain invertebrate species.

Although normal concentrations of calcium augment release, black widow spider venom can exert its effect even in calcium-free solutions,[18,127,207] implying that the release may be through a calcium-independent mechanism, or that intracellular calcium is utilized. The venom probably also prevents endocytosis of vesicle membrane.[127] These effects on the nerve terminal may be related to the venom's ability to insert itself into the membrane to form permanent ionic conductance channels. Brown widow spider (*Latrodectus geometricus*) venom has similar properties but causes discontinuous release of acetylcholine.[61]

Treatment is empiric, consisting of warming and calcium gluconate infusions to reduce muscle cramping. The administration of magnesium sulfate intravenously may help to reduce transmitter release and to control convulsions.[96] It is not certain whether these measures are effective, however. In addition, 2.5 ml of reconstituted antiserum should be administered and this dose repeated if necessary. Atropine may also be beneficial.[97]

The Sydney funnel-web spider (*Atrax robustus*) is a large aggressive spider which produces in its victims nausea, vomiting, abdominal pain, diarrhea, diaphoresis, salivation, lacrimation, hypertension, muscle fasciculations and coma.[92,110,256] Death may occur from asphyxia or cardiac arrest.[110] The toxin produced by male spiders is several times more potent than that of females.[17,207] The toxin (atraxotoxin) produces a repetitive response to single nerve stimulation in nerve-muscle preparations[207] and also the release of transmitter at adrenergic sites.[207] Atraxotoxin affects neuromuscular transmission by promotion of transmitter release without depletion and without anticholinesterase activity.[207]

Paralysis may also occur in human as a result of a salivary toxin elaborated by female ticks[48,260] (Fig. 7.5). Tick paralysis occurs rapidly, is generalized, and may lead to respiratory depression if the offending tick is not found and removed. Patients show severe motor weakness but do not fatigue and do not respond to anticholinesterase drugs.[48,260] Electromyographic studies reveal slowing of motor and sensory nerve conduction[48,182,185,260] One report of a decremental response to repetitive stimulation at 30 Hz has appeared.[182] Terminal motor nerve twigs are believed to be especially vulnerable.[84, 185,260] Endplate potentials at neuromuscular junctions poisoned with toxin from North American ticks (*Dermacentor andersoni* and *Dermacentor variabilis*) are normal,[170] but toxin from an Australian tick (*Ixodes holocylus*) has produced temperature-dependent reduction in evoked transmitter release, suggesting that presynaptic inhibition of acetylcholine release may contribute to paralysis in certain cases.[51]

Scorpion toxin increases acetylcholine release at the neuromuscular junction only secondarily by inducing repetitive potentials in nerve terminal membrane.[288] This effect occurs by delaying the normal sodium channel inactivation during the action potential. Acetylcholine release may be increased as much as 86% and is prevented by tetrodotoxin.[1] Similar effects occur in muscle membrane. The scorpion sting results in serious visceral effects, but clinical disturbances of neuromuscular transmission are not prominent.

A syndrome resembling ocular myasthenia gravis has been reported in a patient within 24 hours of having been stung by wasps.[30] The syndrome persisted for weeks and appeared to be responsive to anticholinesterase drugs and prednisone. Bee,[107] wasp,[107] and hornet[137] venoms have been reported to cause neuromuscular junction disturbances in arthropods, and to produce direct effects on muscle in mammals.[107] However, neuromuscular transmission disturbances are not a regular feature of human envenomation by these species.

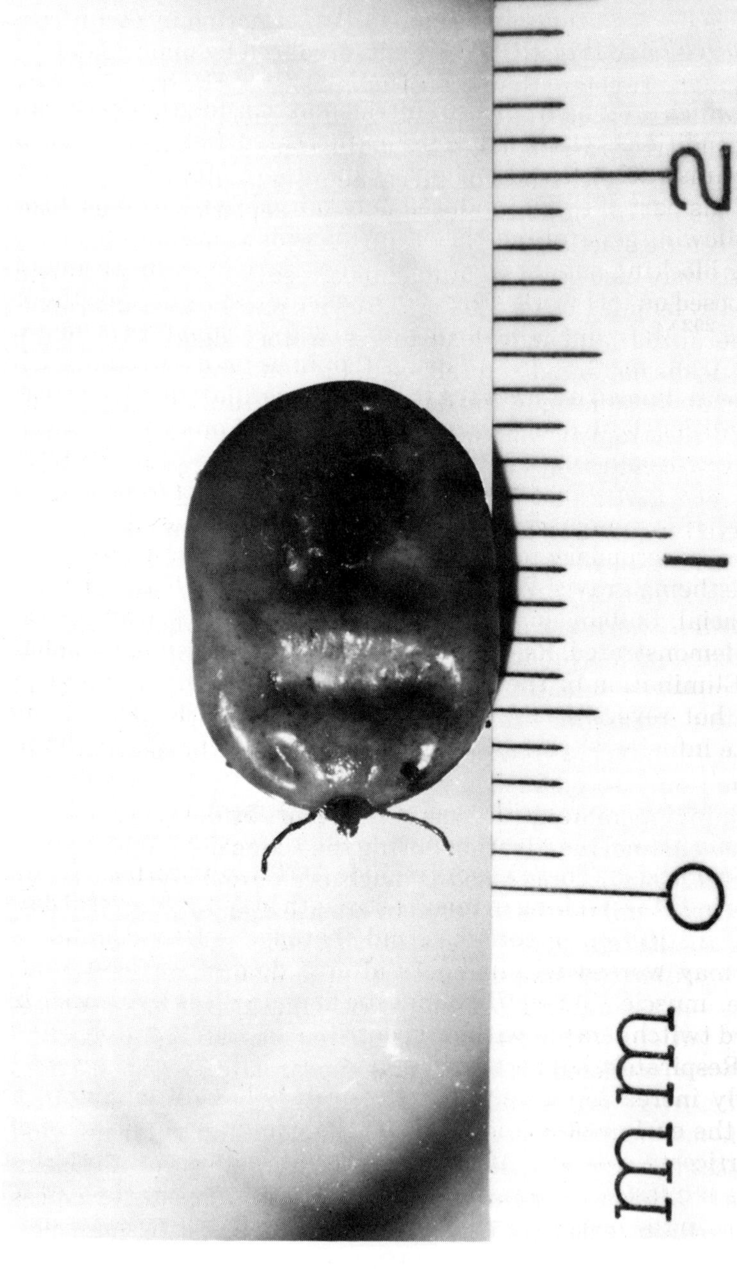

Figure 7.5. Tick (*Dermacentor andersonii*) removed from the occipital region of a five-year-old boy with tick paralysis.

Exogenous Disorders Induced
by Pharmacologic Agents

Presynaptically Acting Drugs

Drugs which alter neuromuscular transmission do so under certain clinical conditions: (1) in patients at increased risk of coincident drug administration, renal or hepatic disease or electrolyte disturbance; (2) as part of a drug-induced generalized immunologic disorder; (3) following general anesthesia during which concomitant neuromuscular blocking agents may or may not have been used; and (4) superimposed on and worsening of myasthenia gravis or myasthenic syndrome.[292] Many drugs have a potential deleterious effect on neuromuscular transmission, and all drugs should be used with caution in patients with known disorders at the neuromuscular junction.[11] This section will deal with drugs which appear to affect presynaptic mechanisms of neuromuscular transmission; however, most drugs affect both pre- and postsynaptic processes. (See also Chapter 4.)

Clinically, symptoms in patients with disturbed neuromuscular transmission secondary to drugs resemble those in naturally occurring myasthenia gravis. Weakness is most commonly found in extraocular, facial, bulbar, or proximal extremity muscles. Fatigue can often be demonstrated. Respiratory weakness may occur early and be severe. Elimination of the suspected offending agent is the major therapy, but reversing the block may be attempted with calcium gluconate infusion,[11] potassium supplementation,[52] and anticholinesterases.[11]

Agents which have been used in the treatment of autoimmune myasthenia gravis have been shown to alter presynaptic neuromuscular transmission. These agents include ACTH, corticosteroids, and azathioprine. A worsening in muscle strength may occur several days after the institution of corticosteroid therapy.[178] Decremental responses may worsen within hours after a dose of corticosteroids. Likewise, muscle contractility may be impaired (as evidenced by decreased twitch tension without a decrease in muscle action potential).[177] Respiratory support may be necessary if the block is severe.[94] Gradually increasing doses of corticosteroids have been shown to prevent the early worsening.[232] From their immunosuppressive effects, corticosteroids and ACTH often result in eventual partial or complete remission of myasthenic symptoms.[32,282] (See chapter 6.) Reduction in the level of circulating antiacetylcholine receptor antibody levels has been shown.[69] The effects of corticosteroids on neuromuscular transmission observed experimentally include depolarization of nerve terminals with reduction in transmitter release,[124] repetitive activity in motor nerve terminals,[62] changes in endplate potentials,[62,74,259,294] changes in choline transport,[160] antagonism of neuromuscular blocking agents,[16,297] and intracellular potassium depletion.[74] The clinical significance of these effects are unknown.[124,192]

Azathioprine, which has been used in immunosuppressive treatment of myasthenia gravis, has been shown to act presynaptically in antagonizing the effects of neuromuscular blocking drugs. This drug inhibits the action of phosphodiesterase. This increases transmitter release from the nerve terminal by allowing cyclic AMP to persist in the nerve terminal for a longer duration.[72]

Recently the calcium channel blocker verapamil was reported by Krendel and Hopkins to have exacerbated weakness in the Lambert-Eaton myasthenic syndrome,[259] possibly by interfering with calcium influx into presynaptic nerve terminals.

Postsynaptically Acting Drugs

Several commonly used drugs have their primary effects on neuromuscular transmission through action restricted to the postsynaptic membrane.

Some patients treated with D-penicillamine have developed signs and symptoms typical of myasthenia gravis (see chapter 6). This complication has occurred in patients treated for rheumatoid arthritis,[7,8,35] Wilson's disease,[169] and scleroderma.[37] The syndrome is associated with circulating antiacetylcholine receptor antibodies.[8,22,169,223,278] The drug has been shown to bind to acetylcholine receptor and induce structural changes that may result in an alteration of the receptor protein as an antigen, and trigger autoimmunity.[22] This results in an increased rate of degradation of receptors.[22] Decremental responses to repetitive stimulation have been demonstrated clinically and in experimental animals.[8,38,155] Strength improves over several weeks to months after the drug is discontinued as the antibody level falls.[8,35,169,223,278] Remission occurs in 70% of patients within one year of withdrawal.[8] The drug has no direct neuromuscular blocking activity.[9] To determine the incidence of this complication, patients with rheumatoid arthritis being treated with or without D-penicillamine[7,12] have been examined for electrophysiologic changes of defective neuromuscular transmission. These studies suggest that most patients treated with D-penicillamine do not develop clinical or electrophysiological changes or antiacetylcholine receptor antibodies.[12]

The ganglionic blocking agent trimethaphan produces hypotension through blockade of acetylcholine receptors in ganglia. The drug may have a direct curare-like effect at the neuromuscular junction.[214] Plasma pseudocholinesterase is also inhibited by the drug and can prolong and augment the neuromuscular blockade induced by depolarizing agents.[210] Oculobulbar signs and acute respiratory paralysis have been reported in patients treated with this drug.[55]

Generalized weakness which is corrected by anticholinesterase drugs has been reported with phenothiazines (chlorpromazine and promazine).[172,215] Experiments have shown that these drugs antagonize the action of applied acetylcholine and may worsen myasthenia gravis.[172] Prolonged apnea from succinylcholine occurred in a patient treated with concomitant phenothiazine.[215] Characteristic decremental responses with repetitive nerve stimulation have been found.[172]

Carnitine plays a role in transport of long-chain fatty acids into mitochondria. It has been used to treat certain lipid storage myopathies[79] and in some hemodialysis patients to correct high plasma triglyceride levels. Neuromuscular blocking activity has been demonstrated for certain carnitine derivatives in nerve-muscle preparations.[126] Only recently, however, have patients been described who developed weakness as a result of carnitine treatment.[79] These patients were being treated for hypertriglyceridemia secondary to hemodialysis. Electrophysiologic studies showed decrement, increased jitter, and blocking.[58] Partial correction with edrophonium was noted.

Pre- and Postsynaptically Acting Drugs

A syndrome similar to myasthenia gravis has been reported in patients on anticonvulsant drugs including phenytoin,[31, 123,195,249] mephenytoin,[123,216] and trimethadione.[23,205] The weakness may resolve quickly when the drug is discontinued, implying a direct effect at the neuromuscular junction.[31,123,216] At the nerve terminal phenytoin has been shown to block release of stimulus-evoked acetylcholine quanta; however, spontaneously released acetylcholine may be increased.[300] The amplitude of miniature endplate potentials has been shown to be reduced, probably by desensitizing the endplate.[300]

Anticonvulsants may produce neuromuscular blockade by promoting an autoimmune reaction against the neuromuscular junction.

This notion is supported by the finding of antithymic, antimuscular, and antinuclear antibodies,[23,205] as well as the protracted course for recovery after some agents are discontinued.[23,205]

Certain cardiovascular agents have been found to worsen or unmask myasthenia gravis or to exacerbate postoperative respiratory depression. Quinidine and procainamide, when used as antiarrhythmic drugs, have produced this clinical problem[70,291] and procainamide was shown to induce myasthenic weakness in a patient with uremic polyneuropathy.[191] These changes in strength may not be reversed by anticholinesterse drugs.[70,291] Quinidine and procainamide are similar to the parent compounds—procaine, quinine, and lidocaine—in that the effect produced may be a curariform effect on acetylcholine receptors,[70,112] and perhaps a local anesthetic action to impair propagation of nerve terminal action potentials.[70] These drugs have been used in the treatment of myotonia[162] and have a direct effect of reducing propagation of muscle action potentials.

The beta-adrenergic blocking agents have been reported to produce myasthenic weakness or to unmask or exacerbate myasthenia gravis.[118,233] These agents have a curariform action and are reversible with anticholinesterase drugs. These effects have been reported with propranolol, oxyprenolol, practolol and timolol.[118,128,233] At high concentrations these drugs also have an effect on presynaptic mechanisms.[295]

Lithium has been reported to potentiate neuromuscular blocking agents,[24] and in a patient who subsequently developed myasthenia gravis, produced profound weakness.[189] Lithium may interfere with acetylcholine synthesis[281] and has an effect on transmitter release from nerve terminals, both spontaneous and evoked.[26] Lithium has also been shown to reduce the number of acetylcholine receptors.[201]

Chloroquine has been reported to disturb neuromuscular transmission and to cause postoperative respiratory depression.[133] The drug has a local anesthetic effect on nerve and directly suppresses the excitability of muscle fiber membranes.[273] It may also act by reducing the amplitude of the endplate potential. Thyroid hormone may exacerbate weakness in myasthenia,[68,193,213] possibly by an effect on the amplitude of the endplate potential. Likewise, hypothyroid patients may show disorders of neuromuscular transmission.[68,143,194,263] A disease similar to the myasthenic syndrome with marked facilitation has been reported in association with hypothyroidism.[263] In patients with thyroid disease, most neuromuscular transmission abnormalities are due to coexistent myasthenia gravis.[237]

Antibiotics and Neuromuscular Transmission Disorders

Antibiotics can alter neuromuscular transmission by either pre- and/or postsynaptic mechanisms. The clinical toxicity and mechanisms of action have been reviewed elsewhere[248] and will only briefly be presented here. The polymyxin antibiotics are capable of producing weakness most frequently in the presence of renal disease[11,171,208] or myasthenia gravis[125,171,208] or when used in combination with other antibiotics or muscle relaxants,[11,171,208] and only occasionally in normal subjects.[171,208] Of this group of antibiotics, the ones that most commonly produce neuromuscular transmission disturbances are polymyxin A and B, colistimethate, and colistin. When severe, the weakness may lead to respiratory depression and apnea. Muscles frequently involved include the levator palpebrae, extraocular and bulbar muscles. Paresthesias may also occur.[171,208] Strength may be improved with calcium infusions or anticholinesterase drugs,[208,247] but these may have no effect or actually worsen the blockade.[171,208,244,246] By increasing transmitter release, 4-aminopyridine may reverse the neuromuscular blockade.[244] Improvement usually occurs when the polymyxins are withdrawn. The major neuromuscular effects are a result of noncompetitive postsynaptic blockade of acetylcholine receptors[244,246,299] and reduction in muscle contractility. Repetitive nerve stimulation studies have demonstrated reduced amplitude of compound muscle action potentials which will decline at both low and high rates of stimulation.[171] Facilitation of the motor response has not been observed.[119,171,208]

Aminoglycoside antibiotics have been known for over 25 years to produce neuromuscular weakness with respiratory depression resembling myasthenia gravis.[171,208,245,287,290] Weakness may occur when the drugs are administered by a variety of routes including oral, intramuscular, intravenous and intraperitoneal.[171,287] Antibiotics in this group include streptomycin, dihydrostreptomycin, neomycin, kanamycin, gentamicin, tobramycin, and amikacin. Pupillary abnormalities have been reported.[171] The degree of weakness is proportional to the dose and to the serum concentrations.[167] Strength may be improved in part by anticholinesterase agents, and to a much greater extent by calcium.[171,208] Neomycin has the greatest potential for producing weakness, whereas tobramycin has the least.[65] Microelectrode studies have demonstrated that these drugs act like toxic levels of magnesium[60] by decreasing transmitter release, both spontaneous and that evoked by nerve stimulation or high potassium solutions.[77,]

[245,246] Reduction in the endplate potential occurs due to both a reduced number of quanta released and a diminished effect of the acetylcholine on the postsynaptic membrane.[77,245,246] A new drug related to the aminoglycosides, spectinomycin, acts in a similar fashion.[247]

Other antibiotics which produce disorders of neuromuscular transmission include the monobasic amino acid antibiotics, lincomycin and clindamycin. With both drugs the neuromuscular blockade is not readily reversed by anticholinesterase drugs.[88,224] Both drugs produce this effect by pre- and postjunctional mechanisms and cause a reduction in miniature endplate potential frequency, evoked transmitter release, and postjunctional acetylcholine sensitivity.[221,246] Lincomycin blockade may be reversed by raising the calcium concentration or by the addition of 3,4-diaminopyridine,[244] but may actually be worsened by neostigmine.[246] Clindamycin appears to block muscle contractility directly and may have a local anesthetic effect.[246] In the tetracycline group, neuromuscular blockade has been reported with tetracycline,[243] oxytetracycline,[243] and rolitetracycline.[299] Studies on nerve-muscle preparations suggest that these actions have an effect like d-tubocurarine in competitively inhibiting the postjunctional acetylcholine receptors.[243,299] Although experimental studies have shown a competitive receptor block, tetracyclines are known to chelate calcium and might be expected to reduce transmitter release. The drugs may also have a direct effect on muscle contractility. Exacerbation of myasthenia gravis has been reported with oxytetracycline and rolitetracycline.[208]

Miscellaneous Agents

A small number of case reports have documented several other drugs to cause defective neuromuscular transmission: tetanus antitoxin,[129] methoxyflurane, aprotinin, and oxytocin.[8] The underlying mechanism for these disorders is unclear.

Magnesium Intoxication

Calcium and magnesium act antagonistically at the neuromuscular junction. Transmitter release varies in proportion to calcium concentration and is inversely related to magnesium concentration. Low calcium concentrations impair transmitter release; however, clinically this effect is overshadowed by the fasciculations, tetany, muscle spasms, and marked excess excitability of peripheral nerve and muscle. In contrast, high concentrations of magnesium produce a clinically obvious disturbance of neuromuscular transmission by altering transmitter release mechanisms[104,253,257] as well as by reducing end-plate sensitivity to applied acetylcholine.[60,87]

Magnesium toxicity occurs in three clinical settings: (1) patients with renal failure, (2) in eclamptic women treated with parenteral magnesium, and (3) in patients given magnesium cathartics who already have defective neuromuscular transmission.[87,104,252,253,257,284]

Other clinical manifestations of magnesium intoxication include altered levels of consciousness ranging from sedation to coma, electrocardiographic changes, cardiac rhythm disturbances, and dry mouth.[284] Decreased muscle stretch reflexes and weakness occur and may lead to paralysis as the magnesium level rises above 4.0 mEq/L.[252] Newborn infants of mothers treated with magnesium for eclampsia may develop weakness.[164] Normal individuals given oral or rectal magnesium may absorb enough of the ion to produce neuromuscular toxicity.[252]

Electrodiagnostic studies are similar to those of other conditions in which transmitter release is impaired. The initial muscle action potential is of low amplitude and decrements further at low rates of nerve stimulation. Marked facilitation of the muscle action potential will occur with exercise or at rates of stimulation above 10 Hz.[257]

Treatment of magnesium intoxication[164,252] involves administering intravenous calcium gluconate. If magnesium has been administered orally or rectally, elimination from the bowel should be assisted. Some clinical improvement has been shown with anticholinesterase drugs.[257] Agents which have been experimentally shown to produce an increase in transmitter release, such as guanidine or 4-aminopyridine, reverse the blockade by magnesium,[141,197,267] but these agents have not been used clinically for this disorder.

Anticholinesterase Agents

Toxicity from anticholinesterase agents carries the potential of a major public health hazard. Toxicity occurs in occupational or accidental exposure to insecticides,[71,116,270,285] in homicides or suicides,[134] and in overmedication with anticholinesterase drugs.[144] Chemical warfare "nerve gases" are a potential hazard.[144] The agents are structurally similar to acetylcholine and bind to cholinesterase.

They produce their effect by blocking the hydrolysis sites for acetylcholine.[144] By doing so, released acetylcholine will escape hydrolysis and have a longer duration of action. This produces an increase in transmitter effect at muscarinic (glands, smooth muscle), nicotinic (ganglionic, neuromuscular junction), and central cholinergic sites. Acetylcholine in high concentrations will produce a depolarizing block at nicotonic receptor sites. The clinical manifestations of anticholinesterase toxicity include increased glandular secretions and gastrointestinal motility, pupillary constriction, alterations in heart rate and blood pressure, muscular weakness, fasciculations,[168] and changes in sensorium including delerium and coma. Quaternary ammonium drugs, such as those used to treat myasthenia gravis (see chapter 6), do not penetrate the central nervous system and also have a unique direct effect on muscle and nerve, resembling applied acetylcholine.[144]

Electrophysiologic studies of patients with anticholinesterase toxicity reveal evidence of an excess acetylcholine effect.[113,116,285] A single nerve stimulation will produce repetitive muscle action potentials. A decremental response to repetitive stimulation occurs, which may become worse if additional anticholinesterase is given.[113,134,276,285] The diagnosis depends on the history, clinical signs, low serum cholinesterase levels and the characteristic electromyographic findings.

Treatment includes oxygenation and endotracheal intubation as needed. Muscarinic and central nervous system effects must be reversed with large doses of atropine (2–4 mg intravenously and repeated as necessary).[116,144,176] In patients poisoned with anticholinesterase agents that bind irreversibly, spontaneous improvement is slow and must await new enzyme synthesis which proceeds at a rate of 1% per day.[144] However, skeletal muscle weakness may be treated with pralidoxime (1 gm intravenously repeated in 20 minutes if necessary). This agent produces its effect by displacing the drug from the cholinesterase and regenerating the enzyme.[144] Rapid reversal may occur and the motor response to nerve stimulation may appear within minutes.

Agents commonly responsible for anticholinesterase poisoning include organophosphorus and carbamate insecticides (parathion, malathion, mipafox, EPN, Bagon, Isopestox, IMPA, carbaryl, Lammate, trichlorfon and Divipan),[276] drugs used in treatment of neuromuscular transmission disorders (pyridostigmine, physostigmine, ambenonium, edrophonium),[144] and drugs used to treat other conditions (ecothiophate).[95] Other neuromuscular effects from organophosphorus drugs include peripheral neuropathy and myopathy.[4,270]

References

1. Abdul-Ghani A, Coutinho-Netto J, Bradford HF: *In vivo* release of acetylcholine evoked by brachial plexus stimulation and tityustoxin. *Biochem Pharmacol* 29:2179–2182, 1980.
2. Achari AN, Trontelj JV, Campos RJ: Multiple sclerosis and myasthenia gravis: A case report with single fiber electromyography. *Neurology* (Minneapolis) 26:544–546, 1976.
3. Agoston S, Van Weerden P, Broekert A: Effects of 4-aminopyridine in Eaton-Lambert syndrome. *Br J Anaesth* 50:383–385, 1978.
4. Ahlgren JD, Manz HJ, Harvey JC: Myopathy of chronic organophosphate poisoning: a clinical entity. *South Med J* 72:555–563, 1979.
5. Ahuja ML, Singh G: Snakebite in India. In Buckley EE, Porges N (eds): *Venoms.* American Association for the Advancement of Sciences, Washington, DC, 1956, pp 341–351.
6. Aita JF, Snyder DH: Myasthenia gravis and multiple sclerosis: An unusual combination of diseases. *Neurology* (Minneapolis) 24:72–75, 1974.
7. Albers JW, Beals CA, Levine SP: Neuromuscular transmission in rheumatoid arthritis, with and without penicillamine treatment. *Neurology* 31:1562–1564, 1981.
8. Albers JW, Hodach RT, Kimmel DW, Treacy WL: Penicillamine-associated myasthenia gravis. *Neurology* 30:1246–1249, 1980.
9. Aldrich MS, Kim YI, Sanders DB: Effects of D-penicillamine on neuromuscular transmission in rats. *Muscle Nerve* 2:180–185, 1979.
10. Almon RR, Andrew CG, Appel SH: Serum globulin in myasthenia gravis: inhibition of alpha-bungarotoxin binding to acetylcholine receptors. *Science* 186:55–57, 1974.
11. Argoz Z, Mastaglia FL: Disorders of neuromuscular transmission caused by drugs. *N Engl J Med* 301:409–413, 1979.
12. Argoz Z, Nicholson L, Fawcell PRW, Mastaglia FL, Hall M: Neuromuscular transmission and acetylcholine receptor antibodies in rheumatoid arthritis patients on D-penicillamine. *Lancet* 1:203, 1980.
13. Arnon SS, Damus K, Chin J: Infant botulism: epidemiology and relation to sudden infant death syndrome. *Epidemiol Rev* 3:45–66, 1981.
14. Arnon SS, Midura TF, Clay SA, Wood RM, Chin J: Infant botulism. *JAMA* 237:1946–1951, 1977.
15. Arnon SS, Midura TF, Damus K, Wood RM, Chin J: Intestinal infection and toxin production by *Clostridium botulinum* as one cause of sudden death syndrome. *Lancet* 1:1273–1276, 1978.
16. Arts WF, Oosterhuis HJ: Effect of prednisolone on neuromuscular blocking in mice in vivo. *Neurology* (Minneapolis) 25:1088–1090, 1975.
17. Atkinson RK: Comparisons of the neurotoxic activity of the venom of several species of funnel web spiders (Atrax). *Aust J Exp Biol Med Sci* 59:307–316, 1981.
18. Baba A, Cooper JR: The action of black widow spider venom on cholinergic mechanisms in synaptosomes. *J Neurochem* 34:1369–1379, 1980.
19. Baginsky RG: A case of peripheral polyneuropathy displaying myasthenic EMG patterns. *Electroencephalogr Clin Neurophysiol* 25:397, 1968.

20. Ball AP, Hopkinson RB, Farrell ID, Hutchinson JGP, Paul R, Watson RDS, Page AJF, Parker RGF, Edwards CW, Snow M, Scott DK, Leone-Ganado A, Hastings A, Ghosh AC, Gilbert RJ: Human botulism caused by *Clostridium botulinum* type E: the Birmingham outbreak. *Q J Med Series* 48:473–491, 1979.

21. Bernstein LP, Antel JP: Motor neuron disease: Decremental responses to repetitive nerve stimulation. *Neurology* 31:202–204, 1981.

22. Bever C, Chang HW, Penn AS, Jaffe IA, Bock E: Chemical alteration of AChR by penicillamine: A mechanism for the induction of myasthenia gravis. *Neurology* 31(2):84, 1981.

23. Booker HE, Chun RE, Sanguino M: Myasthenia gravis syndrome associated with trimethadione. *JAMA* 212:2262–2263, 1970.

24. Borden H, Clarke M, Katz H: The use of pancuronium bromide in patients receiving lithium carbonate. *Can Anaesth Soc J* 21:79–82, 1974.

25. Bowman JR: Myasthenia gravis in young children. *Pediatrics* 1:472–477, 1948.

26. Brainisteanu DD, Volle RL: Modification by lithium of transmitter release at the neuromuscular junction of the frog. *J Pharmacol Exp Ther* 194:362–372, 1975.

27. Brooke MH: Myasthenic syndrome (Eaton-Lambert Syndrome). In *A Clinician's View of Neuromuscular Disease*. Baltimore, Williams and Wilkins, 1977, pp 89–91.

28. Brown JC, Johns RJ: Clinical and physiological studies of the effect of guanidine on patients with myasthenia gravis. *Johns Hopkins Med J* 124:1–8, 1969.

29. Brown JW, Nelson JR, Herrmann C Jr: Sjogren's syndrome with myopathic and myasthenic features. *Bull Los Angeles Neurol Soc* 33:9–20, 1968.

30. Brumlik J: Myasthenia gravis associated with wasp sting. *JAMA* 235:2120–2121, 1976.

31. Brumlik J, Jacobs RS: Myasthenia gravis associated with diphenylhydantoin therapy for epilepsy. *Can J Neurol Sci* 1:127–129, 1974.

32. Brunner NG, Namba T, Grob D: Corticosteroids in management of severe, generalized myasthenia gravis: effectiveness and comparison with corticotropin therapy. *Neurology* (Minneapolis) 22:603–610, 1972.

33. Brunton TL, Rayrer J: On the nature and physiological action of the poison of *Naja tripudians* and other Indian venomous snakes. *Proc R Soc London* 22:68–113, 1874.

34. Buchthal F, Honcke P: Electromyographical examination of patients suffering from poliomyelitis anterior acuta up to six months after the acute stage of disease. *Acta Med Scand* 116:148–164, 1943.

35. Buchnall RC, Dixon AStJ, Glick EN, Woodland J, Zutshi DW: Myasthenia gravis associated with penicillamine treatment for rheumatoid arthritis. *Br Med J* 1:600–602, 1975.

36. Bundey S: A genetic study of infantile and juvenile myasthenia gravis. *J Neurol Neurosurg Psychiatry* 35:41–51, 1972.

37. Burres SA, Kanter ME, Richman DP, Aranson BGW: Studies on the pathophysiology of chronic D-penicillamine-induced myasthenia. *Ann N Y Acad Sci* 377:640–651, 1981.

38. Burres SA, Richman DP, Crayton JW, Aranson BGW: Penicillamine-induced myasthenic responses in the guinea pig. *Muscle Nerve* 2:186–190, 1979.
39. Campa JF, Johns TR, Adelman LS: Familial myasthenia with "tubular aggregates." *Neurology* (Minneapolis) 21:449, 1971.
40. Campbell CH: The effects of snake venoms and their neurotoxins on the nervous system of man and animals. In Hornabrook RW (ed): *Topics on Tropical Neurology*. Philadelphia, FA Davis, 1975, pp 259–293.
41. Carey JE, Wright EA: The site of action of the venom of the sea snake *Enhydrina schistosa*. *Trans R Soc Trop Med Hyg* 55:153–160, 1961.
42. Cendrowski W: A case of multiple sclerosis associated with defective neuromuscular transmission. *Acta Neurol Belg* 75:11–14, 1975.
43. Chang CC, Chen TF, Lee CY: Studies of the presynaptic effect of β-bungarotoxin on neuromuscular transmission. *J Pharmacol Exp Ther* 184:339–345, 1973.
44. Chang CC, Lee CY: Electrophysiological study of the neuromuscular blocking action of cobra neurotoxin. *Br J Pharmacol* 28:172–181, 1966.
45. Chelmicka-Schorr E, Bernstein LP, Surbrugg EG, Huttenlocher PR: Eaton-Lambert syndrome in a 9-year-old girl. *Arch Neurol* 36:572–574, 1979.
46. Cherington M: Botulism: Ten-year experience. *Arch Neurol* 30:432–437, 1974.
47. Cherington M: Guanidine and germine in Eaton-Lambert syndrome. *Neurology* (Minneapolis) 26:944–946, 1976.
48. Cherington M, Snyder R: Tick paralysis, neurophysiologic studies. *N Engl J Med* 278:95–97, 1968.
49. Conomy JP, Levinsohn M, Fanaroff A: Familial infantile myasthenia gravis: A cause of sudden death in young children. *J Pediatr* 87:428–429, 1975.
50. Conti-Tronconi BM, Morgutti M, Albizzati MG, Clementi F: Lymphocyte stimulation by acetylcholine receptor in polymyositis. *J Neurol* 217: 281–286, 1978.
51. Cooper BJ, Spence I: Temperature-dependent inhibition of evoked acetylcholine release in tick paralysis. *Nature* 263:693–695, 1976.
52. Critchley M, Herman KJ, Harrison M, Shields RA, Liversedge LA: Value of exchangeable electrolyte measurement in the treatment of myasthenia gravis. *J Neurol Neurosurg Psychiatry* 40:250–252, 1977.
53. Cushny AR, Yagi S. On the action of cobra venom, Parts I and Parts II. *Philos Trans R Soc London* [Biol] 208:1–36, 1918.
54. Dahl DS, Sato A: Unusual myasthenic state in a teenage boy. *Neurology* (Minneapolis) 24:897–901, 1974.
55. Dale RC, Schroeder ET: Respiratory paralysis during treatment of hypertension with trimethaphan camsylate. *Arch Intern Med* 136:816–881, 1976.
56. Dau PC, Denys EH: Plasmapheresis and immunosuppressive drug therapy in the Eaton-Lambert syndrome. *Ann Neurol* 11:570–575, 1982.
57. Davis FA, Schauf CL: Neural blocking activity of multiple sclerosis and EAE sera. United States–Japan Conference on Multiple Sclerosis, Abstract No. 15. *Neurology* (Minneapolis) 26:43–44, 1976.

58. DeGrandis D, Mezzina C, Fiaschi A, Pinelli P, Buzzato G, Morachiello M: Myasthenia due to carnitine treatment. *J Neurol Sci* 46:365–371, 1980.

59. DeJesus PV, Slater R, Spitz LK, Penn AS: Neuromuscular physiology of wound botulism. *Arch Neurol* 29:425–431, 1973.

60. DelCastillo J, Engbaek L: The nature of the neuromuscular block produced by magnesium. *J Physiol* (London) 124:370–384, 1954.

61. DelCastillo J, Pumplin DW: Discrete and discontinuous action of brown widow spider venom on the presynaptic nerve terminals of frog muscle. *J Physiol* (London) 252:491–508, 1975.

62. Dengler R, Rudel R, Warelas J, Birnberger KL: Corticosteriods and neuromuscular transmission. *Pfluegers Arch* 380:145–151, 1979.

63. Dennis MJ, Miledi R: Non-transmitting neuromuscular junctions during an early stage of end-plate reinnervation. *J Physiol* (London) 239:553–570, 1974.

64. Denys EH, Dau PC, Hofman WW: Plasmapheresis and immunosuppression in myasthenic syndrome: (Lambert-Eaton Syndrome). *Ann N Y Acad Sci* 377:828–829, 1981.

65. DeRosayro M, Healey TEJ: Tobramycin and neuromuscular transmission in the rat-isolated phrenic nerve-diaphragm preparation. *Br J Anaesth* 50:251–254, 1978.

66. Donadio JA, Gangarosa EJ, Faich GA: Diagnosis and treatment of botulism. *J Infec Dis* 124:108–112, 1971.

67. Dowdall MJ, Fohlman JP, Eaker D: Inhibition of high-affinity choline transport in peripheral cholinergic endings by presynaptic snake venom neurotoxins. *Nature* 269:700–702, 1977.

68. Drachman DB: Myasthenia gravis and the thyroid gland. *N Engl J Med* 266:330–333, 1962.

69. Drachman DB: Myasthenia gravis. *N Engl J Med* 298:136–142, 186–193, 1978.

70. Drachman DB, Skom JH: Procainamide—a hazard in myasthenia gravis. *Arch Neurol* 13:316–320, 1965.

71. Drenth HJ, Ensberg IFG, Roberts DV, Wilson A: Neuromuscular function in agricultural workers using pesticides. *Arch Environ Health* 25:395–398, 1972.

72. Dretchen KL, Morgenroth VH, Standaert FG, Walts LF: Azathioprine: effects on neuromuscular transmission. *Anesthesiology* 45:604–609, 1976.

73. Duchen LW: An electronmicroscopic study of the changes induced by botulinum toxin in the motor end-plates of slow and fast skeletal muscle fibers of the mouse. *J Neurol Sci* 14:47-60, 1971.

74. Dudel J, Birnberger KL, Toyka KV, Schlegel C, Besinger U: Effects of myasthenic immunoglobulins and of prednisone on spontaneous miniature end-plate potentials in mouse diaphragms. *Exp Neurol* 66:365–380, 1979.

75. Eaton LM, Lambert EH: Electromyography and electric stimulation of nerves in diseases of the motor unit. *JAMA* 163:1117–1124, 1957.

76. Eisen A, Yufe R, Trop D, Campbell I: Reduced neuromuscular transmission safety factor in multiple sclerosis. *Neurology* (Minneapolis) 28:598–602, 1978.

77. Elmqvist D, Josefsson JO: The nature of the neuromuscular block produced by neomycine. *Acta Physiol Scand* 54:105–110, 1962.
78. Engel AG: Morphologic and immunopathologic findings in myasthenia gravis and in congenital myasthenic syndromes. *J Neurol Neurosurg Psychiatry* 43:577–589, 1980.
79. Engel AG, Angelini C: Carnitine deficiency of human skeletal muscles with associated lipid storage myopathy—A new syndrome. *Science* 173: 899–902, 1973.
80. Engel AG, Lambert EH, Gomez MR: A new myasthenic syndrome with end-plate acetylcholinesterase deficiency, small nerve terminals, and reduced acetylcholine release. *Ann Neurol* 1:315–330, 1977.
81. Engel AG, Lambert EH, Mulder DM, Gomez MR, Whitaker JN, Hart Z, Sahashi K: Recently recognized congenital myasthenic syndromes. *Ann N Y Acad Sci* 377:614–637, 1981.
82. Engel AG, Lambert EH, Mulder DM, Torres CF, Sahashi K, Bertorini TE, Whitaker JN: A newly recognized congenital myasthenic syndrome attributed to a prolonged open time of the acetylcholine-induced ion channel. *Ann Neurol* 11:553–569, 1982.
83. Engel AG, Santa T: Motor endplate fine structure. Quantitative analysis in disorders of neuromuscular transmission and prostigmine-induced alterations. In Desmedt, JE (ed): *New Developments in Electromyography and Clinical Neurophysiology.* Basel, Karger, 1973, pp 196–228.
84. Esplin DW, Philip CB, Hughes LE: Impairment of muscle stretch reflexes in tick paralysis. *Science* 132:958–959, 1969.
85. Faich FA, Graebner RW, Sato S: Failure of guanidine therapy in botulism A. *N Engl J Med* 285:773–776, 1971.
86. Fenichel GM: Clinical syndromes of myasthenia in infancy and childhood. *Arch Neurol* 35:97–103, 1978.
87. Fishman RA: Neurological aspects of magnesium metabolism. *Arch Neurol* 12:562–569, 1965.
88. Fogdall RP, Miller RD: Prolongation of a pancuronium-induced neuromuscular blockade by clindamycin. *Anesthesiology* 41:407–408, 1974.
89. Fohlman J, Eaker D, Karlsson E, Thesleff S: Taipoxin, an extremely potent presynaptic neurotoxin from the venom of the Australian snake taipan (Oxyuranus s. scutellatus). *Eur J Biochem* 68:457–469, 1976.
90. Fritz LC, Tzeng MC, Mauro A: Different components of the black widow spider venom mediate transmitter release of vertebrate and lobster neuromuscular junctions. *Nature* 283:486–489, 1980.
91. Fukunaga H, Engel AG, Osame M, Lambert EH: Paucity of presynaptic membrane active zones in the Lambert-Eaton myasthenic syndrome revealed by freeze-fracture electronmicroscopy. *Neurology* 32(2): A222, 1982.
92. Gage PW, Spence I: The origin of the muscle fasciculation caused by funnel-web spider venom. *Aust J Exp Biol Med Sci* 55:453–461, 1977.

93. Gath I, Kayan A, Leegaard J, Sjaastad O: Myasthenia congenita, electromyographic findings. *Acta Neurol Scand* 46:323–330, 1970.
94. Genkins G, Kornfeld P, Osserman KE, Namba T, Grob D, Brunner NG: The use of ACTH and corticosteroids in myasthenia gravis. *Ann N Y Acad Sci* 183:369–374, 1971.
95. Gesztes T: Prolonged apnoea after suxamethonium injection associated with eye drops containing anticholinesterase agent: A case report. *Br J Anaesth* 38:408–409, 1966.
96. Gilbert EW, Stewart CM: Effective treatment of arachnoidism by calcium salts. *Am J Med Sci* 189:532–536, 1935.
97. Gotlieb A: Spider bites. *Lancet* 1:246, 1970.
98. Greer M, Schotland M: Myasthenia gravis in the newborn. *Pediatrics* 26:101–108, 1960.
99. Gundersen CB: The effects of botulinum toxin on the synthesis, storage and release of acetylcholine. *Prog Neurobiol* 14:99–119, 1980.
100. Gundersen CB, Jenden DJ: Notoxin preferentially inhibits the release of newly synthesized acetylcholine from rat brain synaptosomal fractions. *J Neurosci* 1:1113–1117, 1981.
101. Gurwith MJ, Langston C, Citron DM: Toxin-producing bacteria in infants. *Am J Dis Child* 135:1104–1106, 1981.
102. Gutmann L, Crosby TW, Takamori M, Martin JD: The Eaton-Lambert syndrome and autoimmune disorders. *Am J Med* 53:354–356, 1972.
103. Gutmann L, Pratt L: Pathophysiologic aspects of human botulism. *Arch Neurol* 33:175–179, 1976.
104. Gutmann L, Takamori M: Effect of magnesium on neuromuscular transmission in the Eaton-Lambert syndrome. *Neurology* (Minneapolis) 23:977–980, 1973.
105. Haaland KY, Davis LE: Botulism and memory. *Arch Neurol* 37:657–658, 1980.
106. Habermann E: Actions of botulinum and tetanus toxin. In Lewis GE (ed): *Biomedical Aspects of Botulism*. New York, Academic Press, 1981, pp 129–141.
107. Habermann E: Bee and wasp venoms. *Science* 177:314–322, 1972.
108. Hall ED: Glucocorticoid enhancement of guanidine neuromuscular facilitation. *Exp Neurol* 68:581–588, 1980.
109. Harris JB, Karlsson E, Thesleff S: Effects of an isolated toxin from Australian tiger snake (*Notechis scutatus scutatus*) venom at the mammalian neuromuscular junction. *Br J Pharmacol* 47:141–146, 1973.
110. Harris JB, Sutherland S, Zar MA: Actions of the crude venom of the Sydney funnel-web spider (*Atrax robustus*) on autonomic neuromuscular transmission. *Br J Pharmacol* 72:335–340, 1981.
111. Hart Z, Sahashi K, Lambert EH, Engel AG, Lindstrom JM: A congenital familial myasthenic syndrome caused by a presynaptic defect of transmitter resynthesis or mobilization. *Neurology* 29:556–557, 1979.
112. Harvey AM: The actions of procaine on neuromuscular transmission. *Bull Johns Hopkins Hosp* 65:223–238, 1939.

113. Harvey AM, Lilienthal JL, Talbot SA: On the effects of the intra-atrial injection of acetylcholine and prostigmine in normal man. *Bull Johns Hopkins Hosp* 69:529–546, 1941.

114. Hatheway CL, McCroskey LM: Laboratory investigation of human and animal botulism. In Lewis, GE (ed): *Biomedical Aspects of Botulism.* New York, Academic Press, 1981, pp 165–180.

115. Hawgood BJ, Smith JW: The mode of action at the mouse neuromuscular junction of the phospholipase A-Crotapotin complex isolated from venom of the South American rattlesnake. *Br J Pharmacol* 61:597–606, 1977.

116. Hayes WJ: *Pesticides Studied in Man.* Baltimore, Williams and Wilkins, 1982, pp 284–413.

117. Henriksson KG, Nilsson O, Rosen I, Schiller HH: Clinical, neurophysiological and morphological findings in Eaton-Lambert syndrome. *Acta Neurol Scand* 56:117–140, 1977.

118. Herishanu Y, Rosenberg P: Beta-blockers and myasthenia gravis. *Ann Intern Med* 83:834–835, 1975.

119. Herishanu Y, Taustein I: The electromyographic changes induced by antibiotics: a preliminary study. *Confin Neurol* 33:41–45, 1971.

120. Hildebrand J, Joffroy A, Coers C: Myoneural changes in experimental isoniazide neuropathy. *Arch Neurol* 19:60–70, 1968.

121. Hirokawa N, Heuser JE, Evans L: Structural evidence that botulinum toxin blocks neuromuscular transmission by impairing the calcium influx that normally accompanies nerve depolarization. *J Cell Biol* 88: 160–171, 1980.

122. Hodes R: Electromyographic study of defects of neuromuscular transmission in human poliomyelitis. *Arch Neurol Psychiatry* 60: 457–473, 1948.

123. Hoefer PF, Aranow H, Rowland LP: Myasthenia gravis and epilepsy. *Arch Neurol Psychiatry* 80:10–17, 1958.

124. Hofman WW: Antimyasthenic action of corticosteroids. *Arch Neurol* 34:356–360, 1977.

125. Hokkanen E: The aggravating effect of some antibiotics on the neuromuscular blockade in myasthenia gravis. *Acta Neurol Scand* 40:346– 352, 1964.

126. Hosein EA, Booth SJ, Gasdi I, Kato G: Neuromuscular blocking activity and other pharmacologic properties of various carnitine derivatives. *J Pharmacol Exp Ther* 156:565–572, 1967.

127. Howard BD, Gundersen CB Jr: Effects and mechanisms of polypeptide neurotoxins that act presynaptically. *Ann Rev Pharmacol Toxicol* 20: 307–336, 1980.

128. Hughes RO, Zacharias FJ: Myasthenic syndrome during treatment with practolol. *Br Med J* 1:460–461, 1976.

129. Ionescu-Drinca M, Serbanescu G, Nicolau C, Vioculescu V: Association of myasthenic and neuritic symptoms following administration of anti-tetanic serum. *Rev Roum Neurol* 1C, 3:239–243, 1973.

130. Ishikawa K, Engelhardt JK, Frijisana T, Okamoto T, Katsuki H: A neuromuscular block produced by a cancer tissue extract

derived from a patient with myasthenic syndrome. *Neurology* (Minneapolis) 27:140– 143, 1977.

131. Jenzer G, Mumenthaler M, Ludin HP, Robert F: Autonomic dysfunction in botulism B: a clinical report. *Neurology* (Minneapolis) 25:150– 153, 1975.

132. Johnson RO, Clay SA, Arnon SS: Diagnosis and management of infant botulism. *Am J Dis Child* 133:586–593, 1979.

133. Jui-Yen T: Clinical and experimental studies on mechanism of neuromuscular blockade by chloroquine diorotate. *Jpn J Anesth* 20:491–503, 1971.

134. Jusic A, Milic S: Neuromuscular synapse testing in two cases of suicidal organophosphate pesticide poisoning. *Arch Environ Health* 31:240– 243, 1978.

135. Kao I, Drachman DB, Price DL: Botulinum toxin: Mechanism of presynaptic blockade. *Science* 193:1256–1258, 1976.

136. Kaplan JE, Davis LE, Narayan V, Koster J, Katzenstein D: Botulism, Type A, and treatment with guanidine. *Ann Neurol* 6:69–71, 1979.

137. Kawai N, Hori A: Effect of hornet venom on crustacean neuromuscular junction. *Toxicon* 13:103–104, 1975.

138. Keane JR, Hoyt WF: Myasthenic (vertical) nystagmus: Verification by edrophonium tomography. *JAMA* 212:1209–1210, 1970.

139. Kellaway CH, Cherry RO, Williams FE: The peripheral action of the Australian snake venoms. The curare-like action in mammals. *Aust J Exp Biol Med Sci* 10:181–194, 1932.

140. Keynes G: Surgery of the thymus gland: Second (and third) thoughts. *Lancet* 1:1197–1202, 1954.

141. Kim YI, Goldner MM, Sanders DB: Facilitatory effects of 4-aminopyridine on normal neuromuscular transmission. *Muscle Nerve* 3:105– 111, 1980.

142. Kim YI, Goldner MM, Sanders DB: Facilitatory effects of 4-aminopyridine on neuromuscular transmission in disease states. *Muscle Nerve* 3:112–119, 1980.

143. Kissel P, Schmitt J, Duc M, Duc ML: Myasthenia and thyrotoxicosis. In Walton JN, Canal N, Scarlato G (eds): *Muscle Diseases.* Amsterdam, Excerpta Medica, 1970, pp 464–481.

144. Koelle GB: Anticholinesterase agents. In Goodman LS, Gilman A (eds): *The Pharmacologic Basis of Therapeutics.* New York, Macmillan, 1975, pp 445–466.

145. Koenig MG, Drutz D, Mushlin AI, Schaffner W, Rogers DE: Type B botulism in man. *Am J Med* 42:208–219, 1967.

146. Kugelberg E, Traverner D: Comparison between voluntary and electrical activation of motor units in anterior horn cell diseases: On "central synchronization" of motor units. *Electroencephalogr Clin Neurophysiol* 2:125–132, 1950.

147. Kulifowski Z: Sclerose en plaques avec signes pseudomyastheniques. *Rev Neurol* (Paris) 70:347–348, 1938.

148. Lambert EH: Defects of neuromuscular transmission in syndromes other than myasthenia gravis. *Ann N Y Acad Sci* 135:367–384, 1966.

149. Lambert EH, Elmqvist D: Quantal components of end-plate potentials in the myasthenic syndrome. *Ann N Y Acad Sci* 183:183–199, 1971.
150. Lambert EH, Engel AG, Cherington M: End-plate potentials in human botulism. In Bradley WG (ed): *Third International Congress on Muscle Disease*, Series No. 334. Amsterdam, Excerpta Medica, 1974, p 65.
151. Lambert EH, Rooke ED: Myasthenic state and lung cancer. In Brian L, Norris FH Jr (eds): *The Remote Effects of Cancer on the Nervous System*. New York, Grune & Stratton, 1965, pp 67–80.
152. Lambert EH, Rooke ED, Eaton LM, Hodgson CH: Myasthenic syndrome occasionally associated with bronchial neoplasm: neurophysiological studies. In Viets HR (ed): *Myasthenia Gravis*. Springfield, IL, Charles C. Thomas, 1961, pp 362–410.
153. Lang B, Newsom-Davis J, Wray D, Vincent A: Autoimmune aetiology for myasthenic (Eaton-Lambert) syndrome. *Lancet* 2:224–226, 1981.
154. Lauritzen M, Smith T, Fischer-Hansen B, Sparup J, Olesen J: Eaton-Lambert syndrome and malignant thymoma. *Neurology* 30:634–638, 1980.
155. Lava NS, Vicker JM, Ringel SP, Mittag TW: D-penicillamine-induced neuromuscular disease in guinea pigs. *Neurology* 29:564, 1979.
156. Lee CY: Chemistry and pharmacology of polypeptide toxins in snake venom. *Ann Rev Pharmacol Toxicol* 12:265–286, 1972.
157. Lee CY: Elapid neurotoxins and their mode of action. *Clin Toxicol* 3:457–472, 1970.
158. Lee CY, Chang CC: Modes of actions of purified toxins from elapid venoms on neuromuscular transmission. *Mem Inst Butantan* 33:555–572, 1966.
159. Lester HA: Postsynaptic action of cobra toxin at the myoneural junction. *Nature* 227:727–728, 1970.
160. Leuwin RS, Wolters ECMJ: Effect of corticosteroids on sciatic nerve-tibialis anterior muscle of rats treated with hemicholinium-3. *Neurology* (Minneapolis) 27:171–177, 1977.
161. Levin PM: Congenital myasthenia in siblings. *Arch Neurol* 62:745–748, 1949.
162. Leyburn P, Walton JN: The treatment of myotonia: a controlled clinical trial. *Brain* 82:81–91, 1959.
163. Lindstrom J, Seybold ME, Lennon VA, Whittingham S, Duane DD: Antibody to acetylcholine receptor in myasthenia gravis. *Neurology* (Minneapolis) 26:1054–1059, 1976.
164. Lipsitz PJ, English IC: Hypermagnesemia in the newborn infant. *Pediatrics* 40:856–862, 1967.
165. Lundh H, Nilsson O, Rosen I: 4-Aminopyridine—a new drug tested in the treatment of Eaton-Lambert syndrome. *J Neurol Neurosurg Psychiatry* 40:1109–1112, 1977.
166. Margolis LH, Graves RW: Occurrence of myasthenia gravis in a patient with multiple sclerosis. *N C Med J* 6:243–244, 1945.
167. Markalous P: Respiration and the intraperitoneal application of neomycin and neolymphin. *Anesthesiology* 17:427–437, 1962.
168. Masland RL, Wigton RS: Nerve activity accompanying fasciculation produced by Prostigmin. *J Neurophysiol* 3:269–275, 1940.

169. Masters CL, Dawkins RL, Zilko PJ, Simpson JA, Leedman RJ, Lindstrom J: Penicillamine-associated myasthenia gravis, anti-acetylcholine receptor and antistriational antibodies. *Am J Med* 63:689–694, 1977.
170. McLennan H, Oikawa I: Changes in function of the neuromuscular junction occurring in tick paralysis. *Can J Physiol Pharmacol* 50:53–58, 1972.
171. McQuillen MP, Cantor HE, O'Rourke JR: Myasthenic syndrome associated with antibiotics. *Arch Neurol* 18:402–415, 1968.
172. McQuillen MP, Gross M, Johns RJ: Chlorpromazine-induced weakness in myasthenia gravis. *Arch Neurol* 8:286–290, 1963.
173. Mehta SS, Kelkar PN, Parikh PN: Respiratory failure after snake bite poisoning successfully treated with prolonged artificial ventilation. *Indian J Anaesth* 6:273,1968.
174. Merson MH, Dowell VR: Epidemiologic, clinical and laboratory aspects of wound botulism. *N Engl J Med* 289:1005–1010, 1973.
175. Metral S, Tchernia G, Tran TL: Preliminary observations on the effects of repetitive stimulation during neuropathies induced by vincristine. *Electroencephalogr Clin Neurophysiol* 30:368, 1971.
176. Milby TH: Prevention and management of organophosphate poisoning. *JAMA* 216:2131–2133, 1971.
177. Miller RG, Maxfield M, Mirka A, Milner-Brown HS: Acute inhibition of neuromuscular function by corticosteroids in myasthenia gravis. *Neurology* 31(2):97, 1981.
178. Millikan CH, Eaton LM: Clinical evaluation of ACTH and cortisone in myasthenia gravis. *Neurology* (Minneapolis) 1:145–152, 1951.
179. Mittag TW, Caroscio J: False-positive immunoassay for acetylcholine-receptor antibody in amyotrophic lateral sclerosis. *N Engl J Med* 302:868, 1980.
180. Morgan-Hughes JA, Lecky BRF, Landon DN: Kinetic evidence for abnormal AChRs in myasthenia gravis (MG) and congenital myasthenic diseases (CMD). *Neurology* 31(2):89, 1981.
181. Morgan-Hughes JA, Lecky BRF, Landon DN, Murray NMF: Alterations in the number and affinity of junctional acetylcholine receptors in a myopathy with tubular aggregates. *Brain* 104:279–295, 1981.
182. Morris H: Tick paralysis: electrophysiologic measurements. *South Med J* 70:121–122, 1977.
183. Motoki R, Havada M, Chiba A, Houde K: A case of myasthenia gravis in identical twin brothers. *Int J Surg* 45:674–677, 1966.
184. Mulder DW, Lambert EH, Eaton LM: Myasthenic syndrome in patients with amyotrophic lateral sclerosis. *Neurology* (Minneapolis) 9:627–631, 1959.
185. Murnaghan M: Conduction block of terminal somatic motor fibers in tick paralysis. *Can J Biochem Physiol* 38:287–295, 1960.
186. Murray N, Newsom-Davis J: Treatment with oral 4-aminopyridine in disorders of neuromuscular transmission. *Neurology* 31:265–271, 1981.
187. Namba T, Brunner NG, Brown SB, Muguruma M, Grob D: Familial myasthenia gravis: report of 27 patients in 12 families and review of 164 patients in 73 families. *Arch Neurol* 25:49–60, 1971.

188. Naphade RW, Shetti RN: Use of neostigmine after snake bite. *Br J Anaesth* 49:1065–1068, 1977.
189. Neil JR, Himmelhoch JM, Licata SM: Emergence of myasthenia gravis during treatment with lithium carbonate. *Arch Gen Psychiatry* 33: 1090–1092, 1976.
190. Newsom-Davis J, Lang B, Wray D, Murray N, Vincent A, Gwilt M: Clinical and experimental evidence for a humoral factor in myasthenic (Eaton-Lambert) syndrome. *Neurology* 32(2):A221, 1982.
191. Niakan E, Bertorini TE, Acchiardo S, Werner MF: Procainamide-induced myasthenia-like weakness in a patient with peripheral neuropathy. *Arch Neurol* 38:378–379, 1981.
192. Nobel MD, Peacock JH, Lacher JA, Hofman WW: Prednisone-neostigmine interactions at cholinergic junctions. *Muscle Nerve* 2:155–157, 1979.
193. Norris FH Jr: Neuromuscular transmission in thyroid disease. *Ann Intern Med* 64:81–86, 1966.
194. Norris FH, Calanchini PR, Fallat RT, Panchari S, Jewett B: The administration of guanidine in amyotrophic lateral sclerosis. *Neurology* 24:721–728, 1974.
195. Norris FH, Colella JAB, McFarlin D: Effect of diphenylhydantoin on neuromuscular synapse. *Neurology* (Minneapolis) 14:869–876, 1964.
196. Oh SJ, Halsey JH: Guanidine in Type B botulism. *Arch Intern Med* 135:726–728, 1975.
197. Otsuka M, Endo M: The effect of guanidine on neuromuscular transmission. *J Pharmacol Exp Ther* 128:273–282, 1960.
198. Patrick J, Lindstrom J: Autoimmune response to acetylcholine receptor. *Science* 180:871–872, 1973.
199. Patten BM: Myasthenic syndromes. In Tyler HR, Dawson DM (eds): *Current Neurology Volume 2*. Boston, Houghton Mifflin, 1979, pp 26–35.
200. Patten BM, Hart A, Lovelace R: Multiple sclerosis associated with defect in neuromuscular transmission. *J Neurol Neurosurg Psychiatry* 35:383–394, 1972.
201. Pestronk A, Drachman DB: Lithium reduces the number of acetylcholine receptors in skeletal muscle. *Science* 210:342–343, 1980.
202. Pestronk A, Drachman DB: Reduction of acetylcholine receptors (AChRs) in polymyositis. *Neurology* 32(2):A120, 1982.
203. Pestronk A, Drachman DB, Griffin JW: Effect of botulinum toxin on trophic regulation of acetylcholine receptors. *Nature* 264:787–788, 1976.
204. Petajan JH: Polymyositis and a myasthenic syndrome. *Ann N Y Acad Sci* 377:864–866, 1981.
205. Peterson H: Association of trimethadione therapy and myasthenia gravis. *N Engl J Med* 274:506–507, 1966.
206. Pickett J, Berg B, Chaplin E, Brunstetter-Shafer M: Syndrome of botulism in infancy: Clinical and electrophysiologic study. *N Engl J Med* 295:770–772, 1976.
207. Piek T: Arthropod venoms as tools for the study of neuromuscular transmission. *Comp Biochem Physiol* 68C:75–84, 1981.

208. Pittinger CB, Eryasa Y, Adamson R: Antibiotic-induced paralysis. *Anesth Analg* (Cleveland) 49:487–501, 1970.
209. Polley EH, Vick JA, Chinchta HP, Fischetti DA, Macchitelli FJ, Montanarelli N: Botulinum toxin type A. Effects on central nervous system. *Science* 147:1036–1037, 1965.
210. Poulton TJ, James FM, Lockridge O: Prolonged apnea following trimethaphan and succinylcholine. *Anesthesiology* 50:54–56, 1979.
211. Price DL, Griffin JW, Peck K: Tetanus toxin: evidence for binding of presynaptic nerve endings. *Brain Res* 121:379–384, 1977.
212. Puggaiari M, Cherington M: Botulism and guanidine. Ten years later. *JAMA* 240:2276–2277, 1978.
213. Puvanendran K, Cheah JS, Naganathan N, Yeo PPB, Wong PK: Neuromuscular transmission in thyrotoxicosis. *J Neurol Sci* 43:47–57, 1979.
214. Randall LO, Peterson WG, Lehmann G: The ganglionic blocking action of thiophanium derivatives. *J Pharmacol Exp Ther* 97:48–57, 1949.
215. Regan AG, Aldrete JA: Prolonged apnea after administration of promazine hydrochloride following succinylcholine infusion. *Anesth Analg* (Cleveland) 46:315–318, 1967.
216. Regli F, Guggenheim P: Myasthenisches Syndrom als seltene Komplikation unter Hydantoinbehandlung. *Nervenarzt* 36:315–318, 1965.
217. Reid HA: Antivenom in sea-snake bite poisoning. *Lancet* 1:622–623, 1975.
218. Reid HA: Myoglobinuria and sea-snake bite poisoning. *Br Med J* 1:1284–1289, 1961.
219. Reid HA: Cobra-bites. *Br Med J* 2:540–545, 1964.
220. Robertson WC, Chun RWM, Kornguth SE. Familial infantile myasthenia. *Arch Neurol* 37:117–119, 1980.
221. Rubbo JT, Gergis SD, Sokoll MD: Comparative neuromuscular effects of lincomycin and clindamycin. *Anesth Analg* (Cleveland) 56:329–332, 1977.
222. Rubenstein AE, Horowitz SH, Bender AN: Cholinergic dysautonomia and Eaton-Lambert syndrome. *Neurology* 29:720–723, 1979.
223. Russell AS, Lindstrom JM: Penicillamine-induced myasthenia gravis associated with antibodies to acetylcholine receptor. *Neurology* 28:847–849, 1978.
224. Samuelson RJ, Giesecke AJ Jr, Kallus RT, Stanley VF: Lincomycin-curare interaction. *Anesth Analg* (Cleveland) 54:103–105, 1975.
225. Satoyoshi E, Kinoshita M, Nakazato H, Saku A: Evaluation of four cases with clinical characteristics of myasthenia gravis and multiple sclerosis. *Clin Neurol* (Tokyo) 15:888–894, 1975.
226. Satyamurti S, Drachman DB, Slone F: Blockade of acetylcholine receptors: a model of myasthenia gravis. *Science* 187:955–957, 1975.
227. Schiller HH, Stalberg E: Human botulism studied with single-fiber electromyography. *Arch Neurol* 35:346–349, 1978.
228. Schmitt A, Dreyer F, John C: At least three sequential steps are involved in the tetanus toxin-induced block of neuromuscular transmission. *Naunyn-Schmeidebergs Arch Pharmacol* 317:326–330, 1981.
229. Schwartz MS, Stalberg E: Myasthenic syndrome studied with single fiber electromyography. *Arch Neurol* 32:815–817, 1975.

230. Schwartz MS, Stalberg E: Myasthenia gravis with features of the myasthenic syndrome. *Neurology* (Minneapolis) 25:80–84, 1975.
231. Sellin LC: Postsynaptic effects of botulinum toxin at the neuromuscular junction. In Lewis GE (ed): *Biomedical Aspects of Botulism.* New York, Academic Press, 1981, pp 81–92.
232. Seybold ME, Drachman DB: Gradually increasing doses of prednisone in myasthenia gravis. *N Engl J Med* 290:81–84, 1974.
233. Shaivitz SA: Timolol and myasthenia gravis. *JAMA* 242:1611–1612, 1979.
234. Shapira Y, Cividalli G, Szabo G, Rosin R, Russel A: A myasthenic syndrome in childhood leukemia. *Dev Med Child Neurol* 16:668–671, 1974.
235. Simpson JA: The clinical physiology of the lower motor neurone. *Dev Med Child Neurol* 4:55–64, 1962.
236. Simpson JA: Disorders of neuromuscular transmission. *Proc R Soc Med* 59:993-998, 1966.
237. Simpson JA: The correlation between myasthenia gravis and disorders of the thyroid gland. In *Research in Muscular Dystrophy. Proceedings of the Fourth Symposium.* Edited by Research Committee of Muscular Dystrophy Group. London, Pitmans, 1968, pp 31–34.
238. Simpson JA: Myasthenia gravis and myasthenic syndromes. In Walton JN (ed): *Disorders of Voluntary Muscle.* London, Churchill Livingstone, 1974, pp 653–692.
239. Simpson JA, Lenman JAR: The effect of frequency of stimulation in neuromuscular disease. *Electroencephalogr Clin Neurophysiol* 11:604–605, 1959.
240. Simpson L: Pharmacologic studies on the cellular and subcellular effects of botulinum toxin. In Lewis GE (ed): *Biomedical Aspects of Botulism.* New York, Academic Press, 1981, pp 35–46.
241. Simpson LL: Pharmacological studies on the subcellular site of action of botulinum toxin type A. *J Pharmacol Exp Ther* 206:661–669, 1978.
242. Simpson LL: Kinetic studies on the interaction between botulinum toxin type A and the cholinergic neuromuscular junction. *J Pharmacol Exp Ther* 212:16–21, 1980.
243. Singh YN, Harvey AL, Marshall IG: Antibiotic-induced paralysis of the mouse phrenic nerve-hemidiaphragm preparation, and reversibility by calcium and by neostigmine. *Anesthesiology* 48:418–424, 1978.
244. Singh YN, Marshall IG, Harvey AL: Reversal of antibiotic-induced muscle paralysis by 3,4-diaminopyridine. *J Pharm Pharmacol* 30:249–250, 1978.
245. Singh YN, Marshall IG, Harvey AL: Some effects of the aminoglycoside antibiotic amikacin on neuromuscular and autonomic transmission. *Br J Anaesth* 50:109–117, 1978.
246. Singh YN, Marshall IG, Harvey AL: Depression of transmitter release and post-junctional sensitivity during neuromuscular block produced by antibiotics. *Br J Anaesth* 51:1027–1033, 1979.
247. Singh YN, Marshall IG, Harvey AL: The neuromuscular blocking action of spectinomycin on the mouse hemidiaphragm preparation. *Clin Exp Pharmacol Physiol* 6:159–163, 1979.
248. Singh YN, Marshall IG, Harvey AL: The mechanisms of the muscle paralysing actions of antibiotics, and their interaction with neuromus-

cular blocking agents. *Q Rev Drug Metab Drug Interact* 3:130–153, 1980.

249. So EL, Penry JK: Adverse effects of phenytoin on peripheral nerves and neuromuscular junction: A review. *Epilepsia* 22:467–473, 1981.

250. Southcott RV: The neurologic effects of noxious marine creatures. In Hornabrook RW (ed): *Topics on Tropical Neurology*. Philadephia, FA Davis, 1975, pp 165–258.

251. Spitzer N: Miniature end-plate potentials at mammalian neuromuscular junctions poisoned by botulinum toxin. *Nature New Biol* 237:26–27, 1972.

252. Stevens PJ, Wolff HG: Magnesium intoxication: absorption from the intact gastrointestinal tract. *Arch Neurol Psychiatry* 63:749–759, 1950.

253. Streib E: Adverse effects of magnesium salt cathartics in a patient with the myasthenia syndrome (Lambert-Eaton syndrome). *Ann Neurol* 2:175–176, 1977.

254. Streib EW, Rothner AD: Eaton-Lambert myasthenic syndrome: Long term treatment of three patients with prednisone. *Ann Neurol* 10:448–453, 1981.

255. Sugiyama H: *Clostridium botulinum* neurotoxin. *Microbiol Rev* 44:419–448, 1980.

256. Sutherland SK: The management of bites by the Sydney funnel web spider *Atrax robustus*. *Med J Aust* 1:148–150, 1978.

257. Swift TR: Weakness from magnesium containing cathartics: electrophysiologic studies. *Muscle Nerve* 2:295–298, 1979.

258. Swift TR: Disorders of neuromuscular transmission other than myasthenia gravis. *Muscle Nerve* 4:334–353, 1981.

259. Swift TR, Daroff RB, Drachman DB, Lennon VA: Advances in myasthenia gravis: Proceedings of the Myasthenia Gravis Foundation Medical Advisory Board. *Muscle Nerve* 6:317–318, 1983.

260. Swift TR, Ignacio OJ: Tick paralysis: Electrophysiologic studies. *Neurology* (Minneapolis) 25:1130–1133, 1975.

261. Swift TR, Sackellares JC, Harper KE: The effect of temperature on neuromuscular transmission in myasthenic syndrome. *Electroencephalogr Clin Neurophysiol* 45:18P, 1978.

262. Takamori M, Gutmann L: Intermittent defect of acetylcholine release in myasthenia gravis. *Neurology* (Minneapolis) 21:47–54, 1971.

263. Takamori M, Gutmann L, Crosby TW, Martin JD: Myasthenic syndromes in hypothyroidism. *Arch Neurol* 26:326–335, 1972.

264. Takamori M, Ishii N, Mori M: The role of cyclic 3′,5′-adenosine monophosphate in neuromuscular transmission. *Arch Neurol* 29:420–424, 1973.

265. Takamori M, Iwanaga S: Experimental myasthenia due to alpha-bungarotoxin. *Neurology* (Minneapolis) 26:844–848, 1976.

266. Teng P, Osserman KE: Studies in myasthenia gravis: neonatal and juvenile types. A report of 21 and a review of 188 cases. *J Mt Sinai Hosp N Y* 23:711–727, 1956.

267. Thesleff S: Acetylcholine utilization in myasthenia gravis. *Ann N Y Acad Sci* 135:195–206, 1966.

268. Thesleff S: Aminopyridines and synaptic transmission. *Neuroscience* 5:1413–1419, 1980.
269. Thiele B, Stalberg E: Single fiber EMG findings in polyneuropathies of different etiology. *J Neurol Neurosurg Psychiatry* 38:881–887, 1975.
270. Travers PR: The result of intoxication with orthocresylphosphate absorbed from contaminated cooking oil, as seen in 4029 patients in Morocco. *Proc R Soc Med* 55:57–60, 1962.
271. Tsujihata M, Engel AG, Lambert EH: Motor end-plate fine structure in acrylamide dying-back neuropathy. *Neurology* (Minneapolis) 24:849–856, 1974.
272. Tsujihata M, Hazama R, Ishii N, Ide Y, Takamori M: Ultrastructural localization of acetylcholine receptor at the motor end-plate: myasthenia gravis and other neuromuscular diseases. *Neurology* 30:1203–1211, 1980.
273. Vartanian GA, Chinyanga HM: The mechanism of acute neuromuscular weakness induced by chloroquine. *Can J Physiol* 50:1099–1103, 1972.
274. Vasilescu C, Bucur G, Petrovici A, Florescu A: Myasthenia in patients with dermatomyositis. *J Neurol Sci* 38:129–144, 1978.
275. Vasilescu C, Florescu A: Clinical and electrophysiological studies of carbon disulphide polyneuropathy. *J Neurol* 224:59–70, 1980.
276. Vasilescu C, Florescu A: Clinical and electrophysiological study of neuropathy after organophosphorous compounds poisoning. *Arch Toxicol* 43:305–315, 1980.
277. Vincent A, Cull-Candy SG, Newsom-Davis J, Trautman A, Molenaar PC, Polak RL: Congenital myasthenia: endplate acetylcholine receptors and electrophysiology in five cases. *Muscle Nerve* 4:306–318, 1981.
278. Vincent A, Newsom-Davis J, Martin V: Anti-acetylcholine receptor antibodies in D-penicillamine-associated myasthenia gravis. *Lancet* 1:1254, 1978.
279. Vital-Brazil O: Venoms: Their inhibitory action on neuromuscular transmission. In Cheymol J (ed): *Neuromuscular Blocking and Stimulating Agents*. New York, Pergamon Press, 1972, pp 145–167.
280. Vital-Brazil O, Prado-Franceschi J, Laure CJ: Repetitive muscle response induced by crotamine. *Toxicon* 17:61–67, 1979.
281. Vizi ES, Illes P, Ronai A, Knoll J: The effect of lithium on acetylcholine release and synthesis. *Neuropharmacology* 11:521–530, 1972.
282. Von Reis G, Liljestrand A, Marell G: Treatment of severe myasthenia gravis with large doses of ACTH. *Ann N Y Acad Sci* 135:409–416, 1966.
283. Vroom FQ, Engel WK: Nonneoplastic steroid responsive Lambert-Eaton myasthenic syndrome. *Neurology* 19:281, 1969.
284. Wacker WEC, Parisi AF: Magnesium metabolism. *N Engl J Med* 278:772–776, 1968.
285. Wadia RS, Sadagopan C, Amin RB, Sardesai HV: Neurological manifestations of organophosphorus insecticide poisoning. *J Neurol Neurosurg Psychiatry* 37:841–847, 1974.
286. Ward CD, Murray MF: Effect of temperature on neuromuscular transmission in the Eaton-Lambert syndrome. *J Neurol Neurosurg Psychiatry* 42:247–249, 1979.

287. Warner WA, Sanders E: Neuromuscular blockade associated with gentamicin therapy. *JAMA* 215:1153–1154, 1971.
288. Warnick JE, Albuquerque EX, Diniz CR: Electrophysiological observations on the action of the purified scorpion venom, Tityustoxin, on nerve and skeletal muscle of the rat. *J Pharmacol Exp Ther* 198:155–167, 1976.
289. Warrier CBE, Pillai TDG: Familial myasthenia gravis. *Br Med J* 3:839–840, 1967.
290. Waterman PM, Smith RB: Tobramycin-curare interaction. *Anesth Analg* (Cleveland) 56:587–588, 1977.
291. Way WL, Katzung BG, Larson CP: Recurarization with quinidine. *JAMA* 200:153–154, 1967.
292. Weisman SJ: Masked myasthenia gravis. *JAMA* 141:917–918, 1949.
293. Whiteley AM, Schwartz MS, Sachs JA, Swash M: Congenital myasthenia gravis: Clinical and HLA studies in two brothers. *J Neurol Neurosurg Psychiatry* 39:1145–1150, 1976.
294. Wilson RW, Ward MD, Johns TR: Corticosteroids: A direct effect at the neuromuscular junction. *Neurology* (Minneapolis) 24:1091–1095, 1974.
295. Wislicki L, Rosenblum I: Effects of propanolol on the action of neuromuscular blocking drugs. *Br J Anaesth* 39:939–942, 1967.
296. Wohlfart G: Collateral regeneration from residual motor nerve fibers in amyotrophic lateral sclerosis. *Neurology* (Minneapolis) 7:124–134, 1957.
297. Wolters ECMJ, Leevwin RS: Effect of corticosteroids on the phrenic nerve diaphragm preparation treated with hemicholinium. *Eur J Pharmacol* 29:165–167, 1974.
298. Woolf AL, Alberca-Serrano R, Johnson AG: The intramuscular nerve endings and muscle fibers in amyotrophic lateral sclerosis: A biopsy study. In Norris FJ, Kurland LT (eds): *Motor Neuron Diseases*. New York, Grune & Stratton, 1969, pp 166–174.
299. Wright JM, Collier B: The site of the neuromuscular block produced by polymyxin-B and rolitetracycline. *Can J Physiol Pharmacol* 54:926–936, 1976.
300. Yaari Y, Pincus JH, Argoz Z: Depression of synaptic transmission by diphenylhydantoin. *Ann Neurol* 1:334–338, 1977.

Appendix

Intravenous Edrophonium Test (Tensilon® Test)

Test items

Atropine
Nicotinic acid
Normal saline (for injection)
Edrophonium chloride (Tensilon®)
Intravenous solution bottle (normal saline or 5 percent dextrose in
  water)
Needles, syringes
Stopwatch
Wright respirometer or inspiratory force gauge
Resuscitation equipment

Procedure

The following agents should be drawn into four similar-sized syringes and labeled: atropine, 0.5 mg (labeled "A"); nicotinic acid, 50 mg (labeled "B"); normal saline, 2 ml (labeled "C"), and edrophonium, 10 mg per 2 mL (labeled "D").

With the patient in the supine position, an intravenous infusion is started. Parameters for gauging success or failure of the test are identified: for example, the disappearance of ptosis or restored strength after weakness has been produced by repetitive movement. The physician must make positive statements about the effectiveness of each injection.

NOTE: The solutions should be administered in the order given above because muscarinic side effects of abdominal cramps and nausea, excessive salivation, lacrimation, diarrhea, bowel or bladder incontinence, bradycardia or asystole, and hypotension may occur after administration of an anticholinesterase agent unless the patient is premedicated with atropine.

Beginning with solution "A," inject 0.1 mL through the intravenous tubing for a period of 15 seconds. Rapidly inject the remaining amount of solution "A" 45 seconds later. The physician should appear disappointed if no improvement occurs. After a two-minute interval, solution "B" is injected in a similar manner, and subsequently solutions "C" and "D" are given. Note: Often, in a known myasthenic patient, injection of as little as 5 mg of edrophonium (1.0 mL) will produce clinical improvement.

Interpretation

A dramatic transient improvement in function of the selected parameter should be noted only after the injection of edrophonium. Improvement begins approximately 30 seconds after completion of the injection and lasts for two to five minutes, although occasionally it may last up to 20 minutes. Improvement after atropine, nicotinic acid or saline injection, or effects occurring before 30 seconds or after two minutes with the edrophonium, should be viewed with suspicion.

Generalized Curare Test

Test items

Standard *d*-tubocurarine chloride solution (3 mg per mL)
Normal saline (for injection)
Edrophonium chloride (Tensilon®)
Atropine
Neostigmine (Prostigmin®)
Intravenous solution bottle (normal saline or 5 percent dextrose in
   water)
Needles, syringes
Stopwatch
Wright respirometer or inspiratory force gauge
Resuscitation equipment

Procedure

The curare test dose is formulated according to the patient's weight—0.1 mL of *d*-tubocurarine per 40 lb. of body weight. The appropriate amount is drawn into a 1-mL syringe. The test dose of curare is then injected through the hub opening of a 10-mL syringe. Normal saline is added, making a total volume of exactly 8.0 mL. This syringe is thoroughly mixed by repeated inversion and is labeled "curare test solution." Atropine (0.5 mg), neostigmine (1.5 to 2.0 mg) and edrophonium (15 mg) are also drawn into separate syringes and labeled.

With the patient supine, an intravenous infusion of normal saline or dextrose in water is started, preferably in the nondominant arm; subsequently, the curare test solution will be injected through the intravenous tubing. A baseline recording in tabular form is made of the clinical parameters to be assessed, including pulmonary function and ocular motility.

After the baseline recording is completed, 1.0 mL of the curare test solution is injected every two minutes, with a maximum of eight injections. Timing is critical—the intervals must be exactly 120 seconds and should be monitored with a stopwatch. The clinical parameters are reassessed exactly one minute after each injection. If the baseline parameters definitely change—that is, if weakness develops—the test is terminated by ceasing injection of curare test solution and injecting, in order, 0.5 mg of atropine intravenously, 15 mg of edrophonium intravenously and 1.5 to 2.0 mg of neostigmine intramuscularly. The patient should remain under close observation for at least 24 hours. If weakness does not occur, the curare test is continued until all of the curare solution is given.

Interpretation

The test is positive (and terminated) if there is a gradual onset of weakness, which is reversible with edrophonium and neostigmine. Only a definite change in the clinical parameters is acceptable. Each 1.0 mL of the curare test solution equals 1/80 of the curarizing dose. Weakness developing after 1/80 to 5/80 of the curarizing dose indicates myasthenia gravis. The test is equivocal if 6/80 to 7/80 of the curarizing dose provokes weakness. For equivocal results, the differential diagnosis includes amyotrophic lateral sclerosis, adult-onset acid maltase deficiency, myotonic dystrophy and thyrotoxicosis. The test is considered normal if 8/80 of the curarizing dose, or 8.0 mL of the *d*-tubocurarine solution, is utilized without producing any distinct change from the baseline recording.

Anticholinesterase Medication in the Treatment of Myasthenia Gravis

Drug	Dosage forms available	Equivalent dosages	Onset of action	Duration of action	Usual dosages	Comments
Neostigmine (Prostigmin®)	*Solution:* 0.25 mg. per mL. 0.5 mg. per mL. 1.0 mg. per mL.	0.5 mg. IM 0.5 mg. IV	< 20 minutes 4–8 minutes	2–4 hours 2–4 hours	*Diagnostic test:* 0.4 mg. per kg. IM *or* 0.02 mg. per kg. IV *To reverse curare-induced weakness:* 0.2 mg. per kg. IV	Bromide-sensitive persons may be intolerant to bromide salt form (oral). The methyl-sulfate form (solution) should be used with caution in asthmatic persons.
	Scored tablets: 15 mg.	15 mg. PO	45–75 minutes	3–6 hours	15–60mg. every 6 hours	
Pyridostigmine bromide (Mestinon®)	*Solution:* 5 mg. per mL.	2 mg. IM 2 mg. IV	< 15 minutes 2–5 minutes	2–4 hours 2–4 hours	2 mg. every 4 hours 2 mg. every 4 hours	Oral pyrido-stigmine usual drug of choice for maintenance therapy. Bro-mide-sensi-tive persons may be intol-erant to bro-mide salt form; chlo-ride salt form availa-
	Syrup: 12 mg. per mL.	60 mg. PO	20–30 minutes	3–6 hours	30–60 mg. every 4 hours	
	Scored tablets: 60 mg.	60 mg. PO	20–30 minutes	3–6 hours	30–60 mg. every 4 hours	
	Timed-release tablets: 180 mg.	180 mg. PO	20–60 minutes	6–12 hours	180 mg. every 12 hours	

							ble from manufacturer. Timed-release tablets usually taken only at bedtime; variable rate of dissolution and absorption may cause fluctuating symptoms.
Ambenonium chloride (Mytelase®)	*Scored tablets:* 10 mg.	25 mg.	PO	20–30 minutes	4–8 hours	5–40 mg. every 6 hours	Accumulation in body due to variable metabolism common
Edrophonium chloride (Tensilon®)	*Solution:* 10 mg. per mL.	10 mg. IV 10 mg. IM	20–40 seconds 2–10 minutes	5–20 minutes 10–40 minutes		*Diagnostic test:* 2.5 mg. IV over 15 seconds, followed by 2.5–7.5 mg. 45 seconds later; to confirm IV test, give 10 mg. IM *To reverse curare-induced weakness:* 10 mg. IV every 5–10 minutes, up to 40 mg. *Myasthenic crisis:* Same dose as in diagnostic test should improve strength; increased weakness suggests cholinergic crisis	

*Reprinted by permission from Brumback RA: The neuromuscular junction. Part II: mysasthenia gravis. *Am Fam Physician* 23(2):126–133, 1981, published by the American Academy of Family Physicians.

Index

Acetate, 147
Acetylcholine (ACh), 7–15, 17, 19,
25, 49, 65, 67–69, 71, 73, 75, 76,
79, 90, 94, 96, 100–102, 121, 122,
123, 127, 128, 130–139, 143–149,
151, 153, 154, 161, 162, 167, 169,
205, 213, 218–220, 224, 225, 236,
240, 260–262, 296, 297, 298, 300,
301, 307, 312, 313, 315, 319
Acetylcholinesterase (AChE), 25, 26,
38, 42, 43, 56, 121, 123, 130, 131,
146, 147, 151, 154, 161, 169, 240
Acetylcholine receptor (AChR), 1,
31, 37, 42, 43, 49, 54, 56, 66, 68,
70, 77, 78, 102, 122, 144, 213, 214,
219, 275, 277–281, 286, 296,
302–305, 312, 318, 319, 320, 321
Acoustic impedance, 271, 272
Acrylamide, 244, 296, 304, 308, 309
ACTH, 277, 317
Actin, 67, 240
Actinomycin-D, 214
Action potential, 14, 19, 83, 88, 97,
99, 101, 121, 135, 136, 138, 140,
141, 159, 210, 268, 297, 298, 300,
302, 303, 306, 308, 311, 317, 320,
321
Adenosine, 138
Adenylate cyclase, 136, 142
Adrenaline, 4
Alpha-adrenergic (α-adrenergic)
drugs, 126
Alpha-bungarotoxin (α-
bungarotoxin; α-BuTx), 31, 37,
38, 43, 55, 66, 67, 83, 139, 214,
219, 220, 223, 277, 279, 303, 304,
312

Ambenonium, 284, 324
Amikacin, 321
Aminoglycoside, 143, 321, 322
4-Aminopyridine, 130, 131, 137, 140,
141, 300, 302, 308, 321, 323
Amobarbital, 79
Ammonia, 2
Amyotrophic lateral sclerosis, 235,
236, 303, 304
Anesthetic, 79, 82, 126, 129, 133,
140, 143, 151, 164, 217, 218, 320
Anionic site, 147, 169
Anoxia, 94, 218
Anterior horn cell disease, 234, 304
Anti-acetylcholine receptor
antibodies (AChR-Ab), 259, 260,
274, 275, 277, 280–283, 286, 304,
305, 312, 317–319
Antibiotics, 126, 129, 143, 296, 321,
322
Anticholinesterase, 19, 133, 147–
150, 153, 159, 168–170, 266, 300–
304, 308, 311, 312, 315, 317,
319–324
Antimetabolites, 285
Antinuclear factor, 276, 320
Antiporter, 145
Antitoxin, 307, 310, 322
Aplysia, 86
Aprotinin, 322
Arthropod envenomation, 313–316
ATPase, 100, 133, 145
Atracurium, 152, 160, 161, 167
Atraxotoxin, 315
Atrax robustus, 314
Atropine, 8, 9, 10, 148, 169, 170, 314,
324